Substance Use Disorders

H. Thomas Milhorn

Substance Use Disorders

A Guide for the Primary Care Provider

Springer

H. Thomas Milhorn, MD, PhD
Director, Didactics Section
East Central HealthNet Family Medicine Residency Program
Meridian, Mississippi

Formerly Professor of Family Medicine, Professor of Physiology and Biophysics, and Associate Professor of Psychiatry and Human Behavior
University of Mississippi School of Medicine
Jackson, Mississippi

ISBN 978-3-319-63039-7 ISBN 978-3-319-63040-3 (eBook)
DOI 10.1007/978-3-319-63040-3

Library of Congress Control Number: 2017947158

Printed on acid-free paper

This Springer imprint is published by Springer Nature
The registered company is Springer International Publishing AG
The registered company address is: Gewerbestrasse 11, 6330 Cham, Switzerland

Preface

This book was written for primary care physicians, who almost daily come into contact with substance-dependent individuals and their families. However, it also should be helpful to primary care nurse practitioners and physician assistants, as well as medical students, primary care residents, emergency medicine physicians, ASAM- and APA-certified addictionists and those studying for certification in those specialties, psychiatrists, psychologists, and alcohol/drug counselors.

Primary care physicians are in excellent position to diagnose substance use disorders and to help the families of these patients get them into treatment. In addition, primary care physicians can detoxify patients as needed. On return from treatment, they can participate in the patients' recovery programs to help prevent relapse.

The book is divided into four parts: (1) The Basics; (2) Psychoactive Substance Dependencies; (3) Diagnosis, Treatment, Recovery, Relapse, and the Family; and (4) Special Groups.

Part 1 (The Basics) consists of an overview, the various definitions of substance dependence, and the pharmacology of addictive substances. Chapter 1 "Overview" is an introductory chapter that covers material common to the entire field of substance dependence, such as classification of psychoactive substances based on their effects on the central nervous system, primitive survival brain concept, criteria for substance dependence, addiction medicine specialists, denial, abstinence syndromes, 12-step programs, prescription drug addiction, and DEA drug schedules. Chapter 2 covers the various definitions of substance dependence, and Chap. 3 covers the pharmacology of addictive substances.

Part 2 (Psychoactive Substance Dependencies) covers the various drug dependencies—alcohol dependence, sedative-hypnotic dependence, opioid dependence, stimulant dependence, nicotine dependence, cannabis dependence, dissociative dependence, inhalant dependence, hallucinogen dependence, and anabolic steroid dependence.

Part 3 covers diagnosis, treatment, recovery, relapse, and the family.

Part 4 (Special Groups) covers women, adolescents, the elderly, ethnic minority groups, co-occurring disorders, LGBT patients, HIV-positive patients, and the impaired physician.

To keep from repeatedly saying "his or her," I have used the generic "he" to mean all addicts regardless of sex.

I would like to thank Toby Milhorn who did some of the typing and put the references into the appropriate format, my wife Kay for her patience and understanding while I worked on the manuscript, and the residents in the EC-HealthNet Family Medicine Residency Program for giving me the inspiration to write the book.

Meridian, MS, USA H. Thomas Milhorn

Abbreviations

AA	Alcoholics Anonymous
ACOA	Adult Children of Alcoholics
ADH	Alcohol dehydrogenase
ADM	Addiction medicine
AIDS	Acquired immune deficiency syndrome
ALDH	Aldehyde dehydrogenase
ALS	Amyotrophic lateral sclerosis
ALT	Alanine aminotransferase
AMA	American Medical Association
ASAM	American Society of Addiction Medicine
AST	Aspartate aminotransferase
AUDIT	Alcohol Use Disorders Identification Test
BAC	Blood alcohol concentration
BAL	Blood alcohol level
BBB	Blood-brain barrier
C_o	Zero concentration
cAMP	Cyclic adenosine monophosphate
CBD	Cannabidiol
CDT	Carbohydrate-deficient transferrin
CIWA-Ar	Clinical Institute Withdrawal Assessment for Alcohol—Revised Version
CMRO	Certified medical review officer
CNS	Central nervous system
CT	Computed tomography
D_o	Initial dose
DAST	Drug Abuse Screening Test
DEA	Drug Enforcement Administration
DHHS	Department of Health and Human Services
DSM	*Diagnostic and Statistical Manual of Mental Disorders*
DUI	Driving under the influence
ED	Emergency department
EEG	Electroencephalogram
EMIT	Enzyme multiplied immunoassay technique
EtG	Ethyl glucuronide
FAE	Fetal alcohol effects
FAS	Fetal alcohol syndrome
FDA	US Food and Drug Administration

GABA	Gamma-aminobutyric acid
GBL	Gamma-butyrolactone
GC/MS	Gas chromatography/mass spectrometry
GGT	Gamma-glutamyl transpeptidase
GHB	Gamma-hydroxybutyrate
HALT	Hungry, angry, lonely, or tired
HIV	Human immunodeficiency virus
HPPD	Hallucinogen persisting perception disorder
KCl	Potassium chloride
LAAM	Levo-alpha-acetylmethadol
LSD	Lysergic acid diethylamide
MAO	Monoamine oxidase
MAST	Michigan Alcoholism Screening Test
MCV	Mean cell volume
MDMA	3,4-Methylenedioxymethamphetamine
MEOS	Microsomal ethanol oxidizing system
MME	Morphine milligram equivalents
MRI	Magnetic resonance imaging
NAD	Nicotinamide adenine dinucleotide
NADPH	Nicotinamide adenine dinucleotide phosphate
NIAAA	National Institute on Alcohol Abuse and Alcoholism
NIDA	National Institute on Drug Abuse
NMDA	N-Methyl-D-aspartate
NSAID	Nonsteroidal anti-inflammatory drug
OBOT	Office-based opioid therapy
OTC	Over the counter
PAWS	Post-acute withdrawal syndrome
PCP	Phencyclidine
PDMP	Prescription drug monitoring program
PT	Prothrombin time
REM	Rapid eye movement
SAMHSA	Substance Abuse and Mental Health Services Administration
SIDS	Sudden infant death syndrome
SMAST	Short Michigan Alcoholism Screening Test
T_o	Time zero
THC	Tetrahydrocannabinol
V_d	Volume of distribution
VTA	Ventral tegmental area

Contents

Part IV Special Groups

Part I

The Basics

1 Overview

Key Chapter Points

- Substance abuse can be costly, both financially and health wise.
- Primary care physicians are not well prepared to deal with substance dependence.
- Psychoactive substances differ from other drugs in a number of ways.
- Drugs are usually divided into seven categories according to how they most prominently affect the central nervous system.
- With dependence, the primitive survival brain seizes control from the cerebral cortex.
- Denial is a major component of substance dependence.
- An abstinence syndrome may occur after cessation or cutting down the dose of a psychoactive substance.
- Primary care physicians need to be aware of the prescription-dependent addict.
- Addiction medicine specialists are certified by the American Society of Addiction Medicine and the American Psychiatric Association.
- The American Psychiatric Association spells out the criteria for substance dependence in DSM-5.
- The Drug Enforcement Administration sets the regulations for prescribing controlled substances.

A primary care physician is a specialist in family medicine, internal medicine, or pediatrics who provides care to patients at the point of first contact and provides continuing and comprehensive care of that patient. Care provided by primary care physicians may include chronic, preventive, and acute care in both inpatient and outpatient settings. As a result, primary care physicians are in an excellent position to identify and treat substance use disorders and thereby reduce the associated adverse health, family, and societal effects. However, minimal attention in medical schools and residencies has been given to educating primary care physicians to respond to the needs of individuals and their families affected by substance use problems [1, 2]. The information provided in this book is intended, in part, to improve that situation.

When talking about individuals who are addicted to alcohol or other drugs we need a name. The first thing we should agree on is that alcohol is a drug. Therefore, a *drug addict* is defined as one who is dependent on alcohol or another drug. A *psychoactive substance* is any drug that acts on the brain to alter its function, resulting in temporary changes in perception, mood, consciousness, or behavior. *Alcoholism* is a lay term for alcohol dependence.

H.T. Milhorn, *Substance Use Disorders*, DOI 10.1007/978-3-319-63040-3_1

The Problem

The Financial Cost of Substance Dependence

The cost to the United States due to crime, lost work productivity, and health care from tobacco, alcohol, and illicit drug use is staggering, exacting more than $700 billion annually in costs.

Tobacco The health-care cost related to tobacco is about $130 billion annually, with the overall tobacco-related cost being about $295 billion.

Alcohol For alcohol, the annual health-care cost is approximately $25 billion, with the overall alcohol-related cost about $224 billion.

Illicit drugs The annual health-care cost related to illicit drugs is on the order of $11 billion, with the overall illicit drug-related cost being $193 billion.

The $700 billion annual cost does not include family expenses for counseling, rehabilitation, theft, car crashes, or the incalculable cost of family despair at the loss of a loved one to drug overdoses, drug-related medical problems, drug-related accidents, or drug-related suicides. Drug overdoses now cause more deaths than traffic accidents [3].

Substance Use Prevalence

Substance use is common in the general population and among persons presenting to primary care physicians. In 2014, 16.3 million Americans over the age of 12 reported heavy alcohol use in the prior month. Six and a half million Americans over the age of 12 reported current, nonmedical use of prescription drugs, such as painkillers, tranquilizers, stimulants, and sedatives. Twenty seven million Americans over the age of 12 reported using illicit drugs. Of these, 1.5 million reported using cocaine [4].

Prevalence of illicit drug use for age 12–17, age 18–25, and age 26 and older is given in Table 1.1.

Table 1.1 Prevalence of illicit drug use for ages 12–17, ages 18–25, and ages 26 and older for 2015 (%) (From [4])

	Ages 12–17	Ages 18–25	Age 26 and older
Lifetime	25.30	57.50	50.10
Past year	17.50	37.50	14.60
Past month	8.80	22.30	8.20

Emergency Department Visits

In 2014, 2.1 million emergency department (ED) visits were related to the use of illicit substances. Of these, more than 27% were caused by the non-medical use of prescription drugs, over-the-counter medications, and supplements, and 21.2% involved illicit drugs. Over 14% involved alcohol in combination with other drugs.

Each day, almost 7000 people are treated in emergency departments for using prescription drugs in a manner other than as directed [4].

Deaths

Every day, 44 people in the United States die from overdose of prescription painkillers; more people die from abusing prescription pain relievers than cocaine and heroin combined. The number of overdose deaths caused by prescription painkillers quadrupled between 1999 and 2010 [4].

Treatment Demographics

Of the 2.5 million who received substance abuse treatment in 2014, 41% of admissions were for alcohol dependence, 20% were for opiate/opioid dependence, and 17% were for of marijuana dependence [4].

Consequences

The consequences of illicit substance use include loss of productivity, increased health-care costs, and increased morbidity and mortality. There is increasing recognition of the similarities between substance use disorders and other common chronic illnesses, such as hypertension and diabetes mellitus. Like those illnesses, substance use disorders also can be identified early when there are fewer sequelae and when less intensive treatments can be successful [5].

Substance Use Disorders and the Primary Care Physician

Less than 20% of primary care physicians described themselves as very prepared to identify alcoholism or illegal drug use. More than 50% of patients with substance use disorders said their primary care physician did nothing to address their substance use [5]. Primary care physicians clearly are in need of improved education in regard to substance use disorders.

How Psychoactive Substances Differ from Other Drugs

Psychoactive substances differ from other drugs (aspirin, acetaminophen, lisinopril, metformin, and so forth) in a number of ways [6]:

- They produce an altered mood state, such as sedation, relaxation, or euphoria.
- These effects reinforce the drug use; that is, the feelings aroused by the drug make the user want to use it again.
- Compulsive use occurs when the user feels as though he must have the drug. Without the drug, the user may feel anxious, nervous, or dysphoric. Use continues despite the known, harmful effects. The alcoholic continues to drink despite severe liver disease. The cocaine addict continues to use cocaine despite numerous arrests for possession and a period of prison time from selling the drug.
- Regular and temporal patterns of use occur. The alcoholic may drink every day and at the same time every day. I had one cocaine addict in treatment who every evening at 6:00 o'clock came to the nurses' station demanding medication for her withdrawal symptoms. There were two problems with the situation: (1) The symptoms she described weren't those of cocaine withdrawal but anxiety, and (2) she was past the time to be having any legitimate withdrawal symptoms. Turned out, her regular pattern of cocaine use had been to come home from work every day and about 6:00 o'clock start smoking crack cocaine. The problem was not cocaine withdrawal but cocaine craving.
- Deprivation increases the desire to use the drug. The cigarette smokers have to go outside for a smoke during intermission of a play.
- Paired stimuli increases use. The sight of a crack pipe on a TV movie may set off an intense desire in a recovering cocaine addict to use crack again.
- Tolerance develops. Over time, more and more of the drug is required to get the same high.
- Physical dependence may develop; that is, regular, prolonged use of a drug may produce withdrawal symptoms on cessation of use.
- The relapse rate is high. Many drug users quit several times before finally achieving permanent sobriety. For example, cigarette smokers who successfully quit do so, on average, after six attempts.

Classification of Psychoactive Substances Based on Their Effects on the Central Nervous System

Drugs are usually divided into seven categories according to how they most prominently affect the central nervous system (Table 1.2 [7]).

In addition to the seven categories of psychoactive substances just discussed, I will cover anabolic steroids in Chap. 13.

Club Drugs and Date Rape Drugs

Club Drugs

Club drugs are chemical substances commonly used at nightclubs, music festivals, raves, and dance parties to enhance social intimacy and sensory stimulation. They include 3,4-methylenedioxymethamphetamine (MDMA), also known as

Table 1.2 Classification of psychoactive substances by their effects on the central nervous system (CNS) (From Milhorn [7]. Approved with permission, Springer)

Drug group	Examples	Effects on the CNS
CNS depressants	Alcohol, barbiturates, benzodiazepines, Z drugs	Decrease inhibitions, relieve anxiety, intoxicate, sedate
Opioids	Heroin, morphine, hydromorphone, hydrocodone, oxycodone	Reduce pain, cause euphoria, sedate
CNS stimulants	Amphetamines, cocaine, methylphenidate	Cause excitement, produce euphoria, depress appetite, decrease need for sleep
Cannabinoids	Marijuana, hashish, hash oil	Produce sense of detachment, euphoria, altered time perception
Dissociatives	PCP, ketamine, dextromethorphan	Produce intoxication and reduced pain; disconnection between thoughts, identity, consciousness, and memory
Inhalants	Paint thinners or removers, degreasers, lighter fluid, correction fluid (Liquid Paper), felt-tip marker fluid, electronic contact cleaners, model glue, spray paint	Produce euphoria, sedate
Hallucinogens	LSD, psilocybin, mescaline, peyote, 5-MeO-DMT, MDMA	Produce hallucinations (usually visual but may be auditory or olfactory)

ecstasy; the naturally occurring neurotransmitter/psychoactive drug gamma-hydroxybutyrate (GHB); the benzodiazepine flunitrazepam (Rohypnol); and the dissociative drug ketamine (Ketalar). These drugs are popular because of their low cost and their pleasant effects. Club drugs usually are taken orally and may be taken with alcohol or with other drugs. Drug screening generally is not available for club drugs [8]. Each club drug will be discussed in its appropriate chapter.

Date Rape Drugs

A date rape drug is a chemical substance slipped into a drink to incapacitate someone for a sexual assault. The drugs often have no color, smell, or taste. Because of the amnesia-producing properties of these drugs, the victim is not able to remember what happened. This reduces the chance of a successful prosecution. Date rape drugs include flunitrazepam (Rohypnol), gamma-hydroxybutyrate (GHB), and ketamine (Ketalar) [9].

The Primitive Survival Brain Concept of Substance Dependence

When we first crawled out of the sea and began to walk on the land, the primitive survival brain was in complete control. It was concerned with survival of the individual and the species, that is, finding food and water, fleeing or fighting when circumstances dictated, and having sex for survival of the species. Over time, the thinking, reasoning cerebral cortex evolved around it (Fig. 1.1).

Within the primitive survival brain is located the reward center of the brain. The reward center is part of the limbic system, which is responsible for feelings. It is the feeling produced by a drug that the user seeks. The cocaine addict, for example, would be just as happy getting a high from stimulation of an electrode placed in the reward center of the brain as from doses of cocaine.

The process of moving from substance use to substance dependence is often described as "crossing the wall," which is illustrated in Fig. 1.2. On the substance use side of the wall using cocaine, for example, is a choice. The thinking, reasoning cerebral cortex is in control. Once the person becomes addicted due to altered brain chemistry (moves across the wall), the primitive survival brain takes charge. Using cocaine is no longer a choice. To the addict it feels like a matter of life and death [10].

Denial

Over a period of time, drug users develop behaviors (manipulation, lying, self-pity, irresponsibility) that allow them to keep using the drug, a phenomenon known as *denial.*

Normal Response to Substance Use

Drug use acts on the reward center of the brain to cause drug craving, which acts on the cerebral cortex to cause the addictive behaviors (Fig. 1.3). The addictive behaviors in turn cause guilt, which by negative feedback reduces or cuts down the drug use as indicated by the dashed line [11].

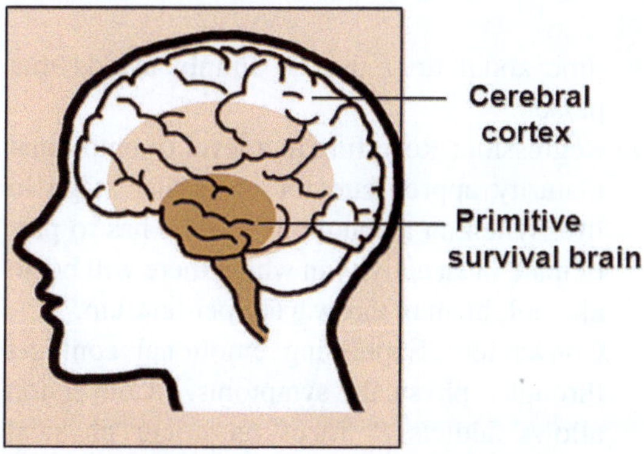

Fig. 1.1 The primitive survival brain (responsible for survival of the individual and the species) and the cerebral cortex (responsible for thinking and reasoning)

Development of Denial

Once drug users develop dependence, the logic center of the brain (cerebral cortex) is unable to control the intense craving for the drug and the drug use. To protect the mind from the psychological pain of the internal conflict between the drug use and the guilt, an elaborate denial system evolves to separate awareness of the addictive behaviors from the drug use, and thereby relieve the guilt (Fig. 1.4). Addictive behaviors no longer cause guilt. The denial system serves to perpetuate the drug use.

Denial can take a number of forms:

- My problems are not due to drug use. "I drink too much because my wife nags me all time; she's the problem."
- Drugs cause adverse consequences in others, but not me. "I know smoking causes lung cancer, but in other people, not me."
- Some ways of using drugs are okay; others are not. "Taking drugs by mouth is okay; doing them I.V. is not."
- Some forms of drugs are okay, others are not. "I can't be an alcoholic; I only drink beer (a case a day)."

Denial is not unique to drug addicts. It occurs in other circumstances. For example, it is the first stage in the grief process: *Denial* leads to *anger* which leads to *bargaining* which leads to *depression* which leads to *acceptance* [12].

Fig. 1.2 Crossing the wall concept of dependence (Based on Milhorn [10])

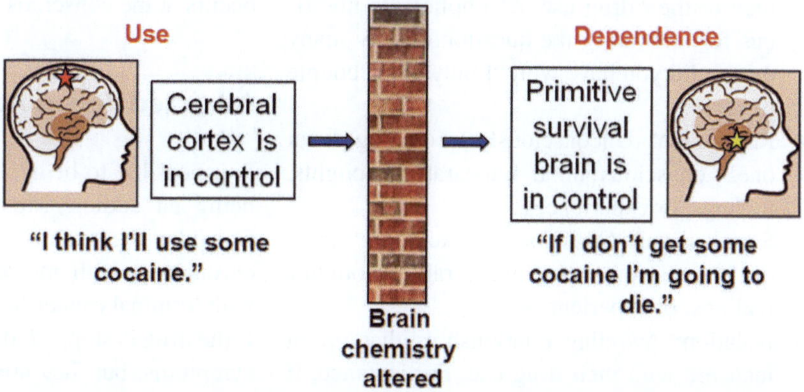

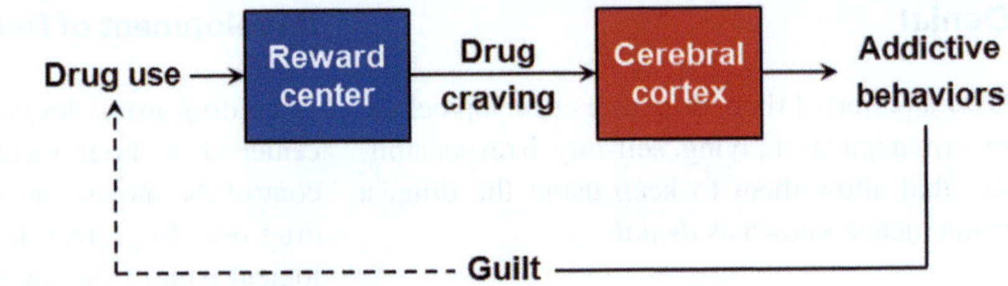

Fig. 1.3 Guilt due to addictive behaviors causes the addict to cut back or stop the drug use (Based on Milhorn [11])

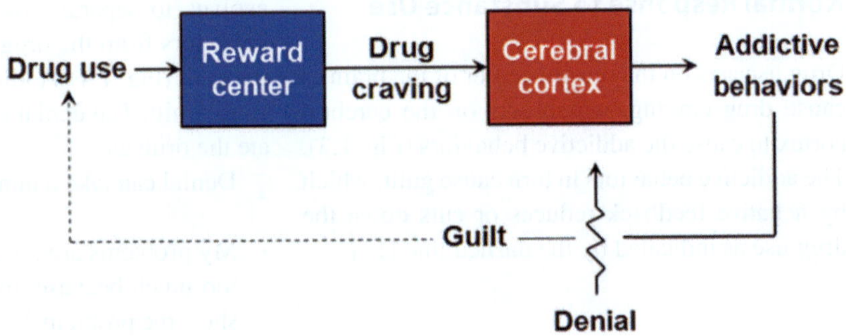

Fig. 1.4 Denial blocks the internal relationship between addictive behaviors and guilt, allowing the addict to continue using drugs (From Milhorn [7]. Approved with permission, Springer)

Tools of Denial

Van Cleave (1987) identified eight tools that addicts use to achieve denial [13]:

1. Rationalization: Using socially acceptable but untrue explanations for inappropriate behavior. "I have to take more pain pills than my doctor prescribed because my back hurts so bad."
2. Projection: Blaming others for one's own failings and inadequacies. "I wouldn't have to drink so much if my wife would just quit nagging me."
3. Minimization: Underestimating the magnitude of their drug use. Alcoholics are notorious for answering the question of how many drinks did you have with "I only had a couple of beers."
4. Repression: Unconsciously excluding from one's conscious mind unbearable thoughts, feelings, or experiences.
5. Suppression: Consciously excluding from one's conscious mind unbearable thoughts, feelings, or experiences
6. Isolation: Avoiding relationships that might interfere with their drug use. For instance, if the addict has a relative who gives him a hard time about drug use he simply avoids that person.
7. Regression: Reverting to a level of emotional maturity appropriate for an earlier stage in life. When an alcoholic is told he has to participate in an activity in which there will be no alcohol, he may throw a temper tantrum.
8. Conversion: Expressing emotional conflicts through physical symptoms. Conversion allows addicts to focus on minor physical problems to avoid dealing with their drug addiction.

All of the mechanisms to achieve denial are subconscious except for suppression, which occurs at the conscious level.

Addicted Versus Addict

Is it possible to be dependent on a drug without being an addict? Most people would say no. Consider the example of people being treated chronically with morphine for pain associated with terminal cancer. They will become addicted. If the drug is stopped, they will suffer withdrawal symptoms, but they are not compulsive users of the morphine and therefore are not addicts.

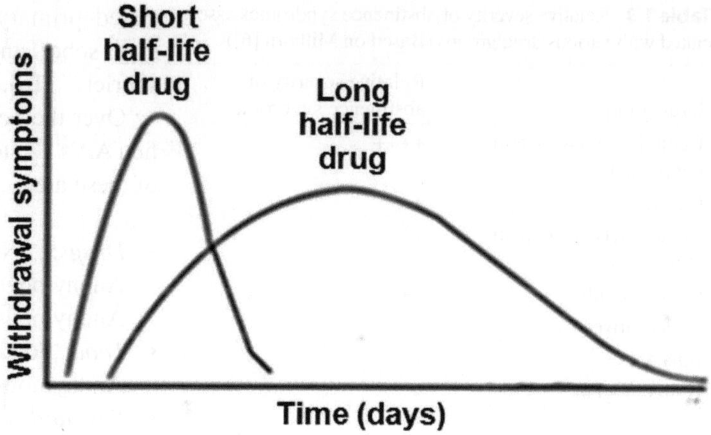

Fig. 1.5 Short half-life and long half-life severity and lengths of withdrawal symptoms

A fellow addictionist described a hypothetical situation to make the distinction. He said, "If I tie you down and give you high doses of I.V. morphine for two weeks, you will become addicted. Then I let you go. If you are not an addict, you will come looking for me to beat me up. If you are an addict you will come looking for me to get some more morphine."

The majority of withdrawal symptoms for short half-life drugs tend to run their course in 5–10 days and to be more severe. The withdrawal symptoms from long half-life drugs may last 2 to 4 weeks and be less severe (Fig. 1.5).

Minor symptoms for some drugs, called *post-acute abstinence syndrome*, may last for weeks to months or more [14].

Abstinence Syndromes

An *abstinence syndrome* (withdrawal signs and symptoms) is a constellation of physical and physiologic changes undergone by individuals who have become physically dependent on a drug and who are abruptly deprived of that substance.

As a rule, the severity of withdrawal symptoms is inversely proportional to the half-life of the drug, and the length of withdrawal symptoms is proportional to the drugs' half-life. For example, a drug with a short half-life will cause a more intense abstinence syndrome, but for a shorter time than a drug with a long half-life, which will have a less intense abstinence syndrome that lasts longer.

Abstinence syndromes are opposite those of dependence. For example, alcohol use causes sedation, whereas withdrawal causes hyperalertness. Opiate use causes constipation, whereas withdrawal causes diarrhea.

Severity of Abstinence Syndromes

Dependence on most drugs of abuse results in an abstinence syndrome when the drug is abruptly stopped. Table 1.3 shows the relative severity of abstinence syndromes associated with various drug groups.

The alcohol abstinence syndrome by far is the worst. Some people still die from delirium tremens despite good medical care. Opioid abstinence syndrome is the next worse. People as a rule do not die from it, although at its peak they may wish they would. The CNS stimulant, cannabinoid, and dissociative drugs have abstinence syndromes that may make the addict very uncomfortable, but do not require detoxification medication. The inhalant and anabolic steroid abstinence syndromes are mild. The hallucinogen group of drugs does not have an abstinence syndrome associated with it [6].

Table 1.3 Relative severity of abstinence syndromes associated with various drug groups (Based on Milhorn [6])

Drug group	Relative severity of abstinence syndrome
Central nervous system depressants	++++
Opioids	+++
Central nervous system stimulants	++
Cannabinoids	++
Dissociatives	++
Inhalants	+
Hallucinogens	–

The Beginning of All 12-Step Programs

Alcoholics Anonymous (AA) began with an idea by William (Bill) Griffith Wilson in Akron, Ohio, in 1935. The principles of AA were based on those of *The Oxford Group*, a nondenominational movement modeled after first-century Christianity. Wilson, using the 12 steps he had put together, remained sober on his own for a period of time before he decided that alcoholics should help other alcoholics stay sober. He made inquiries about any local alcoholics he could talk to and was referred to Dr. Bob Smith, a surgeon. After talking to Wilson, Smith stopped drinking and invited Wilson to stay at his home. Smith relapsed almost a month later while attending a medical conference in Atlantic City.

Returning to Akron, he was given one beer by Wilson the next morning to settle his nerves so he could perform an operation. It proved to be the last drink Smith would take for the rest of his life. He died of colon cancer 15 years later. Wilson stayed sober until his death from emphysema in 1971, 37 years after the founding of AA. He whipped his alcohol problem but could never get control of his nicotine dependence.

To share their method, Wilson and other members of AA wrote the book, *Alcoholics Anonymous,* known as the *Big Book* in AA, which was published in 1939. Bill Wilson and Dr. Bob Smith are considered cofounders of AA. AA's stated primary purpose is "to help alcoholics stay sober and help other alcoholics achieve sobriety" [15].

Over the years, numerous groups have modified AA's 12 steps to meet their own needs. Some of these are:

- *Drugs*: Narcotics Anonymous, Cocaine Anonymous, Nicotine Anonymous, Pills Anonymous
- *Food*: Food Addicts Anonymous, Overeaters Anonymous
- *Sex and Love*: Love Addicts Anonymous, Sexaholics Anonymous
- *Family*: Al-Anon, Alateen, Nar-Anon, Adult Children of Alcoholics, Co-Dependents Anonymous
- *Others*: Gamblers Anonymous, Workaholics Anonymous, Procrastinators Anonymous, Self Mutilators Anonymous

A website that gives information about 56 12-step groups is www.sobernation.com/list-of-12-step-programs [16].

The Prescription Drug-Dependent Patient

Patient Behaviors

Behaviors that occur when patients who are dependent on prescription drugs interact with primary care physicians include drug-seeking behavior, doctor shopping, use of scams to maintain or increase their supply of drugs, and prescription fraud [17].

Drug-Seeking Behavior

Drug-seeking behavior refers to a patient's manipulative, demanding behavior to obtain medication. The patient may insist on receiving a controlled drug prescription on the first visit and claim that nonaddictive medications don't work. The patient may claim to be allergic to all nonaddicting medications for the problem. The patient may claim to have a high tolerance to drugs, to lose prescriptions or drop them in the commode, or to run out of prescriptions early. A new patient may claim to be from out of town and to have left his medications at home.

The patient may sell or forge prescriptions or may use the stolen prescriptions of family members and friends. Nonpharmacologic treatment recommendations, such as nonaddicting medications, behavioral training, psychotherapy, and 12-step recovery programs, are resisted. The patient may offer bribes or sex or may make outright threats of harm to a person or property.

Substance-dependent patients may learn that the physician's enabling instincts and discomfort with confrontation are so great that the physician's initial "no" can be turned into a "yes" if they apply enough pressure.

Doctor Shopping

Doctor shopping describes patients who use at least two and often multiple physicians in attempts to obtain prescriptions to assure a supply of controlled substances. Doctor shopping is a type of behavior common in emergency department settings where the staff may not know the patient.

Doctor shopping has historically been a difficult pattern to identify, but pharmacy networks and managed care companies are making this type of drug-seeking behavior an increasingly difficult option. Physicians should ally with their local pharmacists, who share the legal liability when a controlled drug prescription is filled. By working together, physicians and pharmacists can more effectively identify and monitor drug-abusing patients.

Scams

A scam is a dishonest way to get drugs by deceiving people. Scams are sometimes used to obtain additional medications, more potent or higher dosage formulations, or brand-name drugs because of their higher street value.

Once a scam has worked in a given practice, that scam will likely continue to surface periodically in that office practice until the physician ceases to reinforce the scam.

A common scam is for a person to show up at the emergency department or physician's office with a complaint of having a kidney stone. They often say they know the symptoms because they have had them in the past. They may even prick their finger with a pin in the bathroom and let a drop of blood fall into their urine sample. According to them, nothing works for the pain but a narcotic, usually Dilaudid. Patients have been known to show up in the emergency department complaining of severe left-sided chest pain with radiation down the left arm to get I.V. morphine, and some have even been admitted to the coronary care unit where they get more morphine.

Another common scam is for a drug-dependent person to call the on-call physician at night and claim to be a regular patient of the physician's partner. The person then claims to be out of a prescribed controlled substance because he was unable to come to the office earlier in the day to get it refilled. The excuse may be that his father had a heart attack and he had to take him to the hospital or some similar made-up story.

Prescription Fraud

Prescription fraud is defined as the illegal acquisition of prescription drugs for personal use or profit. Prescription pads may be stolen from physicians' offices and prescriptions are then written for fictitious patients. Some patients, in an effort to obtain additional amounts of legitimately prescribed drugs, alter the physician's prescription by increasing the number of pills/capsule prescribed. Some drug users have prescription pads of a legitimate doctor printed with a different callback number that is answered by an accomplice to verify the prescription. Some drug users call in their own prescriptions and give their own telephone number as a callback confirmation.

Characteristics of Overprescribing Physicians

The American Medical Association describes four mechanisms—the four "Ds"—by which a physician becomes involved in overprescribing. These are (1) dated, (2) duped, (3) dishonest, and (4) disabled [17].

Dated

Dated refers to physicians who are out of date regarding knowledge of pharmacology and the differential diagnosis and management of chronic pain, anxiety, insomnia, and addiction.

Thus, they are less confident in their skills dealing with substance use problems than other physicians.

Duped

Physicians may be duped by patients. Physicians are generally a caring, trusting group of professionals who try to help their patients in an open and honest relationship based on mutual respect. Thus, physicians may be vulnerable to manipulative patients.

Dishonest

Dishonest physicians are uncommon. However, there are a few physicians in every geographic area who are willing to write prescriptions for controlled substances in exchange for financial gain. These physicians are sometimes referred to as "Dr. Feelgood," or in the case of celebrities "Drug dealers to the stars." Such physicians should be reported to the state medical board or other law enforcement agencies and appropriately investigated.

Disabled

Disabled physicians are defined in this context as physicians with a medical, psychiatric, or substance dependence problem. These physicians may be "loose" prescribers of controlled substances and may be less likely to confront patients who are abusing substances out of fear of turning suspicion on themselves.

Addiction Medicine Specialists

A physician who specializes in addiction medicine is called an addictionist. Two groups of physicians treat substance use disorders in the United States—physicians certified by the American Society of Addiction Medicine and physicians certified by the American Psychiatric Association.

American Society of Addiction Medicine

The American Society of Addiction Medicine (ASAM) is a professional society representing over 4000 physicians, clinicians, and associated professionals in the field of addiction medicine. The organization was admitted to the American Medical Association House of Delegates as a voting member in June 1988. In 1990, the AMA added addiction medicine (ADM) to its list of designated specialties.

To become certified in addiction medicine by ASAM, one must complete an ACGME-approved residency (family medicine, internal medicine, pediatrics, etc.), complete a 1-year fellowship in addiction medicine, and then pass a certification exam given by the American Society of Preventive Medicine [18].

American Psychiatric Association

Addiction psychiatry was founded in 1991. It is a medical subspecialty within the specialty of psychiatry that focuses on the evaluation, diagnosis, and treatment of people with substance dependence. To become a certified addiction psychiatrist, one must first be certified as a general psychiatrist by the American Psychiatric Association. Next, these general psychiatrists must commit themselves to an ACGME-accredited fellowship in addiction psychiatry. Addiction psychiatry fellowships are 1 year in length and are set in a hospital or clinical setting where the fellows can learn to diagnose and treat substance use disorders as well as potential coexisting psychiatric disorders. They must then pass a certification exam given by the American Society of Psychiatry and Neurology [19].

DSM-5 Criteria for Substance Dependence

The American Psychiatric Association's DSM-5, published in 2013, gives specific criteria for the diagnosis of substance dependence. The term abuse is no longer used. Instead, DSM-5 combines substance abuse and substance dependence into a single disorder measured on a continuum from mild to severe. Each specific substance is addressed as a separate use disorder, that is, alcohol use disorder, stimulant use disorder, hallucinogen use disorder, and so forth. In DSM-5, the diagnosis of substance dependence includes 11 different criteria [20]:

1. Taking the substance in larger amounts or for longer than you meant to.
2. Wanting to cut down or stop using the substance but not managing to.
3. Spending a lot of time getting, using, or recovering from use of the substance.
4. Cravings and urges to use the substance.
5. Not managing to do what you should at work, home, or school, because of substance use.
6. Continuing to use, even when it causes problems in relationships.
7. Giving up important social, occupational, or recreational activities because of substance use.
8. Using substances again and again, even when it puts you in danger.
9. Continuing to use, even when you know you have a physical or psychological problem that could have been caused or made worse by the substance.
10. Needing more of the substance to get the effect you want.
11. Development of withdrawal symptoms, which can be relieved by taking more of the substance.

A score of 2–3 indicates mild substance dependence (formerly called substance abuse), a score of 4–5 indicates moderate dependence, and a score of 6 or more indicates severe dependence. In this book, I will use the term *abuse* not as a diagnostic term. Instead, I will use it to mean alcohol use in access or any drinking by those under the legal age or those who are pregnant. Abuse of illicit drugs will mean any use of amphetamine, cocaine, heroin, and so forth. Abuse of prescription drugs will mean using prescription medications not prescribed for the person or using a greater amount of medication than was prescribed.

Besides the ICD-10 codes for dependence, primary care physicians also can use ICD-10 to code:

- ***In early remission***: None of the criteria for dependence have been present for at least 3 months and less than 12 months, with the exception of craving for the substance.
- ***In sustained remission***: None of the criteria for dependence have been present for a period of 12 months or longer, with the exception of craving for the substance.
- ***On maintenance therapy***: Methadone, buprenorphine, naltrexone, disulfiram, acamprosate.
- ***In a controlled environment*****:** Halfway house, residential program.

DEA Drug Schedules and Prescribing Regulations

A prescription for a controlled substance must include the patient's full name, the patient's address, and the practitioner's full name, address, and DEA (Drug Enforcement Administration) registration number. There are no specific federal limits to quantities of drugs dispensed via a prescription.

DEA Drug Schedules

- Schedule I includes substances with no currently accepted medical use and a high potential for abuse. Schedule I drugs include the most dangerous drugs of all the drug schedules. They potentially can cause severe psychological or physical dependence.
- Schedule II includes substances with a high potential for abuse, with use potentially leading to severe psychological or physical dependence. These drugs have accepted medical uses.
- Schedule III includes substances with a moderate to low potential for physical and psychological dependence. Abuse potential is less

than drugs in Schedule I and Schedule II, but more than those in Schedule IV.

- Schedule IV includes substances with a low potential for abuse and low risk of dependence.
- Schedule V includes substances with lower potential for abuse than Schedule IV and consists of preparations containing limited quantities of certain narcotics. Schedule V drugs are generally used for antidiarrheal, antitussive, and analgesic purposes [21].

Examples of drugs in each schedule are given in Table 1.4.

Prescribing Regulations

Schedule III–V Substances

A prescription for controlled substances in Schedules III-V may be communicated either orally, in writing, or by facsimile (electronically) to the pharmacist. Schedule III-V controlled substances may be refilled if authorized on the prescription; however, the prescription may only be refilled up to five times within 6 months after the date on which the prescription was issued [22].

Schedule II Substances

Schedule II controlled substances require a written prescription, which must be signed by the practitioner. There is no federal time limit within which a Schedule II prescription must be filled after being signed by the practitioner. The refilling of a prescription for a controlled substance listed in Schedule II is prohibited.

While some states and many insurance carriers limit the quantity of controlled substance dispensed to a 30-day supply, there are no specific federal limits to quantities of drugs dispensed via a prescription. An individual practitioner may issue multiple prescriptions authorizing the patient to receive a total of up to a 90-day supply of a Schedule II controlled substance.

For Schedule II controlled substances, an oral order is only permitted in an emergency situation.

Exceptions for Schedule II Facsimile Prescriptions

The facsimile of a Schedule II prescription may serve as the original prescription as follows:

- A practitioner prescribing Schedule II narcotic controlled substances to be compounded for the direct administration to a patient by intravenous, intramuscular, subcutaneous, or intraspinal infusion may transmit the prescription by facsimile.
- A practitioner prescribing a Schedule II narcotic controlled substance for a patient enrolled in a hospice care program certified and/or paid for by Medicare under Title XVIII or a hospice program which is licensed by the state may transmit a prescription to the dispensing pharmacy by facsimile. The practitioner or the practitioner's agent may transmit the prescription to the pharmacy. The practitioner or agent will note on the prescription that it is for a hospice patient. The facsimile serves as the original written prescription. The pharmacy will

Table 1.4 Examples of drugs in various DEA schedules (From [22])

DEA schedule	Examples
Schedule I	Heroin, lysergic acid diethylamide (LSD), marijuana (cannabis), 3,4-methylenedioxymethamphetamine (ecstasy), methaqualone, and peyote
Schedule II	Combination products with less than 15 mg of hydrocodone per dosage unit (Vicodin), cocaine, methamphetamine, methadone, hydromorphone (Dilaudid), meperidine (Demerol), oxycodone (OxyContin), fentanyl, Dexedrine, Adderall, and Ritalin
Schedule III	Products containing less than 90 mg of codeine per dosage unit (Tylenol with codeine), ketamine, anabolic steroids, testosterone
Schedule IV	Xanax, Soma, Darvon, Darvocet, Valium, Ativan, Talwin, Ambien, Tramadol
Schedule V	Cough preparations with less than 200 mg of codeine per 100 ml (Robitussin AC), Lomotil, Motofen, Lyrica, Parepectolin

consider the facsimile prescription a "written prescription" and no further prescription verification is required.

- Practitioners prescribing Schedule II controlled substances for residents of long-term care facilities may transmit a prescription by facsimile to the dispensing pharmacy. The practitioner's agent may also transmit the prescription to the pharmacy. The facsimile prescription serves as the original written prescription for the pharmacy [22].

The primary care physician should realize that treating a substance-abusing patient and seeing that patient return to normal life functioning makes the effort worthwhile [23].

Summary

A *drug addict* is defined as one who is dependent on alcohol or another drug. The cost to the United States due to crime, lost work productivity, and health care from tobacco, alcohol, and illicit drug use is staggering, exacting more than $700 billion annually in costs.

Primary care physicians are not well prepared to deal with substance dependence. Psychoactive substances differ from other drugs in a number of ways. Drugs are usually divided into seven categories according to how they most prominently affect the central nervous system. With dependence, the primitive survival brain seizes control from the cerebral cortex. Denial is a major component of substance dependence.

An abstinence syndrome may occur after cessation or cutting down the dose of a psychoactive substance. Primary care physicians need to be aware of the prescription-dependent addict.

Addiction medicine specialists are certified by the American Society of Addiction Medicine and the American Psychiatric Association. The American Psychiatric Association spells out the criteria for substance dependence in DSM-5. The term *abuse* is no longer used. The Drug Enforcement Administration sets the regulations for prescribing controlled substances.

References

1. Curley B. Drug Free website. http://www.drugfree.org/news-service/few-medical-students-learn-about-addiction. May 31, 2001.
2. Milhorn HT. Chemical dependency: is medical education falling short? Mississippi State Medical Association Impaired Physicians' Newsletter. April 1989.
3. Trends and statistics. National Institute of Drug Abuse (NIDA) website. https://www.drugabuse.gov/related-topics/trends-statistics. 2015.
4. Behavioral health trends in the United States: results from the 2014 national survey on drug use and health. Substance Abuse and Mental Health Substance Abuse Administration (SAMHSA) website. https://www.samhsa.gov/data/sites/default/files/NSDUH-FRR1-2014/NSDUH-FRR1-2014.pdf. September 2015.
5. Shapiro B, Coffa D, McCance-Katz EF. A primary care approach to substance misuse. Am Fam Physician. 2013;88(2):113–21.
6. Milhorn HT. Drug and alcohol abuse: the authoritative guide for parents, teachers, and counselors. New York: Da Capo Press; 2003.
7. Milhorn HT. Chemical dependence: diagnosis, treatment, and prevention. New York: Springer-Verlag; 1990.
8. Gahlinger P. Illegal drugs: a complete guide to their history, chemistry, use, and abuse. New York: Plume Publishing; 2003.
9. Date rape drugs fact sheet. Womens Health website. http://www.womenshealth.gov/publications/our-publications/fact-sheet/date-rape-drugs.html. July 16, 2012.
10. Milhorn HT. Understanding chemical dependence. J Miss State Med Assoc. 1992;33(4):123–8.
11. Milhorn HT. Introduction to biological control systems. In: The application of control theory to physiological systems. Philadelphia: WB Saunders; 1966. p. 113–137.
12. Kubler-Ross E. On death and dying. New York: The Macmillan Company; 1969.
13. Van Cleave S, Byrd W, Revel K. If drugs are so bad, why do people keep using them: how denial and guilt perpetuate drug abuse. In: Counseling for substance abuse and addiction. Waco: Word Books; 1987. p. 63–7.
14. Post-acute withdrawal syndrome (PAWS). UCLA Dual Diagnosis Program website. http://www.semel.ucla.edu/dual-diagnosis-program/News_and_Resources/PAWS
15. History of alcoholics anonymous. The Alcoholism Guide website. http://www.the-alcoholism-guide.org/history-of-alcoholics-anonymous.html
16. Stoddart T. List of 12 step programs. Sober Nation website. https://sobernation.com/list-of-12-step-programs. September 23, 2011.

17. Longo LP, Parran T, Johnson B, Kinsey W. Management of the drug-seeking patient. Am Fam Physician. 2000;61(8):2401–8.
18. Paths to certification. American Society of Addiction Medicine (ASAM) website. http://www.asam.org/membership/paths-to-certification
19. Addiction psychiatry. American Psychiatric Association (APA) website. https://psychiatry.org/psychiatrists/practice/professional-interests/addiction-psychiatry. February 2000.
20. DSM-5. Arlington: American Psychiatric Association (APA) Publishing; 2013.
21. Drug schedules. Drug Enforcement Administration (DEA) website. http://www.dea.gov/druginfo/ds.shtml
22. Section V – valid prescription requirements. Drug Enforcement Administration (DEA). US Department of Justice, Office of Diversion Control. Practitioner's Manual. 2006.
23. Weaver M, Jarvis MAE, Schnoll SH. Role of the primary care physician in problems of substance abuse. Archiv Intern Med. 1999;159(9):913–24.

2 Definitions of Substance Dependence

Key Chapter Points

- The Oxford Dictionary defines dependence as "the state of relying on or being controlled by someone or something else."
- The biopsychosocial definition views substance dependence as continuing to use a drug despite significant biological, psychological, or social problems.
- The disease concept of dependence allows primary care physicians to use familiar techniques to make a diagnosis, form a treatment plan, educate a patient about drugs, and discuss prognosis.
- The AMA's definition recognizes substance dependence to be a primary, chronic disease with genetic, psychosocial, and environmental factors influencing its development and manifestations.
- ASAM's definition recognizes substance dependence to be a primary, chronic disease of brain reward, motivation, memory, and related circuitry.

Addiction is a lay term for *dependence*. The Oxford Dictionary defines dependence as "the state of relying on or being controlled by someone or something else [1]." For our purpose, the definition becomes "the state of relying on or being controlled by a drug (including alcohol)." I will use addiction and dependence as synonyms in this book.

Other definitions of substance dependence include the biopsychosocial definition, the disease concept definition, the American Medical Association definition, and the American Society of Addiction Medicine (ASAM) definition.

The Biopsychosocial Definition of Substance Dependence

According to the biopsychosocial model, substance dependence is defined as having significant biological, psychological, or sociological problems and continuing to use the drug that is causing the problem(s). It should be noted that the word "or" is used instead of "and." By this model, you do not have to have problems in all three areas, or even two, to be considered substance dependent.

Biological Factors

The fundamental etiological assumption of the biological view of substance dependence is that individuals who become dependent on a chemical substance are in some significant way biologically different from those who do not become dependent. This factor, whatever it is, makes these individuals more susceptible to becoming dependent. Genetic studies do in fact confirm that the tendency to become dependent on alcohol, cocaine, and opioids is inherited.

H.T. Milhorn, *Substance Use Disorders*, DOI 10.1007/978-3-319-63040-3_2

Changes in the neurotransmitters in the reward center of the brain during the addictive process causes craving for the drug. Withdrawal symptoms may occur.

Medical problems from substance use include lung cancer and emphysema from smoking cigarettes; alcoholic hepatitis and cirrhosis from drinking alcohol; hepatitis B and C from intravenous drug use; HIV/AIDS from unprotected sex; myocardial infarction, seizures, and stroke from cocaine or methamphetamine use; and bacterial endocarditis of the heart valves from intravenous drug use [2].

Psychological Factors

The psychological view of substance dependence once argued that certain personality types, personality traits, or other psychopathology generated aversive emotional states that a person then relieved by substance use. Substance use was viewed as a form of self-medication to treat a deeper, underlying psychological disorder. According to this view, substance abuse would be expected to stop once its cause had been effectively treated.

Support for this position rested on studies showing significantly increased incidences of psychopathologies among substance-dependent individuals. However, the vast majority of these studies were conducted on addicts after they had already become substance dependent, so that their psychopathologies were at least as likely to be the product of substance dependence as its cause.

Prior to 1980, *addictive personality* was a concept used by physicians to explain addiction as the result of preexisting character defects in individuals. In general, studies looking at personality characteristic of individuals in recovery from substance dependence show no difference from those who have never been substance dependent. In other words, you can't tell which person will become substance dependent and which will not by looking at their personality profiles.

The term, addictive personality, is still used by the lay public, and the Internet is replete with questionnaires for you to take to determine if you have this affliction.

Traditional psychotherapy, when aimed at psychopathology other than substance dependence, generally has not been effective in eliminating substance dependence.

Personality characteristics probably do play a role in the development of substance dependence in some individuals, such as those with antisocial, borderline, and paranoid personality disorders. However, these individuals account only for a small percentage of the substance-dependent population.

That said, there is sufficient evidence that the mentally ill may use drugs to alleviate some of their symptoms. For example, the use of tobacco products by patients with schizophrenia is believed to lessen the symptoms of the disease and improve cognition. If a person's mind is racing because of a manic state, alcohol may slow it down. If a person has intense sadness or hopelessness because of depression, cocaine or amphetamines may improve this for a period of time [3].

Psychological problems due to substance dependence include depression, anxiety, mood swings, confusion, hallucinations, impaired judgment, desire to engage in risky behavior, decrease in pleasure in everyday life (anhedonia), impulsiveness, and loss of self-control.

Social learning due to patterns of use in the addict's family (smoking, casual drinking, marijuana use), peer pressure, and advertising and media influence play a role in who will use drugs and who will not.

Denial is an extremely important psychological aspect of substance dependence. It is a defense mechanism postulated by Sigmund Freud. Denial is defined most simply as not recognizing or admitting to one's self that a problem exists. This is despite the fact that the problem is evident to others. Denial was discussed in Chap. 1.

Sociological Factors

Sociological problems associated with substance dependence include (1) family problems, (2) financial problems, (3) legal problems, and (4) isolation.

Family Problems

Substance dependence causes many problems in the family. Addicts often neglect children, both physically and emotionally. They may become violent with family members, leading to spousal or child abuse. The addict can become self-centered and oblivious to other peoples' concerns. He may begin to neglect family responsibilities. Things such as paying the mortgage and bills are no longer important to him. Other members have to pick up the slack. This can lead to resentment.

The addict or the spouse may begin to cheat on the other partner. The problems may lead to separation or divorce [4].

Financial Problems

Drug addicted individuals may struggle economically because of missing work, losing their jobs, making poor financial decisions, or spending large amounts of money on their addictions.

Alcohol or other drug use on the job can cause accidents and decreased productivity. Addicted employees may begin to be late for work, neglect their personal hygiene, and display erratic or unacceptable behaviors. Other problems may include tardiness and sleeping on the job. In addition, theft from the company, trouble with co-workers, illegal activities at work including selling illicit drugs to other employees, and increased disciplinary problems may occur. Substance dependence can make it difficult for a person to find work after losing a job. They may have to settle for low-paying jobs beneath their education or skill sets.

A person with a history of substance use may have to pay higher medical insurance premiums. Illnesses and physical injuries associated with drug use can lead to higher medical expenses. Drug dependence can cause significant medical problems (cirrhosis of the liver, pancreatitis, stroke, myocardial infarction) and can put a person at an increased risk for various cancers. In addition, drug use is associated with higher risks for infections, such as bacterial endocarditis, hepatitis B, and HIV, all of which increases out-of-pocket medical expenses.

Drug-using people who have a difficult time making regular rent or automobile payments always seem to find money to buy their drugs.

Legal Problems

Using alcohol or other drugs slows functioning in the brain, which may lead to automobile accidents or driving under the influence (DUI) infractions. A first DUI offense may require DUI classes and, in some states, license suspensions. Having multiple DUI convictions may be considered a felony, requiring mandatory jail time.

Prescription fraud is a growing problem. It is defined as the illegal acquisition of prescription drugs for personal use or profit. Some of the most abused prescription drugs include hydrocodone plus acetaminophen (Vicodin), oxycodone (OxyContin), diazepam (Valium), oxycodone plus acetaminophen (Percocet), and alprazolam (Xanax). Prescription fraud is often directed at these drugs. For those who are convicted, prescription fraud is a felony punishable by up to 5 years in prison, unless the individual can negotiate drug rehabilitation in lieu of jail time.

Intense drug cravings may drive addicts to commit crimes to get drugs or money to buy them. Property crimes such as theft, larceny, and burglary are among the most common crimes committed by addicts. Theft can be a misdemeanor or a felony, with a wide range of penalties.

The nature of addiction causes men and women to use whatever means necessary to get their drugs, including prostituting their bodies for drugs or drug money [5].

Isolation

Drug dependence progressively leads to isolation, a phenomenon said to be like peeling off the layers of an onion. The first layer to go, the outer layer, is the individual's hobbies, like collecting stamps or sports cards. The next layer to be peeled off is outside activities, like bowling or playing cards. Then the spouse may leave the addicted individual. The last thing to go, the inner layer of the onion, is the job. Then the addict has achieved complete and total isolation—just him and the drug [5].

Disease Concept Definition of Substance Dependence

Over the past several years, there has been considerable debate among the lay public about whether or not alcoholism is a disease, as opposed to a lack of willpower, a bad habit, or immoral behavior. Considerable evidence supports the concept of substance dependence being a disease, including genetic studies and the natural course of alcoholism.

Genetic Studies

The majority of research on the genetics of substance dependence has been on alcoholism. This is because alcoholism has a long and prominent history, is the most common substance dependence problem, and is much easier to study than other drug dependencies.

Family, twin, and adoption studies are the classic techniques for examining the role that genetic factors play in substance dependence. In addition, searches have been done to identify specific genetic markers to identify at an early age those who are likely to develop a substance use disorder should they begin to use alcohol or another drug. Attempts also have been made to identify the specific gene that puts individuals at risk for a substance use disorder.

Family Studies

Family studies analyze transmission of substance use disorders from generation to generation through families. The basic approach determines if family members of substance-dependent individuals are at increased risk for substance dependence.

The association between alcoholic individuals and a family history of alcoholism was first noted over 75 years ago. Since that time it has been shown that the risk of becoming addicted to alcohol, opioids, and cocaine directly relates to the closeness of the genetic relationship to addicted family members [6].

Twin Studies

Twin studies are based on the fact that there are two types of twins—identical twins, which share 100% of their genes and nonidentical twins, which share 50% of their genes. The premise is that if addiction is related to genetic factors, the risk for the disorder should be considerably higher in the identical twin of an addict than in the nonidentical twin of an addict. Studies have borne this out for alcohol, marijuana, and cocaine [7–9].

Adoption Studies

Adoption studies aim to separate the effects of genes and environment by studying the similarity between adopted children, their biological parents, and their adoptive parents. Studies comparing adopted sons and daughters of alcoholics by nonalcoholic families have shown that the adopted sons of alcoholics are almost four times as likely to become alcoholics. Daughters of alcoholics show a similar result but to a lesser degree [10–12].

Genetic Markers

In addition to the above studies, promising genetic markers have been provided by research in electrophysiology, endocrinology, and biochemistry. The idea is that if these markers are positive, the individual has a greater risk of becoming addicted [13–19].

Gene Studies

Several studies have investigated the possibility that a gene might be responsible for the development of alcoholism. Several different genes have been identified [20–22].

Conclusions About Genetic Studies

Research has shown that what is inherited is not substance dependence but a genetic predisposition that renders a person more vulnerable to develop the disorder if that person drinks or uses other drugs. However, one can become substance dependent without a genetic disposition by frequent, heavy drinking, or other drug use. It is believed that 50–60% of the risk for alcoholism is genetically determined for both men and women, while the other 40–50% is due to environmental factors [23].

Natural Course of Alcoholism

Every disease, such as diabetes mellitus or hypertension, left untreated follows a natural course or progression. The same is true of alcoholism and other drug dependences. In 1960, E. M. Jellinek, who is considered by many to be the father of the disease concept of alcoholism, showed that the natural course for many alcoholics can be divided into four phases, each of which is progressively worse than the one before [24].

There is no time limit for the entire course or for any of its phases. Some alcoholics progress more slowly through the phases than others. In some, progression through some phases is prolonged, while progression through others is very brief. For the most part, from the time an individual begins to lose control to the time when he passes into the final phase of alcoholism requires, on average, 15 years for men and 7–8 years for women.

The four phases of Jellinek's alcohol progression are (1) the prealcoholic phase, (2) the prodromal phase, (3) the crucial phase, and (4) the chronic phase.

Prealcoholic Phase

In the prealcoholic phase, the individual's use of alcohol is socially motivated. The prospective alcoholic experiences psychological relief from alcohol. Drinking becomes his means of handling stress.

Prodromal Phase

In the prodromal phase, drinking moves from a means of psychological escape from tensions, problems, and inhibitions. The alcoholic begins to drink more heavily and more often than his friends. When drunk, he may recklessly spend money and boast of real or imagined accomplishments.

Temporary losses of memory after a drinking bout (*blackouts*) begin to occur. Gulping and sneaking drinks become commonplace. He may also fortify himself with a few drinks before going to a party and drink other people's unfinished drinks at the party. Morning after hangovers become more frequent and increasingly painful.

Crucial Phase

In the crucial phase, the drinker's psychological habit becomes a physical addiction. Once he takes a drink he cannot stop, a phenomenon known as *loss of control*. The loss of control induces feelings of guilt and shame, so the alcoholic concocts an elaborate system of reasons or excuses for his drinking—the pressure on the job is too great, his wife yells at him all the time, or a drink will soothe his nerves. The alibis are mostly made to reassure him that his drinking behavior is acceptable.

The alcoholic needs a drink in the morning to start the day right (*eye opener*). The morning drink serves to ease his jangled nerves or soothe a hangover.

By now, the drinker is under pressure from his family, friends, and/or employer to quit drinking, so he tries to break the hold that alcohol has on him. He may try changing the kind of drink—from whiskey to beer or from wine to beer. That does no good. Then he may set up his own rules as to when he will drink and what he will drink. But one sip of alcohol and the heavy drinking starts all over again.

He begins to become *antisocial*. The alcoholic now prefers to drink alone or only with other alcoholics, regardless of their social level. He broods over imagined wrongs inflicted by others and thinks that people are staring at him or talking about him. He is highly critical of others and may become violent or destructive.

The alcoholic's continuing antisocial behavior causes his friends to avoid him. His spouse may leave him. Tension develops among him, his employer, and his fellow workers. Eventually he loses his job.

Physical and mental erosion caused by uncontrolled drinking leads him to make the rounds of hospitals emergency departments, doctor offices, and psychiatrists. But because he will not admit the extent of his drinking, he seldom receives any lasting benefit, in part because he fails to follow the doctor's instructions.

Chronic Phase

In the chronic phase, the last stages of alcoholism, the alcoholic has no choice—he must drink. He gets helplessly drunk for days at a time (*bender*). He disregards everything—family, job, food, and even shelter. He now attempts to escape the problems caused by the drinking by drinking. Tremors and hallucinations may occur (delirium tremens), which are sometimes fatal. If he survives he swears off alcohol forever, only eventually to relapse once more.

Having an available supply of alcohol becomes the most important thing in his life. He will spend every last cent, and if necessary sell the coat off his back to get and keep alcohol. He may hide his bottles so there will always be a drink close at hand (*protecting his supply*).

The alcoholic now shows open hostility toward others. This can be a conscious effort to protect his supply of alcohol or it can be the outward evidence of an unconscious desire for self-punishment. He becomes constantly fearful of things he cannot name—a feeling of impending doom or destruction.

The alcoholic finally realizes that he can no longer make excuses or blame others for his problems. He admits he is licked and that his drinking is out of control and is beyond his ability to control it. All the signposts point to custodial care or death. Death may come in advanced cases of cirrhosis of the liver, pancreatitis, or hemorrhage from esophageal varices. Or the alcoholic may commit suicide.

The Disease Concept and the Primary Care Physician

The disease concept of dependence allows primary care physicians to use familiar techniques to make a diagnosis, form a treatment plan, educate a patient about drugs, and discuss prognosis. It helps differentiate addiction from a bad habit, moral weakness, or a lack of willpower. Most importantly, it obligates primary care physicians to address the problem of addiction in a nonjudgmental way [25].

AMA'S Definition of Substance Dependence

In 1956, the American Medical Association (AMA) declared alcoholism to be a disease and gave the following definition:

> Alcoholism is a primary, chronic disease with genetic, psychosocial, and environmental factors influencing its development and manifestations. The disease is often progressive and fatal. It is characterized by continuous or periodic impaired control over drinking, preoccupation with the drug alcohol, use of alcohol despite adverse consequences, and distortions in thinking, most notably denial. [26]

In 1987, the AMA extended its declaration to all psychoactive substances.

ASAM'S Definition of Substance Dependence

In 2011, the American Society of Addiction Medicine (ASAM) updated its definition of addiction, highlighting that addiction is a chronic brain disorder and not simply a behavioral problem involving too much alcohol or other drugs. The definition also describes addiction as a primary disease [27]. Addiction is also recognized as a chronic disease, like cardiovascular disease or diabetes mellitus. ASAM's definition is as follows:

> Addiction is a primary, chronic disease of brain reward, motivation, memory, and related circuitry. Dysfunction in these circuits leads to characteristic biological, psychological, social and spiritual manifestations. This is reflected in an individual pathologically pursuing reward and/or relief by substance use and other behaviors. Addiction is characterized by inability to abstain consistently, impairment in behavioral control, craving, diminished recognition of significant problems with one's behaviors and interpersonal relationships, and a dysfunctional emotional response. Like other chronic diseases, addiction often involves cycles of relapse and remission. Without treatment or engagement in

recovery activities, addiction is progressive and can result in disability or premature death.

Summary

The biopsychosocial definition views substance dependence as continuing to use a drug despite significant biological, psychological, or social problems. The fundamental etiological assumption of the biological view of substance dependence is that individuals who become dependent on a chemical substance are in some significant way biologically different from those who do not become dependent. Psychological problems due to substance dependence include depression, anxiety, mood swings, confusion, hallucinations, impaired judgment, a desire to engage in risky behavior, a decrease in pleasure in everyday life (anhedonia), impulsiveness, and loss of self-control. Sociological problems associated with substance dependence include (1) family problems, (2) financial problems, (3) legal problems, and (4) isolation.

The disease concept of dependence allows primary care physicians to use familiar techniques to make a diagnosis, form a treatment plan, educate a patient about drugs, and discuss prognosis. Family, twin, and adoption studies are the classic techniques for examining the role that genetic factors play in substance dependence.

The AMA's definition recognizes substance dependence to be a primary, chronic disease with genetic, psychosocial, and environmental factors influencing its development and manifestations.

ASAM's definition recognizes substance dependence to be a primary, chronic disease of brain reward, motivation, memory, and related circuitry.

References

1. Dependence. Oxford Dictionary. https://en.oxforddictionaries.com/definition/dependence
2. Milhorn HT. Screening, assessment, and diagnosis. In: Wilford BB, editor. Review course syllabus. New York: American Society of Addiction Medicine; 1990.
3. Why do drug use disorders often co-occur with other mental illnesses? National Institute on Drug Abuse (NIDA) website. https://www.drugabuse.gov/publications/research-reports/comorbidity-addiction-other-mental-illnesses/why-do-drug-use-disorders-often-co-occur-other-men. September 2010.
4. Lameman BE. Effects on family. Addiction in Family website. http://addictioninfamily.com/family-issues/effects-on-family
5. Milhorn HT. Understanding chemical dependence. J Miss State Med Assoc. 1992;33(4):123–8.
6. Rounsaville BJ, Kosten TR, Weissman MM, et al. Psychiatric disorders in relatives of probands with opiate addiction. Arch Gen Psychiatry. 1991;48(1):33–42.
7. Kaji L. Alcoholism in twins: studies on the etiology and sequels of abuse of alcohol. Stockholm: Almqvist and Wiksell; 1960.
8. Kendler KS, Neale MC, Kessler RC, et al. A test of the equal-environment assumption in twin studies of psychiatric illness. Behav Genet. 1993;23(1):21–7.
9. Kendler KS, Prescott CA. Cocaine use, abuse, and dependence in a population-based sample of female twins. Br J Psychiatry. 1998;173:345–50.
10. Goodwin DW, Schlesinger F, Hermansen L, Guze SB, Winokur G. Alcohol problems in adoptees raised apart from alcoholic biological parents. Arch Gen Psychiatry. 1973;28:238–43.
11. Bohman M. Some genetic aspects of alcoholism and criminality. Arch Gen Psychiatry. 1978;35(3):269–76.
12. Cotton NS. The familial incidence of alcoholism: a review. J Stud Alcohol. 1979;40(1):89–116.
13. Schuckit MA. Self-rating of alcohol intoxication by young men with and without family histories of alcoholism. J Stud Alcohol. 1980;41(3):242–9.
14. Begleiter H, Porjesz B, Bihari B, Kissin B. Event-related potentials in boys at risk for alcoholism. Science. 1984;225(4669):1493–6.
15. Schuckit MA, Gold E, Risch C. Serum prolactin levels in sons of alcoholics and control subjects. Am J Psychiatry. 1987;144(7):854–9.
16. Tabakoff B, Hoffman PL. Genetics and biological markers of risk for alcoholism. Public Health Rep. 1988;103(6):690–8.
17. Ratsma JE, Van der Stelt O, Gunning WB. Neurochemical markers of alcoholism vulnerability in humans. Alcohol Alcohol. 2002;37(6):522–33.
18. Oroszi G, Goldman D. Alcoholism: genes and mechanisms. Pharmacogenomics. 2004;5(8):1037–48.
19. Zalewska-Kaszubska J, Czarneca E. Deficit in beta-endorphin peptide and tendency to alcohol abuse. Peptides. 2005;26(4):701–5.
20. Blum K, Noble EP, Sheridan PJ, et al. Allelic association of human dopamine D_2 receptor gene in alcoholism. JAMA. 1990;263(15):2055–60.
21. Dick DM, Edenberg HJ, Xuei X, et al. Association of GABRG3 with alcohol dependence. Alcohol Clin Exp Res. 2004;28:4–9.

22. Pandey SC, Roy A, Zhang H. Partial deletion of the CREB gene promotes alcohol-drinking behaviors. J Neurosci. 2004;24(21):5022–30.
23. The genetics of alcoholism. National Institute on Alcohol Abuse and Alcoholism (NIAAA) website. https://pubs.niaaa.nih.gov/publications/aa18.htm. October 2003.
24. Jellinek EM. The disease concept of alcoholism. New Haven: Hillhouse; 1960.
25. Milhorn HT. Chemical dependence: diagnosis, treatment, and prevention. New York: Springer-Verlag; 1990.
26. Morse RM, Daniel KF. The definition of alcoholism. JAMA. 1992;268(8):1012–4.
27. ASAM releases new definition of addiction. American Society of Addiction Medicine (ASAM) website. http://www.asam.org/quality-practice/definition-of-addiction. August 15, 2011.

3 Pharmacology of Psychoactive Substances

Key Chapter Points

- Many drugs produce their effects by interacting with specific macromolecules (receptors) that are usually located on a cell's outer membrane.
- A synapse is a specialized junction at which a neuron communicates with a target cell or another neuron.
- The brain recognizes all pleasures in the same way, whether they originate from a psychoactive substance, a sexual encounter, or a good meal. This occurs in the reward center of the brain.
- Upregulation and downregulation involve the development of increased or decreased numbers of postsynaptic receptors in response to a decreased or increased drug level, respectively.
- Drug-receptor interactions are usually discussed in terms of semilogarithmic, dose-response plots of drug plasma concentration versus physiological response.
- If a drug is capable of producing a symptom, regular use of the drug at the original dose level may evoke the symptom not after the first dose but after multiple doses, a phenomenon known as kindling.
- Most, if not all, psychoactive drugs lose some effect with repeated use. Individuals who wish to achieve a specific effect, such as becoming high, must use larger and larger doses, a phenomenon known as tolerance.
- The term physical dependence is used to distinguish drugs that, when patients stop using them, cause an abstinence syndrome.
- The set and setting of using drugs can have an influence on the type of experience a person has.

An understanding of the basic principles of pharmacology is essential to understand how psychoactive substances exert their effects. Pharmacology has two major components—pharmacodynamics and pharmacokinetics [1].

Pharmacodynamics

The study of how drugs exert their effects is called *pharmacodynamics*. It focuses on how the molecules of most drugs interact with specific receptors on target cells, how a biological response occurs, the relationship of the dose and the resultant response to a drug, and the way one drug can alter the response to another.

Receptors

Many drugs produce their effects by interacting with specific macromolecules that are usually located on a cell's outer membrane. These specific interaction sites are called *receptors*. The shape, size, electrical charge, and other properties of the receptor surface must be compatible

H.T. Milhorn, *Substance Use Disorders*, DOI 10.1007/978-3-319-63040-3_3

with those of the specific drug molecules that interact with it. This interaction is often described by a lock and key analogy. *Agonists* interact with the receptor to form a drug-receptor complex, and in doing so alter cell function to cause a response. Agonists whose characteristics exactly match those of the receptor cause a strong response (Fig. 3.1a), while agonists that do not precisely match the receptor cause a weaker response (Figs. 3.1b, c). Some drugs, called *antagonists*, have properties that allow them to bind to a receptor but produce no response. By binding to the receptor, they prevent formation of an agonist-receptor complex and thereby block the response that would ordinarily occur. These may be strong antagonists (Fig. 3.1d) or weak antagonists (Fig. 3.1e).

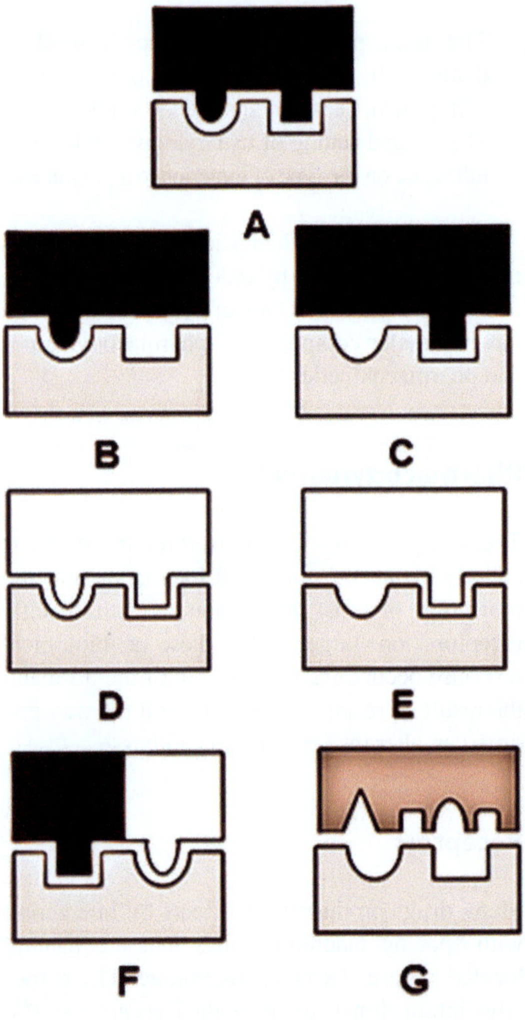

Fig. 3.1 Lock and key analogy: (**a**) strong agonist, (**b**, **c**) weak agonists, (**d**) strong antagonist, (**e**) weak antagonist, (**f**) agonist-antagonist, and (**g**) no reaction

Naloxone (Narcan) and naltrexone (Trexan) are examples of opioid antagonists. They will actually displace drugs such as morphine and hydromorphone (Dilaudid) from receptors. Some analgesic drugs, such as pentazocine (Talwin) and nalbuphine (Nubain), have varying degrees of both agonist and antagonist activity (Fig. 3.1f). They will precipitate withdrawal symptoms in narcotic addicts. Finally, drugs that do not match receptor sites will not interact at all (Fig. 3.1g) [2].

The binding of a drug molecule to its receptor is the first step leading to a response. In many cases this activates a second step. Drugs that cause muscle contraction, for example, do so by first forming a drug-receptor complex on the muscle cell. This activates adenyl cyclase, an enzyme that increases the formation of cyclic adenosine monophosphate (cAMP). In turn, cAMP increases the flow of calcium ions in to the cell, activating the contractile proteins and causing muscle contraction [3].

Synapse

A *synapse* is a specialized junction at which a neuron communicates with a target cell or another neuron. At a synapse, a neuron releases a chemical transmitter that diffuses across a small gap and activates special sites called *receptors* on the target cell or another neuron.

Synaptic Transmission

As a nerve impulse travels from one neuron (presynaptic neuron) to another neuron (postsynaptic neuron) it must cross a gap known as a synapse (Fig. 3.2). The transmission across the synapse requires the action of a chemical substance called a *neurotransmitter*. Neurotransmitters include dopamine, norepinephrine, and serotonin.

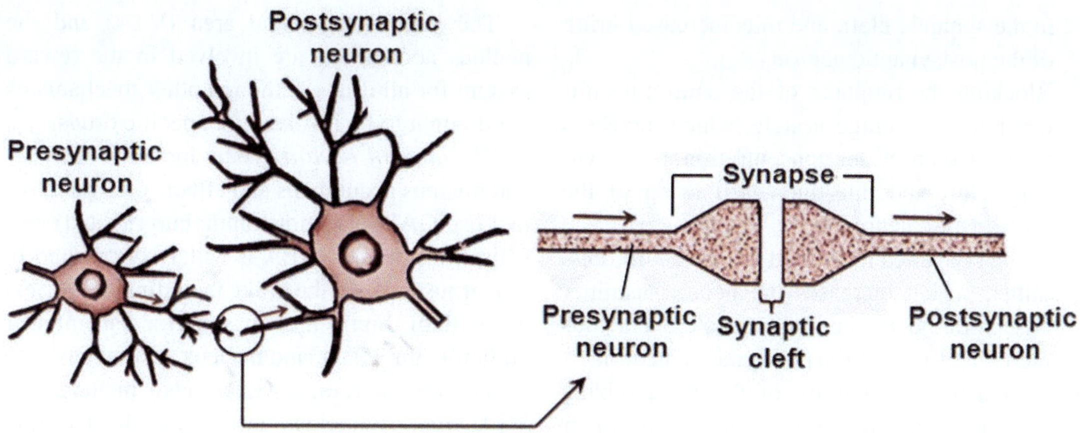

Fig. 3.2 Nerve impulse transmission between two neurons separated by a synapse

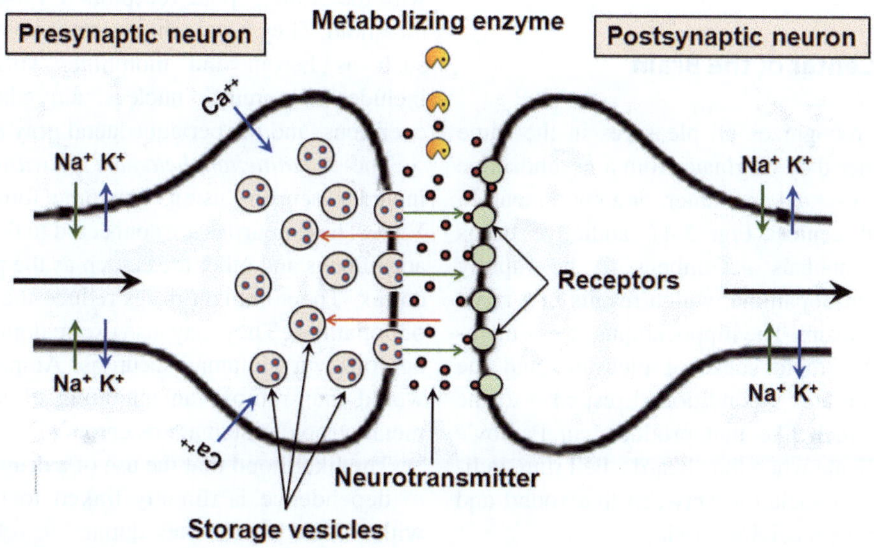

Fig. 3.3 Transmission across a synapse

Synaptic Function

As the action potential moves down the *presynaptic neuron* (Fig. 3.3), it reaches the nerve terminal where it acts on *storage vesicles* to initiate the release of neurotransmitter molecules. The neurotransmitter molecules then cross the *synaptic cleft*, where they momentarily interact with receptors on the *postsynaptic neuron*. Activation of the receptors initiates an action potential in the postsynaptic neuron. After a brief interaction with the *postsynaptic receptors*, the neurotransmitter molecules tend to return to the presynaptic vesicles for storage and reuse. A portion of the neurotransmitter molecules is rendered inactive by a specific enzyme in the synaptic cleft. Synaptic transmission is very rapid, requiring only about 1/1000 of a second [4, 5].

If the synapses are in the reward center of the brain, any drug that greatly increases transmission will produce euphoria, and anything that greatly decreases transmission will cause dysphoria. Drugs can alter synaptic function by [6]:

- Directly stimulating the postsynaptic receptors to increase postsynaptic neuron firing.
- Causing increased release of the neurotransmitter from the storage vesicle, which increases the neurotransmitter concentration

in the synaptic cleft, and thus increased firing of the postsynaptic neuron.

- Blocking the reuptake of the neurotransmitters into the storage vesicle, which increases the neurotransmitter concentration in the synaptic cleft and thus increased firing of the postsynaptic neuron.
- Being converted in the body to the neurotransmitter, which increases the neurotransmitter concentration in the synaptic cleft and thus increased firing of the postsynaptic neuron.
- Decreasing the activity of the metabolizing enzyme, which increases the neurotransmitter in the synaptic cleft, increases the firing rate of the postsynaptic neuron.

Reward Center of the Brain

The brain recognizes all pleasures in the same way, whether they originate from a psychoactive substance, a sexual encounter, or a good meal. In the reward center (Fig. 3.4), addictive drugs cause the nucleus accumbens to be rapidly flooded with dopamine, which results in a rapid sense of pleasure. The hippocampus stores memories of this rapid sense of pleasure, and the amygdala creates a conditioned response to the stimulus, much like that produced in Pavlov's dogs to salivate when they heard a bell ring, indicating their association between that sound and the thought of receiving food.

The ventral tegmental area (VTA) and the nucleus accumbens are involved in the reward system for all drugs, although other mechanisms are thought to be involved for specific drugs.

The alcohol reward system includes the VTA and nucleus accumbens and affects the structures that use GABA (gamma-aminobutyric acid) as a neurotransmitter. GABA is widely distributed in numerous areas of the brain, including the cortex, cerebellum, hippocampus, superior and inferior colliculi, amygdala, and nucleus accumbens.

The *opioid reward system* also includes the VTA and the nucleus accumbens. In addition, opioids affect structures that use brain chemical peptides (endorphins, enkephalins) that react with the brain's opiate receptors to raise the pain threshold. They mimic the action of opioid drugs, such as heroin and morphine. This system includes the arcuate nucleus, amygdala, locus coeruleus, and the periaqueductal gray area.

The *cocaine/amphetamine reward system* includes neurons using dopamine found in the VTA. These neurons are connected to the nucleus accumbens and other areas such as the prefrontal cortex. The stimulant drugs reduce the reuptake of dopamine. They may also excite dopaminergic neurons via glutamate neurons. Amphetamines would thus remove an inhibiting effect due to metabotropic glutamate receptors [7].

The likelihood that the use of a drug will lead to dependence is directly linked to the speed with which it promotes dopamine release and

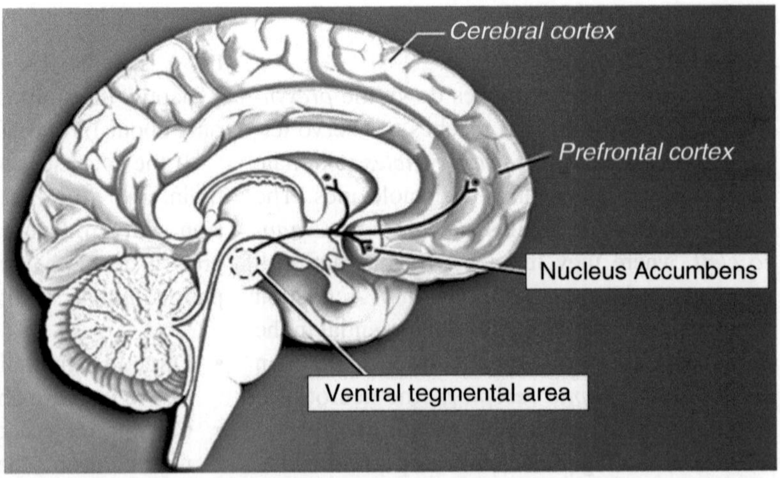

Fig. 3.4 Reward center of the brain

the intensity of that release. Smoking a drug or injecting it intravenously produces a faster, stronger dopamine response than taking a pill orally, and is more likely to lead to repeated drug use.

Addictive drugs can release up to ten times the amount of dopamine that natural rewards do, and they do so more rapidly. As dependence develops, the brain responds by producing less dopamine or decreasing the number of dopamine receptors. As a result, dopamine has less impact on the brain's reward center. The drug no longer causes as much pleasure as it once did. This causes the addict to increase the dose of the drug.

Dopamine not only contributes to the experience of pleasure, but it also plays a role in learning and memory. It interacts with another neurotransmitter, glutamate, to take over the brain's system of reward-related learning. This system has an important role in sustaining life because it links activities needed for human survival, such as eating, drinking, and having sex, with pleasure and reward.

The reward circuit in the brain includes areas involved with motivation and memory as well as with pleasure. Repeated exposure to an addictive substance causes nerve cells in the nucleus accumbens and the prefrontal cortex to communicate in a way that couples enjoying a drug with craving it. This process motivates the drug user to seek out the drug.

The learning process also is important in developing substance dependence. The hippocampus and the amygdala store information about environmental cues associated with the drug. These memories help create intense craving whenever the person encounters an environmental cue, such as a cocaine addict who sees a crack pipe on a television show [8].

Neurotransmitters Affected by Psychoactive Substances

Neurotransmitters affected by psychoactive substances are given in Table 3.1 [9].

Upregulation and Downregulation

Upregulation and downregulation involve the development of increased or decreased numbers of postsynaptic receptors in response to a decreased or increase d drug level, respectively, as illustrated in Fig. 3.5. Figure 3.5a shows a normal synaptic neurotransmitter concentration in the synaptic cleft and a normal number of postsynaptic receptors. As a result, the firing rate of the postsynaptic neuron is normal. Next, the neurotransmitter concentration increases (Fig. 3.5b). In response, the number of postsynaptic receptors decreases in an attempt to return the postsynaptic neuron firing rate back to normal. In Fig. 3.5c, the neurotransmitter concentration in the synaptic cleft decreases. In response, the number of postsynaptic receptors increases in an attempt to return the postsynaptic firing rate back to normal.

As an example of downregulation, consider excessive activation of the postsynaptic receptors as a result of long-term heroin use. A decrease in the number of postsynaptic receptors occurs in an attempt to return the postsynaptic neuron firing rate to normal. If the heroin addict's supply is suddenly cutoff, the postsynaptic neuron firing rate decreases due to the decreased number of postsynaptic receptors. The result is dysphoria.

As an example of upregulation, consider a schizophrenic patient treated with an antipsychotic medication such as chlorpromazine (Thorazine) for a prolonged period of time, producing a blockade of postsynaptic receptors in the basal ganglia. This causes the development of additional postsynaptic receptors in an attempt to return the postsynaptic neuron firing rate to normal. If removal of the neuroleptic blockade occurs, the patient may develop tardive dyskinesia because normal amounts of dopamine now overactivate the excess receptors [1, 4].

Dose-Response Relationships

A dose-response relationship is an association between the dose of a drug administered and its pharmacologic effect.

Table 3.1 Neurotransmitters affected by psychoactive substances (From Sherman [9])

Neurotransmitter	Distribution in the CNS	Functions affected	Drugs that affect the neurotransmitter
Dopamine	Midbrain, ventral tegmental area (VTA), cerebral cortex, hypothalamus	Pleasure and reward, movement, attention, memory	Cocaine, amphetamine, methamphetamine. In addition, virtually all drugs of abuse directly or indirectly augment dopamine in the reward pathway
Serotonin	Midbrain, VTA, cerebral cortex, hypothalamus	Mood, sleep, sexual desire, appetite	MDMA (ecstasy), LSD, cocaine
Norepinephrine	Midbrain, VTA, cerebral cortex, hypothalamus	Sensory processing, movement, sleep, mood, memory, anxiety	Cocaine, methamphetamine, amphetamine
Endogenous opioids (endorphin and enkephalin)	Widely distributed in the brain but regions vary in type of receptors, spinal cord	Analgesia, sedation, rate of bodily functions, mood	Heroin, morphine, oxycodone
Acetylcholine	Hippocampus, cerebral cortex, thalamus, basal ganglia, cerebellum	Memory, arousal, attention, mood	Nicotine
Endogenous cannabinoids (anandamide)	Cerebral cortex, hippocampus, thalamus, basal ganglia	Movement, cognition and memory	Marijuana
Glutamate	Widely distributed in the brain	Neuron activity (increased rate), learning, cognition, memory	Ketamine, phencyclidine, alcohol
Gamma-aminobutyric acid (GABA)	Widely distributed in the brain	Neuron activity (slowed), anxiety, memory, anesthesia	Sedatives, tranquilizers, alcohol

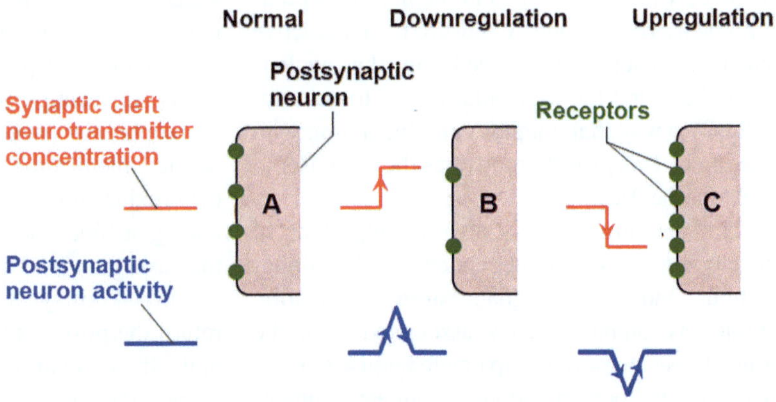

Fig. 3.5 Synaptic transmission: (**a**) normal, (**b**) downregulation, and (**c**) upregulation

Dose-Response Plots

Drug-receptor interactions are usually discussed in terms of semilogarithmic, dose-response plots of drug plasma concentration versus physiological response (Fig. 3.6). The semilogarithmic plot has several advantages. It can display a wide range of doses, and its curves are usually S-shaped with linear middle segments. This implies that binding to the receptors is a first-order process within this linearity, that is, that the amount of a drug binding to the receptors is directly proportional to the drug's concentration. Drugs producing the same effects by the same mechanism produce dose-response curves whose linear segments parallel each other. When two drugs act individually by binding to the same receptors, they produce the same maximum response (plateau). The plateau means that all

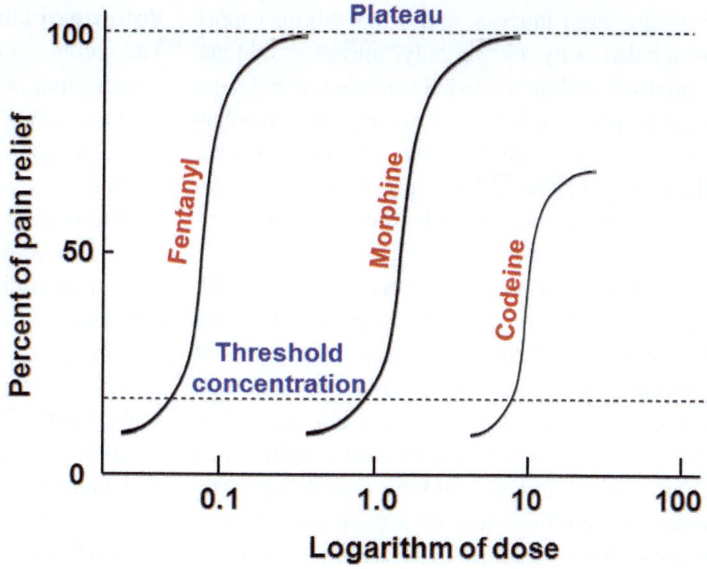

Fig. 3.6 Dose-response curves for fentanyl, morphine, and codeine

receptors have become saturated. In addition, a minimum plasma concentration of a drug is necessary to initiate a response. The amount of drug that produces this minimum concentration is called the *threshold* dose [1, 10].

Affinity, Potency, and Efficacy

The tendency of a drug to be bound at given receptor sites is known as its *affinity*. In Fig. 3.6, fentanyl produces a response at a lower dose than morphine. Therefore, it has a greater affinity for the receptors, and is said to be more potent. *Potency* indicates the dose of a drug needed to produce a given response when compared to the dose of another drug required to produce the same response [1].

Fentanyl and morphine reach the same plateau. They therefore have the same *efficacy* (response-producing ability) despite differing potencies. Drugs that plateau at lower maximum responses than other drugs, such as codeine, are said to be less efficacious. No amount of codeine will produce the efficacy of morphine or fentanyl [11].

Kindling

If a drug is capable of producing a symptom, regular use of the drug at the original dose level may evoke the symptom not after the first dose but after multiple doses, a phenomenon known as *kindling*. The paranoid schizophreniform reaction to cocaine is an example of kindling. It may not occur with the first dose, the second dose, or even the third dose, but it develops after many doses over a period of time [4].

Pharmacokinetics

Pharmacokinetics is the branch of pharmacology concerned with the movement of drugs within the body. Four major processes determine both the intensity and duration of a drug's action: (1) absorption, (2) distribution, (3) metabolism, and (4) excretion [10]. We will limit our discussion to route of administration, distribution, enzymatic reactions, and steady-state relationships.

Route of Administration

Drugs can be ingested orally, insufflated (snorted) via the nasal mucosa, inhaled, or injected. Ingested drugs must cross the intestinal mucosa to reach the bloodstream. Some drugs—alcohol, for example—may be partially absorbed in the stomach. Drugs that are insufflated, such as cocaine, must cross the nasal mucosa, and drugs whose vapors are inhaled (amyl nitrate, butyl nitrite) or that are combusted and then inhaled (nicotine, marijuana, cocaine, phencyclidine) must cross the alveolar-capillary membrane to reach the bloodstream. Many drugs can be injected subcutaneously, intramuscularly, or intravenously (cocaine, methamphetamine, heroin).

The site of absorption can markedly affect the rapidity of onset of a drug's effect as well as the degree of its effect. Cocaine in the form of chewed coca leaf, for example, is slowly absorbed in the buccal mucosa and small intestine. It is absorbed more rapidly and reaches a higher peak when smoked. In fact, smoking cocaine approximates the rapid delivery of intravenous cocaine because drugs that reach the alveoli have rapid access in the bloodstream through the large alveolar-capillary membrane. Because most of the cardiac output passes through the pulmonary capillaries, the delivery of a drug from the alveoli to the brain is further enhanced [3].

Distribution

A drug's distribution depends on its volume of distribution, its protein binding, and its accumulation in adipose tissue.

Volume of Distribution

The *volume of distribution* (V_d) is the theoretical volume that would be necessary to contain the total amount of an administered drug at the same concentration that is observed in the blood plasma.

The simplest compartments of distribution for drugs can be described in terms of extracellular and intracellular water, with a subdivision of extracellular water into plasma (intravascular) and interstitial (extravascular) fluids (Fig. 3.7). Drugs that stay in the plasma distribute to 3 l of body fluid. Charged drugs may distribute only through extracellular fluid (3 + 10 = 13 l), because they cannot readily cross cell membranes. Drugs that are water soluble and cross membranes readily, such as ethanol, may be distributed into all body water (3 + 10 + 27 = 40 l) [5].

The V_d of a drug is a ratio of the amount of drug in the body divided by the concentration of the drug in the plasma at that time. It is usually calculated by dividing the initial dose (D_o) of drug by an extrapolated concentration at time zero (C_o).

$$V_d = \text{Initial dose}(D_o) / \text{Time zero concentration}(C_o)$$

Figure 3.8 is a plot of the logarithm of a drug as a function of time. The beta phase is due to metabolism and excretion. The beta phase line is

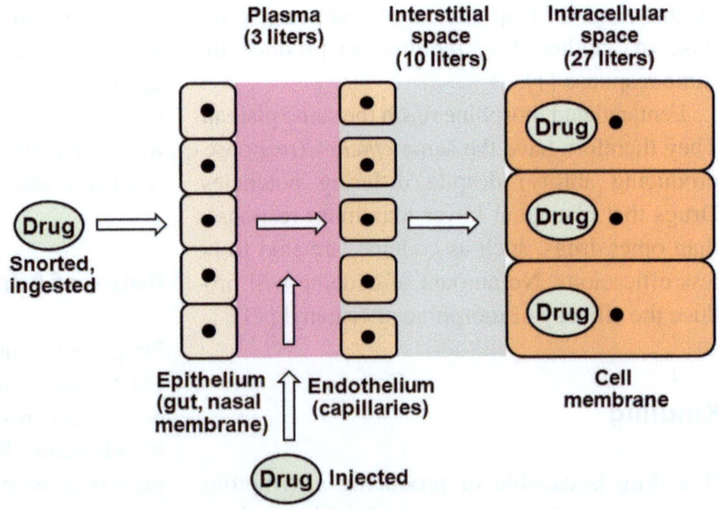

Fig. 3.7 Drug distribution

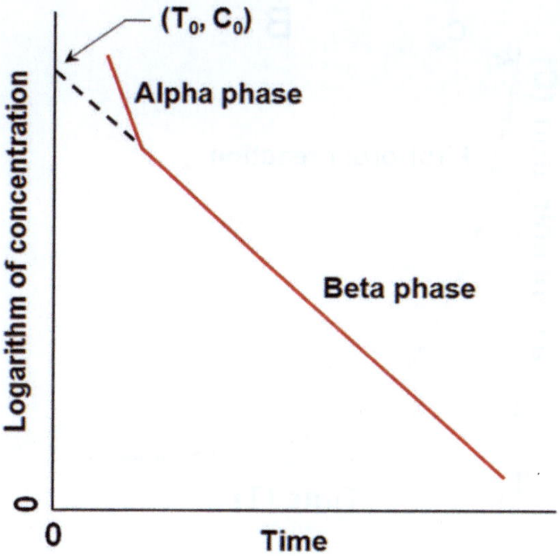

Fig. 3.8 Decline of drug concentration in plasma over time

extrapolated backward in time to time zero (T_0.). The concentration of the drug (C_0) at time T_0 can then be determined. The alpha phase is due to the initial drug distribution.

The volume of distribution is used clinically when trying to determine the loading dose necessary for a desired blood concentration of a drug, and is also used for estimating a blood concentration in the treatment of an overdose.

The volume of distribution is usually further divided by the patient's body weight, and the result expressed in terms of liters per kilogram. Following injection, most drugs will show some distribution into the tissues and extracellular fluid. Some drug will be retained in the plasma, but may be bound to plasma proteins. Remember, only the free drug is able to exert its effect.

Drugs that remain confined to the plasma will exhibit a volume of distribution similar to plasma volume [3].

The Blood-Brain Barrier

The blood-brain barrier (BBB) is a highly selective permeability barrier that separates the circulating blood from the brain extracellular fluid. The capillary endothelial cells of the central nervous system (CNS) greatly reduce the ability of many drug molecules to diffuse across the membrane and reach effective concentrations in the brain. The BBB probably evolved to protect the cells of the CNS against foreign substances. Only drugs that are very lipid soluble can cross the blood-brain barrier well and produce achievable actions in the CNS. Such drugs include anesthetic gases, alcohol, sedatives, and hypnotics. Some portions of the CNS, such as the chemoreceptor trigger zone, which is responsible for nausea, are outside the barrier [5].

Enzymatic Reactions

The two most common types of enzymatic reactions that occur in the body are zero-order reactions and first-order reactions.

Zero-Order Reaction

In a *zero-order reaction*, the binding sites on the enzymes are saturated. The rate of metabolism, therefore, is constant

$$C = C_o - kT$$

in which C is concentration, C_o is the initial concentration, k is the rate constant, and T is time. A zero-order reaction is independent of the concentration of the reactants. The greater the rate constant the more rapid the decline in concentration. Ethanol is an important example of a drug that undergoes a zero-order reaction.

First-Order Reaction

In a *first-order reaction*, a drug's concentration is well below the level that would saturate the binding sites of the enzyme. The drug is, therefore, metabolized at a rate proportional to its concentration

$$C = C_o e^{-kT}$$

in which C is concentration, C_o is initial concentration, k is the rate constant (half-life) of the drug, and T is time [13]. Most drugs undergo first-order reactions, which is independent of dose. Zero-order reaction and first-order reaction are illustrated in Fig. 3.9.

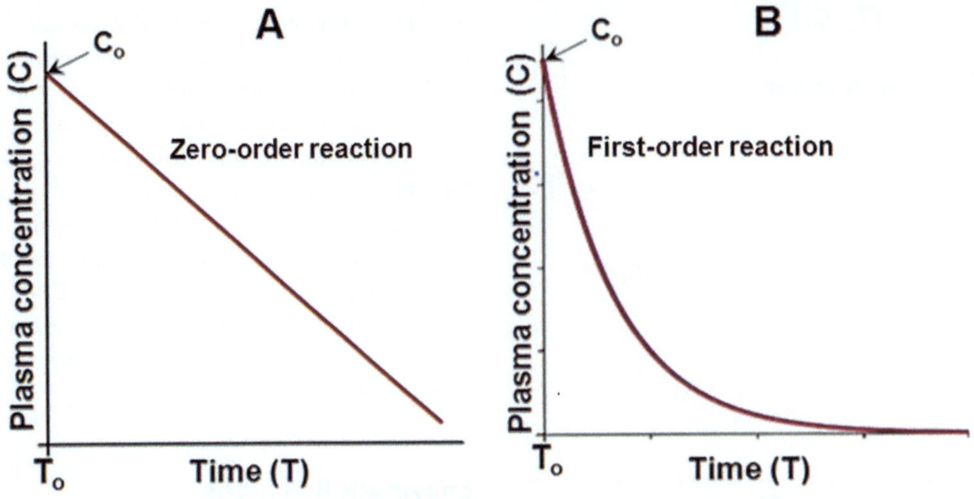

Fig. 3.9 (**a**) Zero-order kinetics and (**b**) first-order kinetics

Some drugs, such as phenytoin (Dilantin), undergo first-order reactions at lower concentrations and zero-order reactions at higher concentrations [3]. Second-order reactions do occur in the body, but they are much less common, so I will not discuss them.

Enzyme Inhibition and Induction

Drug-metabolizing enzymes may be inhibited or induced (stimulated). Inhibition may be competitive or noncompetitive.

Competitive inhibition occurs when another substance of similar structure combines reversibly with an enzyme's active site (Fig. 3.10a). This type of inhibition may be overcome by increasing a drug's concentration. One example of competitive inhibition is the inhibition of acetaldehyde dehydrogenase by disulfiram (Antabuse). Because the toxic acetaldehyde formed by the metabolism of the ethanol cannot be biotransformed, it builds up in the body. This results in a severe reaction when patients ingest ethanol.

Noncompetitive inhibition occurs when an agent, unrelated in structure to the drug, binds in a distorted manner to prevent normal interaction between the drug and the enzyme (Fig. 3.10b). This form of inhibition cannot be overcome by increasing the drug's concentration.

Microsomal enzymes undergo a quantitative increase in metabolizing ability (induction) when persistently exposed to a variety of drugs. Since most drugs that do this are lipid soluble, entering the liver cells is necessary for drugs to cause enzyme induction. Phenobarbital is the most commonly known drug to do this. A few older drugs, such as meprobamate (Equanil, Miltown) and glutethimide (Doriden), may undergo enzyme induction and therefore hasten their own metabolism [3].

Steady-State Relationships

The *half-life* of a drug is defined as the time required for the serum concentration of the drug to fall to 50% of its previous level (Fig. 3.11). Only drugs that undergo first-order reactions can be described in terms of half-life. The time it takes drugs (such as alcohol) that undergo zero-order reactions to fall to 50% of their previous level depends on the dose—the greater the dose, the longer the time required for this to occur. The half-life of a drug is determined by the interaction between absorption, distribution, metabolism, and excretion [5].

When a drug is administered at intervals greater than or equal to its half-life, it will begin

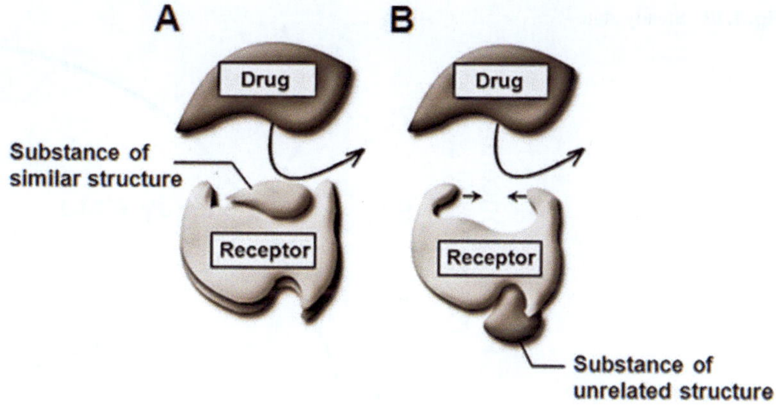

Fig. 3.10 Drug metabolism: (**a**) competitive inhibition and (**b**) noncompetitive inhibition

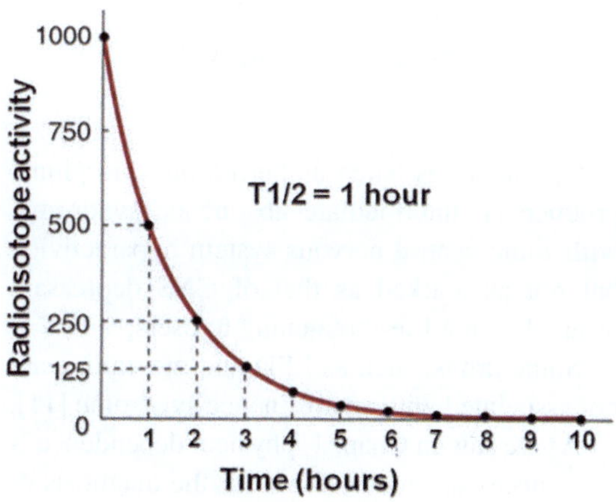

Fig. 3.11 Half-life of a drug

to accumulate in the serum because some of the previous dose is still in the blood when each subsequent dose is taken. Eventually a point of balance (a steady state) is reached in which the rate of excretion and metabolism is equal to the rate of administration (Fig. 3.12). The dose markedly affects the steady-state level but does not affect the time required to reach it, which is a function only of the drug's half-life. The steady-state concentration, whatever it is going to be, will be reached in four or five half-lives of the drug, regardless of dose size [10].

Tolerance

Most, if not all, psychoactive drugs lose some effect with repeated use. Individuals who wish to achieve a specific effect, such as becoming high, must use larger and larger doses, a phenomenon known as *tolerance*. Tolerance is traditionally divided into dispositional and pharmacodynamic tolerance. *Dispositional tolerance* involves an increased rate of metabolism, almost always because of hepatic microenzyme induction. This probably plays a small role in the development of tolerance to drugs. The major cause of tolerance, *pharmacodynamic tolerance*, takes place at the cellular level in the brain, resulting in part from neurotransmitter downregulation.

Dependent individuals simply function better at a given serum level of a drug that nontolerant individuals do. An alcoholic with a blood alcohol level greater than 0.4 gm/100 ml may still be walking and talking, while most nontolerant individuals would be approaching a comatose state at this level.

Tolerance is not an all-or-none phenomenon. Drug users develop it to some aspects of drug actions but not to others. Amphetamine abusers, for example, may develop tolerance to the cardiovascular and euphoric effects of the drug but remain at high risk for the psychotic effects [3].

Cross-Tolerance

The development of tolerance to drugs in the same class as an abused drug, *cross-tolerance*, occurs without actual use of other drugs. Heroin addicts, for example, automatically develop tolerance to other opioid drugs, such as morphine, hydromorphone, or codeine, as they become

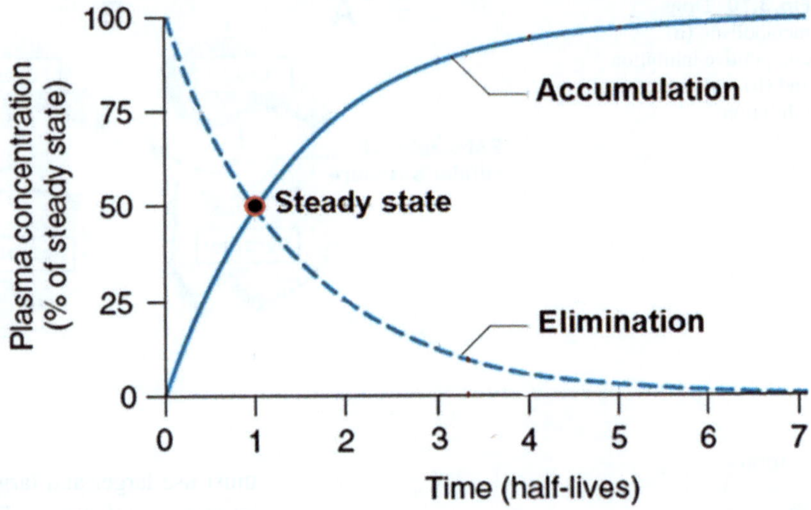

Fig. 3.12 Steady state

tolerant to the effects of heroin. Heroin addicts on methadone maintenance who are injured, for example, will not respond to the usual dose of narcotic pain medication. Alcoholics develop cross-tolerance to other central nervous system depressant drugs, such as barbiturates, benzodiazepines, and gaseous anesthetics [11].

Physical Dependence and Abstinence Syndrome

The term *physical dependence* is used to distinguish drugs that, when patients stop using them, cause an *abstinence syndrome*—that is, they cause patients to develop withdrawal symptoms as discussed in Chap. 1. The most dramatic abstinence syndrome is produced by drugs that depress the central nervous system (alcohol, barbiturates, benzodiazepines). It results from central nervous system hyperactivity, which produces tachycardia, hypertension, anxiety, insomnia, tremer, and sometimes seizures. Death occasionally occurs, particularly when the syndrome develops into delirium tremens.

Drugs like amphetamines and cocaine have much less dramatic withdrawal symptoms. In fact, for many years cocaine was thought not to produce physical dependence because doctors did not recognize its rather mild abstinence syndrome.

Opioid drugs, such as heroin and morphine, produce an intermediate abstinence syndrome, with some central nervous system hyperactivity, but not as marked as that of CNS depressant drugs. It is not life-threatening to users.

Some drugs, such as LSD and mescaline, are not associated with an abstinence syndrome [11].

As we saw in Chap. 1, physical dependence is not a necessary requirement for the diagnosis of substance dependence. Similarly, physical dependence by itself does not mean that a person has the disease of addiction.

Set and Setting

Set and setting refer to the mindset (set) and environment (setting) of the drug experience. The set and setting of using drugs can have an influence on the type of experience a person has. Set and setting are particularly important when using psychoactive drugs, such as LSD, ecstasy, ketamine, and hallucinogenic mushrooms [12].

The term *set and setting* was coined by Timothy Leary who was a Harvard lecturer and researcher who became an advocate for LSD use [13].

Set refers to the state a person brings to the experience. It includes physiological set and psychological set. General health, body size, condition of the liver and kidneys, the amount of food in the stomach, and how well rested the body is are some of the variables that comprise one's *physiological set.* For example, drinking alcohol on an empty stomach leads to more rapid absorption and, consequently, to more rapid intoxication.

The expectation of the user, based on his previous experiences, stories he has heard about the drug, and what he has seen when others have used the same drug are the most important aspects of *psychological set.* These factors account for the well-known placebo effect of drugs.

Setting refers to the environment in which a drug is used. A novice user might experience a somewhat different effect when using a drug at a party where loud rock music is being played as opposed to using it alone in the privacy of his home.

Summary

An understanding of the basic principles of pharmacology is essential to understanding how psychoactive substances exert their effects. Many drugs produce their effects by interacting with specific macromolecules (receptors) that are usually located on a cell's outer membrane. A synapse is a specialized junction at which a neuron communicates with a target cell or another neuron. The brain recognizes all pleasures in the same way, whether they originate from a psychoactive substance, a sexual encounter, or a good meal. This occurs in the reward center of the brain. Dopamine not only contributes to the experience of pleasure, but it also plays a role in learning and memory.

The two most common types of enzymatic reactions that occur in the body are zero-order reactions and first-order reactions. Upregulation and downregulation involve the development of increased or decreased numbers of postsynaptic receptors in response to a decreased or increased drug level, respectively.

Drug-receptor interactions are usually discussed in terms of semilogarithmic, dose-response plots of drug plasma concentration versus physiological response. If a drug is capable of producing a symptom, regular use of the drug at the original dose level may evoke the symptom not after the first dose but after multiple doses, a phenomenon known as kindling.

Most, if not all, psychoactive drugs lose some effect with repeated use. Individuals who wish to achieve a specific effect, such as becoming high, must use larger and larger doses, a phenomenon known as tolerance. The term physical dependence is used to distinguish drugs that, when patients stop using them, cause an abstinence syndrome. The set and setting of using drugs can have an influence on the type of experience a person has.

References

1. Holford NHG. Pharmacokinetics and pharmacodynamics: rational dosing and the time course of drug action. In: Katzung BG, Trevor AJ, editors. Basic and clinical pharmacology. 13th ed. New York: McGraw-Hill Education; 2015. p. 41–55.
2. Von Zastrow M. Drug receptors and pharmacodynamics. In: Katzung BG, Trevor AJ, editors. Basic and clinical pharmacology. 13th ed. New York: McGraw-Hill Education; 2015. p. 20–40.
3. Wilford BB, editor. Pharmacology. In: AMSAODD review course syllabus, AMSAODD, Rockville, MD;1987. p. 13–47.
4. Cohen S. Neurotransmitters, neuropeptides, and neurohormones. In: The chemical brain: the neurochemistry of addictive disorders. Irvine: Care Institute; 1988. p. 11–56.
5. Shafer M, Marieb E, editors. The nurse, pharmacology, and drug therapy. Redwood City: Addison-Wesley; 1989.
6. Milhorn HT. Drug and alcohol abuse: the authoritative guide for parents, teachers, and counselors. New York: Da Capo Press; 2003.
7. The brain's drug reward system. National Institute on Drug Abuse (NIDA). 11(4). https://archives.drugabuse.gov/NIDA_Notes/NNVol11N4/Brain.html. September/October 1996.
8. Howard J. Shaffer. Overcoming addiction: paths toward recovery. Harvard Health Publications. Boston: Harvard Medical School; 2011.
9. Sherman C. Impacts of drugs on neurotransmission. National Institute on Drug Abuse (NIDA) website. https://www.drugabuse.gov/news-events/nida-notes/2007/10/impacts-drugs-neurotransmission. October 1, 2007.
10. Golan DE, Tashjian AH, Armstrong EJ, Armstrong AW. Principles of pharmacology: the pathophysiological basis of drug therapy. 3rd ed. Philadelphia:

Wolters Kluwer Health/Lippincott Williams & Wilkins; 2011.
11. Milhorn HT. Chemical dependence: diagnosis, treatment, and prevention. New York: Springer-Verlag; 1990.
12. Hartney E. What are set and setting in developing addiction? Very Well website. https://www.verywell.com/what-are-set-and-setting-22270. July 14, 2016.
13. Leary T. University of Virginia Library website. https://explore.lib.virginia.edu/exhibits

Part II
Psychoactive Substance Dependencies

Alcohol Dependence

4

Key Chapter Points

- Alcohol is believed to mimic GABA's effect by binding to GABA receptors and thereby inhibiting neuronal signaling.
- Over 90% of consumed alcohol is metabolized in the liver; the rest is excreted unchanged by the lungs and the kidneys.
- The effects of various blood alcohol levels range from feeling warm and relaxed after one to two drinks to death from respiratory depression at much higher levels.
- Excessive drinking includes binge drinking, heavy drinking, and any drinking by pregnant women or people younger than age 21.
- Short-term health risks most often are the result of binge drinking and include injuries, such as motor vehicle crashes, falls, drowning, and burns. Risks also include violence, homicide, suicide, sexual assault, and intimate partner violence.
- Over time, excessive alcohol use can lead to the development of chronic diseases and other serious problems involving virtually every organ system of the body.
- Low to moderate alcohol consumption may have beneficial effects on health.
- The acute phase of the alcohol abstinence syndrome has traditionally been divided into three stages.
- Benzodiazepines are typically used to treat withdrawal symptoms.
- Overdose of ethanol, methanol, and ethylene glycol sometimes occurs.

The common types of alcohol are ethyl alcohol (ethanol), isopropyl alcohol (isopropanol), methyl alcohol (methanol), and ethylene glycol. Ethanol, a sedative-hypnotic, is known as beverage alcohol. It is consumed for a variety of reasons, including partying, getting high, and preventing withdrawal symptoms. Isopropanol, known as rubbing alcohol, is used in hand sanitizers and disinfecting pads. Methanol is widely used as a raw material in the production of other chemicals, particularly formaldehyde, which in turn is used in the production of plastics. Ethylene glycol is mainly used in antifreeze [1].

I will devote the majority of this chapter to ethanol. I will cover the other alcohols at the end of the chapter. Therefore, until then the term alcohol will mean ethanol.

Forms of Alcoholic Beverages

The types of ethanol commonly consumed are divided into three major categories—beer, wine, and spirits. *Beer* is made of a mixture called wort, which is comprised of yeast and a cereal grain like barley, corn, wheat, or rye. The wort is fermented to produce carbon dioxide and alcohol and then flavored with hops, which are the female ripened flower of a perennial climbing vine known as *Humulus lupulus*.

H.T. Milhorn, *Substance Use Disorders*, DOI 10.1007/978-3-319-63040-3_4

The alcohol content in beer varies according to brand and type and usually falls in the range of 4 to 8% alcohol, the exact percentage being determined by state law [2].

Wine is made from different types of grapes or more nontraditional ingredients like fruit or grains. Yeast is added to the crushed ingredients, and then the wine is stored in vats for fermentation. After a full fermentation process, wine goes into barrels to age. Red wines are stored in wooden barrels to add the woody flavor to the wine. White wines are stored in metal barrels to maintain a lighter flavor.

Wine is generally between 10 and 14% alcohol. Yeast stops further fermentation once alcohol reaches about 14%. To obtain a higher percentage of alcohol, the water content is decreased, essentially condensing the alcohol content in the final product [2, 3].

Types of *spirits* include gin, vodka, rum, tequila, whiskey, and brandy. This type of alcohol is made by distilling a fermented grain, fruit, or vegetable that contains alcohol.

Spirits are also called hard liquor or distilled beverages, and often contain between 20 and 65% alcohol, which is 40 to 130 proof, respectively. A brand named Everclear contains 95% alcohol (190 proof).

Whiskey is distilled from malted grains, port wine and sherry are wines that are fortified to boost the alcohol content, and brandy is distilled wine [2].

Twelve ounces of beer contains about the same amount of alcohol as five ounces of wine, three ounces of port or sherry, and 1.5 ounces of 80 proof whiskey or liquor [4].

Prevalence of Alcohol Use and Dependence

Prevalence of Drinking

In 2015, 86.4% of people ages 18 or older reported that they drank alcohol at some point in their lifetime, 70.1% reported that they drank in the past year, and 56.0% reported that they drank in the past month [5].

Prevalence of Binge Drinking and Heavy Drinking

In 2015, 26.9% of people ages 18 or older reported that they engaged in binge drinking in the past month, and 7.0% reported that they engaged in heavy alcohol use in the past month [5].

Prevalence of Alcohol Use Disorder

In the United States, 16.3 million adults ages 18 and older had an alcohol use disorder in 2014. This included 10.6 million men (9.2%) and 5.7 million women (4.6%) [5].

Treatment Statistics

About 1.5 million adults received treatment for an alcohol use disorder at a specialized facility in 2014. This included 1.1 million men and 431,000 women. This was only 8.9% of adults who needed treatment 90 [5].

Alcohol-Related Liver Problems

In 2013, of the 72,559 liver disease deaths, 45.8% involved alcohol. Among males, 46,568 (48.5%) of the liver disease deaths involved alcohol. Among females, 25,991 (41.8%) of the liver disease deaths involved alcohol. Among all cirrhosis deaths in 2011, 48.0% were alcohol related. In 2009, alcohol-related liver disease was the primary cause of almost one in three liver transplants in the United States [5].

Alcohol-Related Deaths

Nearly 88,000 people (62,000 men and 26,000 women) die from alcohol-related causes annually. This makes alcohol the fourth leading preventable cause of death in the United States.

In 2014, alcohol-impaired driving fatalities accounted for 9967 deaths, which represented 31% of overall driving fatalities [5].

The Financial Cost of Alcohol Dependence

Alcohol-related health-care costs amount to about $223.5 billion per year. Almost 75% of those costs($167.6 billion) can be traced to binge drinking [6].

Pharmacology

Pharmacodynamics

Gamma-butyric acid (GABA) is the major inhibitory neurotransmitter in the brain. Alcohol is believed to mimic GABA's effect by binding to GABA receptors and thereby inhibiting neuronal signaling.

Alcohol also inhibits the major excitatory neurotransmitter, glutamate, particularly at the N-methyl-d-aspartate (NMDA) glutamate receptor. In addition, it releases other inhibitory neurotransmitters, such as dopamine and serotonin. Consumption of even small amounts of alcohol increases the amount of dopamine in the nucleus accumbens area of the brain. In fact, multiple neurotransmitters in various parts of the brain combine to make the consumption of small doses of alcohol pleasurable [7].

Pharmacokinetics

Ethanol is a small, water-soluble molecule that is absorbed rabidly and completely, 20% from the stomach and 80% from the small intestine. Ingested alcohol on an empty stomach reaches a peak level within 40 min. Food in the gut delays alcohol consumption.

Distribution is rapid, with tissue levels approximating the blood level. The volume of distribution is about 50 l in a 70 kg person.

Over 90% of consumed alcohol is metabolized in the liver; the rest is excreted unchanged by the lungs and the kidneys.

The rate of oxidation obeys zero-order kinetics; that is, it is independent of concentration. A typical adult can metabolize 7–10 g of alcohol

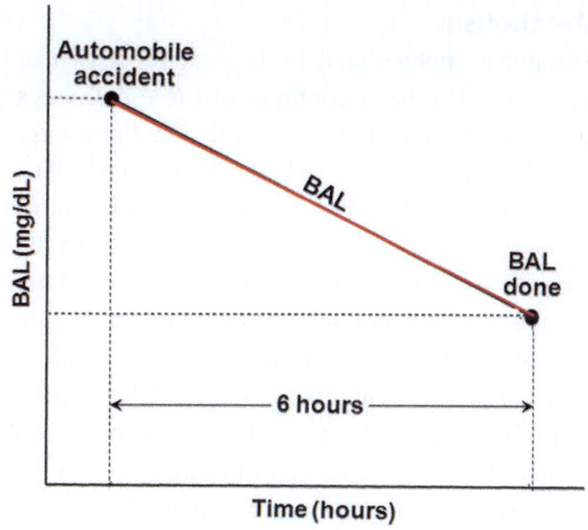

Fig. 4.1 Illustration of how to calculate backward to determine the BAL at an earlier time

(1 ounce of 80 proof whiskey) per hour [8]. That means that, with an estimate of total body water and a blood alcohol level (BAL), one can determine the BAL at a previous time, say at the time of an automobile accident as shown in Fig. 4.1. I was asked to do this calculation once as an expert witness in a trial.

Let's assume that a 70 kg man was detained 6 h after leaving the scene of an automobile accident in which he was involved and that at the time of his detainment his blood alcohol level was 0.07 g/dL or 0.7 g/l, which doesn't qualify as being legally drunk. The question is "What was his blood alcohol level at the time of the accident?" We know that the volume of distribution for this man is 50 l and that alcohol is metabolized at 7–10 g/h (let's take the middle ground and say 8.5 g/h).

His total body alcohol content at the time of detainment would be 0.7 g/l × 50 l = 35 g. In 6 h with an alcohol metabolizing rate of 8.5 g/h, the amount of alcohol he would have metabolized is 6 h × 8.5 g/h = 51 g of alcohol. Therefore, his total body alcohol content at the time of the accident would be 35 g + 51 g = 86 g. His blood alcohol concentration in grams/liter would be 86 g/50 l = 1.72 g/l or 0.172 g/dL. Clearly at the time of the accident his BAL was well above the legally drunk value of 0.08 g/dL.

Metabolism

Alcohol is metabolized by several processes or pathways. The most common of these pathways involves two enzymes—alcohol dehydrogenase (ADH) and aldehyde dehydrogenase (ALDH). These enzymes help break apart the alcohol molecule, making it possible to eliminate it from the body. First, alcohol dehydrogenase (ADH) metabolizes alcohol to acetaldehyde, a highly toxic substance. Then, in a second step, acetaldehyde is further metabolized to another less active by-product called acetate, which is then broken down into water and carbon dioxide by aldehyde dehydrogenase (ALDH) for elimination.

$$\underset{\text{Alcohol}}{CH_3CH_2OH} \xrightarrow{\text{ADH}} \underset{\text{Acetaldehyde}}{CH_3CHO} \rightarrow \underset{\text{Acetate}}{CH_3COOH} \xrightarrow{\text{ALDH}} \underset{\text{Water}}{H_2O} + \underset{\text{Carbon dioxide}}{CO_2}$$

This system of alcohol metabolism uses nicotinamide adenine dinucleotide (NAD) as a cofactor.

The microsomal ethanol oxidizing system (MEOS) is an alternate pathway of ethanol metabolism that occurs in the microsomes in the oxidation of ethanol to acetaldehyde. While playing only a minor role in ethanol metabolism in light drinking, MEOS activity increases after heavy chronic alcohol consumption. The MEOS pathway uses nicotinamide adenine dinucleotide phosphate (NADPH) instead of NAD as a cofactor.

Over 90% of the acetaldehyde formed by both reactions is metabolized by the liver. Enzyme-inducing drugs, such as barbiturates, may enhance the rate of alcohol metabolism [9, 10].

Pharmacological Actions

Alcohol affects most systems of the body, including the central nervous system, circulatory system, gastrointestinal system, urinary system, and thermoregulatory system. In addition, alcohol is responsible for a number of cancers.

Central Nervous System

The central nervous system is more acutely affected by alcohol than any other organ system. Alcohol can cause relief of anxiety, sedation, slurred speech, ataxia, impaired judgment, and uninhibited behavior. The apparent stimulation, which occurs at low doses, results from depression of inhibitory mechanisms [8].

The effects of various blood alcohol levels (BALs), or blood alcohol concentrations (BACs), range from feeling warm and relaxed after one to two drinks (0.02 g/dL) to death from respiratory depression at a BAL greater or equal to 0.4 g/dL. Specific effects at various blood alcohol levels in a nontolerant person are given in (Table 4.1) [11].

Individuals with a history of long, frequent drinking develop tolerance to alcohol so that a much higher BAL must be achieved to obtain the effects of a normally lower BAL. Alcoholics may

Table 4.1 Specific effects at various blood alcohol levels in a nontolerant person (Based on [11])

BAL (g/dL)	Dose-specific effects
0.039	No loss of coordination, slight euphoria, and loss of shyness. Relaxation, but depressant effects are not apparent
0.040–0.059	Feeling of well-being, relaxation, lower inhibitions, and sensation of warmth. Euphoria. Some minor impairment of judgment and memory, lowering of caution
0.06–0.099	Slight impairment of balance, speech, vision, reaction time, and hearing. Euphoria. Reduced judgment and self-control. Impaired reasoning and memory
0.100–0.129	Significant impairment of motor coordination and loss of good judgment. Speech may be slurred; balance, peripheral vision, reaction time, and hearing are impaired
0.130–0.159	Gross motor impairment and lack of physical control. Blurred vision and major loss of balance. Euphoria decreases and dysphoria begins
0.160–0.199	Dysphoria predominates, nausea may appear. The drinker has the appearance of a sloppy drunk
0.200–0.249	Needs assistance in walking; total mental confusion. Dysphoria with nausea and vomiting; possible blackout
0.250–0.399	Alcohol poisoning. Loss of consciousness
0.40 +	Onset of coma, possible death due to respiratory arrest

walk into the emergency department and answer questions reasonably well with a BAL above 0.45, a level that would render nontolerant individuals comatose or dead.

Circulatory System

The immediate effects of alcohol on the circulatory system are relatively minor. Blood pressure, cardiac output, and myocardial contraction do not change greatly in most people after they consume a moderate amount of alcohol. However, a significant decrease in myocardial contractility has been reported in some. Alcohol in moderate doses causes vasodilation, especially of the cutaneous vessels, producing a warm and flushed skin [12].

Gastrointestinal System

Alcohol in a 10% concentration (20 proof) drink stimulates salivary and gastric secretions. In a 20% concentration (40 proof) drink, alcohol depresses gastric secretion. Alcohol in a 40% concentration (80 proof) drink is very irritating to the gastric mucosa and causes congestive hyperemia and inflammation and may produce an erosive gastritis. Consumed to the point of intoxication, alcohol stops gastrointestinal motor function, causing pylorospasm and vomiting [12].

Urinary System

Alcohol exerts a diuretic effect on the kidneys. This most likely is due to a direct effect of alcohol on the neurohypophyseal system to decrease the secretion of antidiuretic hormone (ADH). This effect is directly proportional to the BAL [12].

Thermoregulatory System

Because of the enhanced cutaneous blood flow, increased sweating tends to occur. This causes the body to lose heat more readily so that the internal temperature begins to fall. With ingestion of large amounts of alcohol, the central temperature regulating system becomes depressed, and the fall in body temperature may be pronounced. Heavy alcohol consumption during exposure to cold weather is very dangerous [12, 13].

Interaction of Alcohol with Other Drugs

The impairment of muscular coordination and judgment that is associated with the ingestion of a moderate amount of alcohol is enhanced when people use other sedative-hypnotic drugs or opioids. After drinking alcohol, patients taking some oral hypoglycemics may experience unpleasant symptoms similar to those patients taking disulfiram (Antabuse). Similar interactions may occur with some antibiotics and some anti-inflammatory drugs.

The enhanced hypoglycemic effect of alcohol with some oral hypoglycemic agents is also seen with insulin. Alcohol can interfere with the therapeutic actions of a wide variety of medications by altering their metabolism. For example, acute ingestion of alcohol reduces the clearance of phenytoin (Dilantin) because both drugs compete for the same enzyme in the liver.

In the chronic drinker, enzyme induction by alcohol occurs so that during a period of abstinence an enhanced rate of clearance occurs [14].

Street Names for Alcohol

Street names for alcohol include swish, booze, brew, hard stuff, hooch, jack, juice, sauce, shine, vino, chug, cold one, gargle, goof, and giggle juice.

What Is Excessive Drinking?

According to the Centers for Disease Control and Prevention [15], excessive drinking includes binge drinking, heavy drinking, and any drinking by pregnant women or people younger than age 21. Binge drinking, the most common form of excessive drinking, is defined as consuming:

- For women, four or more drinks during a single occasion
- For men, five or more drinks during a single occasion

Heavy drinking is defined as consuming:

- For women, eight or more drinks per week
- For men, 15 or more drinks per week

Most people who drink excessively may not be alcohol dependent [15].

Subtypes of Alcoholism

Several classifications of subtypes of alcoholism exist. The two most common ones are an observational classification and a genetic classification.

Observational Classification

The observational classification consists of five subtypes: (1) Young adult subtype, (2) young antisocial subtype, (3) functional subtype, (4) intermediate familial subtype, and (5) chronic severe subtype [16].

Young Adult Subtype

The young adult subtype accounts for about 32% of US alcoholics. About 24 years old on average, they usually become heavy drinkers by age 20. They drink less frequently than other alcoholics, but they tend to binge drink when they drink. They rarely seek help for alcohol dependence. This is the largest subtype.

Young Antisocial Subtype

The young antisocial subtype comprises 21% of US alcoholics. They are 26 years old, on average. More than half have antisocial personality disorder. They tend to start drinking at age 15 and become alcoholics by 18. They are more likely to smoke cigarettes and marijuana and do other drugs.

Functional Subtype

The functional subtype accounts for about 19% of US alcoholics. They are generally middle-aged, working adults who tend to have stable relationships, more education, and higher incomes than other alcoholics. On average they tend to drink every other day, often consuming five or more drinks on drinking days.

Intermediate Familial Subtype

The intermediate familial subtype makes up nearly 19% of US alcoholics. Nearly half have close relatives who are alcoholics. Alcoholics in this subtype typically began drinking by age 17 and became alcoholics in their early 30s.

Chronic Severe Subtype

The chronic severe subtype is the rarest subtype, accounting for about 9% of US alcoholics. This subtype mainly includes men, has the highest divorce rate, and frequently includes users of illicit drugs.

Genetic Classification

The genetic classification divides alcoholism into type I and type II [17]. Environment is not an important factor.

Type I Alcoholism

Type I alcoholism is transmitted by females, onset is later in life, and it does not include an antisocial component. These individuals avoid harm.

Type II Alcoholism

Type II alcoholism is transmitted by males, it has an early onset, and there is an antisocial component. These alcoholics are novelty seeking and feel no guilt.

Health Risks

Short-Term Health Risks

Short-term health risks most often are the result of binge drinking and include injuries, such as motor vehicle crashes, falls, drowning, and burns. Risks also include violence, homicide, suicide, sexual assault, and intimate partner violence.

Risky sexual behaviors, including unprotected sex or sex with multiple partners, may occur. These behaviors can result in unintended pregnancy or sexually transmitted diseases, including HIV. Miscarriage and stillbirth or fetal alcohol spectrum disorder among pregnant women may occur. At high BALs, alcohol poisoning, a medical emergency, may occur [15].

Long-Term Health Effects

Over time, excessive alcohol use can lead to the development of chronic diseases and other serious problems involving virtually every organ system of the body, including the neurological system; cardiovascular system; head, ears, eyes, nose, and throat; hematological/immunological system; gastrointestinal system; metabolic and renal systems; endocrine and reproductive systems; nutritional system; and dermatological system. Cancer also is a long-term risk of alcohol consumption.

Neurological System

Long-term neurological consequences of alcoholism include Wernicke-Korsakoff syndrome, alcoholic dementia, hepatic encephalopathy, cerebellar degeneration, and peripheral neuropathy. Rarer disorders include Marchiafava-Bignami disease and central pontine myelinolysis [18–20].

Cardiovascular System

Cardiovascular complications of alcohol dependence include cardiac arrhythmias, hypertension, and cardiomyopathy [21–23].

Head, Eyes, Ears, Nose, and Throat

Heavy alcohol use can cause poor dentition, oropharyngeal lesions, hoarseness, plethoric faces, parotid gland enlargement, injected conjunctiva, and flushed skin [22].

Hematological/Immunological Systems

Hematological abnormalities encountered in alcoholics include anemia, macrocytosis of alcoholism, leukopenia, coagulation disorders, and thrombocytopenia. Immunological abnormalities result in an increased infection rate [22, 23].

Gastrointestinal System

Gastrointestinal manifestations of alcohol dependence may include fatty liver, alcoholic hepatitis, cirrhosis, gastritis, gastric ulcers, and upper GI bleeding. Alcohol dependence also may cause chronic esophagitis and esophageal stricture, lactose intolerance, diarrhea, vitamin B_{12} and folate deficiency, and electrolyte imbalances. It also causes acute and chronic pancreatitis [23–25].

Musculoskeletal System

Musculoskeletal effects of alcohol dependence include myopathy, aseptic necrosis of the femoral head, and gout [26].

Metabolic and Renal Systems

Metabolic disturbances from alcohol dependence include alcoholic ketoacidosis, hypomagnesemia, hypocalcemia, and hypophosphatemia. The major renal effect is the hepatorenal syndrome [27].

Endocrine System

Alcohol causes ADH levels to fall, accounting for the diuretic effect of alcohol. It also can cause a pseudo-Cushing's syndrome. It can deplete glycogen stores from malnutrition, contributing to hypoglycemia [22, 23].

Reproductive System

Alcohol is toxic to the testes, the pituitary, and the hypothalamus, all of which affect the reproductive system. With the development of cirrhosis, feminization of men occurs. Testicular atrophy may occur in severe cases. Menstrual disturbances and infertility may occur in women [22, 23].

Nutritional System

Alcohol impairs nutrition in a variety of ways. It suppresses the appetite, both directly and as a result of gastritis. It damages the organs of digestion, including the liver, the pancreas, and the small intestine. Alcohol is highly caloric—a shot of liquor (1.5 ounces of 80 proof) has 105 calories.

These are said to be "empty calories" because they contain none of the nutrients, vitamins, minerals, or amino acids required for the body to function. It is not unusual for half of an alcoholic's calories to be obtained from alcohol, which contributes to malnutrition in advanced stages of alcohol dependence.

Many specific syndromes resulting from vitamin deficiencies can result from alcohol dependence. These include beriberi, riboflavin deficiency, pellagra, pyridoxine deficiency, and scurvy [22, 28].

Dermatological System

Common dermatologic manifestations of alcohol dependence are reddened face and nose, edematous eyelids, injected conjunctiva, rosacea, and rhinophyma. Scaly skin and seborrheic dermatitis are common. Cigarette burns and bruises are also common. Spider angioma, palmar erythema, and ecchymoses occur with advance liver disease [22, 23].

Cancer

The fact that most alcoholics smoke complicates the question of etiology in many cancers. Oral and esophageal cancers seem to be related more to drinking than smoking. However smoking acts synergistically in producing these tumors. The risk of developing laryngeal cancer is more strongly associated with smoking. Alcohol may act as a co-carcinogen with hepatitis B virus in producing hepatocellular carcinoma (hepatoma).

Alcohol is a known cause or thought to be involved in cancers of the mouth, pharynx, larynx, esophagus, liver, colon and rectum, and breast. Alcohol may also increase the risk of cancer of the pancreas. For each of these cancers, the risk increases with the amount of alcohol consumed [22].

Health Benefits of Drinking Alcohol

Low to moderate alcohol consumption may have beneficial effects on health. Low to moderate use is usually defined as one or two drinks a day for a man or one drink a day for a woman. Health benefits include decreased risk for heart disease and mortality due to heart disease, decreased risk of ischemic stroke, and decreased risk of diabetes.

It is estimated that 26,000 deaths were averted in 2005 because of reductions in ischemic heart disease, ischemic stroke, and diabetes from the benefits attributed to moderate alcohol consumption [29].

Evaluation of the Alcoholic

Evaluation of the alcoholic should include the quantity of alcoholic intake, duration of alcohol use, time since last drink, and previous alcohol withdrawals, including seizures. The physician should assess possible complicating medical conditions, such as arrhythmias, congestive heart failure, coronary artery disease, gastrointestinal bleeding, infections, liver disease, nervous system impairment, and pancreatitis. In addition, he or she should determine the history of concurrent psychiatric conditions and use of other psychoactive substances.

The physician should check blood glucose, CBC, liver function tests, a urine drug screen, blood alcohol level, electrolytes, and magnesium. Aspartate aminotransferase (AST) is typically two times greater than alanine aminotransferase (ALT) in heavy drinkers. Gamma-glutamyl transpeptidase (GGT) is the most sensitive of the liver enzymes for alcoholism. Mean cell volume (MCV) is often elevated.

Carbohydrate-deficient transferrin (CDT) levels appear to be elevated following alcohol consumption of 60–80 g/day for 2 or 3 weeks, and they normalize with a mean half-life of 2 to 4 weeks of abstinence. False-positive CDT results can occur in patients with an inborn error of glycoprotein metabolism or a genetic D variant of transferrin. False positives can also occur in patients with severe nonalcoholic liver diseases, those with diseases characterized by high total transferrin, and individuals who have received combined kidney and pancreas transplants.

Two commercial kits to quantitate CDT in serum are available—CDTect and %CDT. Although CDTect has less sensitivity for females than for males, there does not appear to be a gender effect with %CDT. Despite the fact that the sensitivities of GGT and CDT appear approximately equal, CDT is far more specific than GGT and other liver function tests [28]. CDT may not be available everywhere [30]. Diagnosis is discussed in Chap. 14.

Tolerance

In people who drink large amounts of alcohol on a regular basis, the liver adapts to metabolize the alcohol more rapidly than it normally does. The liver does this by producing larger amounts of the enzymes, which break down alcohol. Because the liver has become more efficient, the individual needs to drink more alcohol to get the same effect.

The brain also has a role in the development of alcohol tolerance. When the neurotransmitter systems in the brain are regularly exposed to large amounts of alcohol, they begin to suppress the functioning of the neurotransmitter systems. The GABA system adapts so that the alcohol is less effective. Because of this adaption, heavy drinkers require more alcohol to get the same effect.

Heavy alcohol consumption over a period of years can lead to reverse tolerance due to the liver damage as a result of the buildup of fat and scar tissue. The reduced ability of the damaged liver to metabolize alcohol means that small amounts can lead to a high blood alcohol concentration and more rapid intoxication [31].

Dependence

Alcohol dependence is defined by the American Psychiatric Association's DSM-5 criteria discussed in Chap. 1.

Abstinence Syndrome

Stages of the Alcohol Abstinence Syndrome

The acute phase of the alcohol abstinence syndrome has traditionally been divided into three stages; however, the signs, symptoms, and temporal sequence of these stages may vary.

Stage 1

Mild alcohol abstinence syndrome consists of anxiety, tremor, insomnia, headache, palpitations, and gastrointestinal disturbances. These symptoms often appear 6 to 12 h after a person stops drinking. Sometimes a person will still have a measurable blood alcohol level when symptoms start. These symptoms may become more pronounced, and patients progress to the second stage.

Stage 2

Moderate alcohol abstinence syndrome consists of the symptoms of Stage 1 symptoms plus diaphoresis, increased systolic blood pressure, tachypnea, tachycardia, confusion, and mild hyperthermia. The visual hallucinations in the presence of a relatively clear mind are called alcoholic hallucinosis. Although this condition is called alcoholic hallucinosis, it's not the same as the hallucinations associated with delirium tremens (DTs). Most patients are aware that the unusual sensations aren't real.

Insomnia occurs, patients are hyperalert and easily startled, and patients crave alcohol. Some patients may experience visual, auditory, or tactile hallucinations. These symptoms usually end within 48 h. These may become more pronounced and patients progress to the third stage.

Stage 3

Severe alcohol abstinence syndrome includes symptoms of delirium tremens, which usually begin between 48 to 72 h after drinking has stopped. Symptoms, which usually peak at 5 days, include pulse rate in the range of 120 to 140 beats/min, elevated blood pressure, perfuse sweating, elevated body temperature, delirium, hallucinations (primarily visual) which the patient cannot distinguish from reality, severe tremors, and seizures.

DTs is associated with significant mortality (between 5 and 20%). Deaths occur from electrolyte disturbances, seizures, aspiration pneumonia, cardiac dysrhythmias, dehydration, and cardiac failure. Risk factors for DTs include a history of withdrawal seizures or DTs, acute medical illness, abnormal liver function, and older age [32, 33].

Differential Diagnosis of Alcohol Withdrawal

The list of disorders that can masquerade as alcohol withdrawal is long. It includes disorders that involve increased sympathetic activity and altered mental status. Some of the more common ones are thyrotoxicosis, anticholinergic poisoning, sedative-hypnotic withdrawal, amphetamine or cocaine use, seizures and associated mental status changes, CNS infections, and CNS hemorrhage.

Treatment of Alcohol Abstinence Syndrome

Drug treatment for detoxification involves two basic principles: (1) substituting another sedative-hypnotic agent for alcohol, usually a benzodiazepine, and (2) gradually tapering the dose. Substituting another agent for alcohol is based on the concept of cross-tolerance; that is, benzodiazepines are pharmacological substitutes for alcohol.

The Clinical Institute Withdrawal Assessment of Alcohol-revised version (CIWA-Ar) is a short test that rates the severity of withdrawal as observed by the clinician and helps to decide the detoxification regimen.

CIWA-Ar covers ten areas: (1) nausea and vomiting, (2) tremor, (3) paroxysmal sweats, (4) anxiety, (5) agitation, (6) tactile disturbances, (7) auditory disturbances, (8) visual disturbances, (9) headache or fullness in head, and (10) orientation and clouding of sensorium.

Each area is rated 1 to 7, except for "orientation and clouding of sensorium" which is rated 1 to 4. One is normal or not present and 7 is severe (4 for orientation and clouding of sensorium).

Scores less than 8 indicate minimal to mild withdrawal. Scores of 8 to 15 indicate moderate withdrawal. Scores of 15 or more indicate severe withdrawal. The maximum score is 67 [34].

Outpatient Detoxification

Outpatient treatment is for mild withdrawal symptoms (Stage1). Patient monitoring is important. In the outpatient setting, the patient who is undergoing withdrawal must be monitored by a person who is committed to staying with the patient throughout the detoxification process. Daily physician visits are necessary until detoxification has been completed and the patient is medically stable.

Detoxification medication may not be needed for very mild symptoms. If medication is needed, several detoxification medication regimens are appropriate for use in the outpatient setting. Chlordiazepoxide (Librium) is an ideal drug. It has a wide therapeutic window and is self-tapering because of its long half-life [35, 36]. Three regimens can be used: (1) rigid, (2) flexible, and (3) front loading (Table 4.2). Doses can be withheld or reduced as needed to prevent excessive drowsiness or increased if not adequate for controlling withdrawal symptoms.

With a rigid schedule, medication dosing is ordered at the beginning of detoxification for all

Table 4.2 Typical alternative detoxification protocols for Stage 1 (mild) alcohol abstinence syndrome using chlordiazepoxide (Based on Prater [35])

Schedule	Day 1	Day 2	Day 3	Day 4
Rigid	25–50 mg four times daily	25–50 mg three times daily	25–50 twice daily	25–50 mg at bedtime
Flexible	25–50 mg every 4–6 h as needed based on symptoms	25–50 mg every 6–8 h as needed	25–50 every 12 h as needed	25–50 mg at bedtime as needed
Front loading	50–100 mg every 2–4 h until sedation is achieved; then 25–50 mg every 4 to 6 h as needed	25–50 mg every 4–6 h as needed	25–50 every 4 to 6 h as needed	None

Table 4.3 Typical alternative outpatient detoxification protocols for alcohol abstinence syndrome using lorazepam or oxazepam (Based on Prater [35])

Medication	Dosage
Lorazepam (Ativan)	1–2 mg every 3 or 4 h for 3–5 days
Oxazepam (Serax)	20–40 mg every 3 or 4 h for 3–5 days

days of the process. With a flexible schedule, medication is ordered on an as-needed basis. With a front loading schedule, the patient is given adequate medication to cause sedation up front, and then small amounts of the drug are added as needed during the detoxification period.

Valium (diazepam) can be used instead of chlordiazepoxide by converting the chlordiazepoxide dose to a diazepam dose by using the conversion 25 mg chlordiazepoxide = 10 mg diazepam.

Because the liver's ability to oxidize substances declines prior to its ability to conjugate substances, medications conjugated by the liver, such as lorazepam (Ativan) and oxazepam (Serax), may be used in place of chlordiazepoxide or diazepam in patients with significant liver disease [35]. Typical detoxification schedules for lorazepam and oxazepam are given in Table 4.3. Doses can be withheld or reduced as needed to prevent excessive drowsiness or increased if not adequate for controlling withdrawal symptoms.

For any detoxification regimen, the physician should give 100 mg of thiamine orally per day for 3 days. Clonidine (Catapres) can be helpful in reducing the increased noradrenergic output that persists in some patients after the completion of detoxification.

Inpatient Detoxification

Indications

Indications for inpatient detoxification include severe withdrawal symptoms, multiple previous detoxifications, and significant medical or psychiatric illnesses. Delirium tremens requires ICU treatment. Phenytoin (Dilantin) and other seizure medications are not effective in preventing withdrawal seizures; the best treatment is adequate

Table 4.4 Typical inpatient detoxification protocols for Stage 2 (moderate) and Stage 3 (severe) alcohol abstinence syndromes using chlordiazepoxide or lorazepam (Based on Miller [36])

Moderate withdrawal	Severe withdrawal
Diazepam: 15–20 mg orally four times daily on day 1; 10–20 mg orally four times daily on day 2; 5–15 mg orally four times daily on day 3; 10 mg orally four times daily on day 4; 5 mg orally four times daily on day 5	Diazepam: 10–25 mg orally as needed every hour while awake until sedation occurs
Or	Or
Lorazepam: 2–4 mg orally four times daily on days 1 and 2; 1–2 mg orally four times daily on days 3 and 4; 1 mg orally twice daily on day 5	Lorazepam: 1–2 mg intravenously as needed every hour while awake for 3–5 days (to sedate)

benzodiazepine dosing. However, if the patient has a history of non-withdrawal seizures, seizure medication should be given in addition to the benzodiazepine. Typical inpatient detoxification protocols for Stage 2 (moderate) and Stage 3 (severe) alcohol abstinence syndromes using chlordiazepoxide or lorazepam are given in Table 4.4. Doses can be withheld or reduced as needed to prevent excessive drowsiness or increased if not adequate for controlling withdrawal symptoms.

Chlordiazepoxide can be substituted for diazepam by converting the diazepam dose to a chlordiazepoxide dose by using the conversion 10 mg diazepam = 25 mg chlordiazepoxide. Lorazepam is the only benzodiazepine that can be given intramuscularly.

Folic acid, 1 mg orally, is given daily to correct any folate deficiency. To prevent precipitation of Wernicke-Korsakoff syndrome, the intramuscular injection of thiamine should be given before administration of a glucose load.

The serum magnesium level should be determined in patients with a history of withdrawal seizures and in those who are malnourished. Magnesium deficiency, in the presence of good renal function, can be corrected by administration of a 50% solution of magnesium sulfate, 2 mL intramuscularly every 6 h for 48 h. Because intramuscular injection of magnesium can be uncomfortable, it is best given intravenously if an intravenous line is present. Although oral magnesium supplements are available, magnesium is not adequately absorbed from the gastrointestinal tract to correct significant deficits.

Some physicians give a multivitamin with zinc once or twice a day. The zinc may ensure continued function of alcohol dehydrogenase.

Serum calcium levels should also be measured, and if hypocalcemia is present, it can be corrected by administering a 10% calcium gluconate solution until the serum calcium level rises above 7.5 mg/dL. No more than 10 mL is usually required.

Hypophosphatemia can be corrected by adding 20 to 40 mmol of potassium phosphate to each liter of intravenous fluid.

Nausea and vomiting can be controlled with promethazine (Phenergan) 25 to 50 mg orally, by intramuscular injection, or by suppository every 6 h as needed. For inpatient detoxification, it can be given intravenously. Alternatively, ondansetron (Zofran) can be used in a dose of 4 to 8 mg every 6 to 8 h.

To control alcoholic hallucinosis, haloperidol (Haldol) in small doses (one to 2 mg every 4 h) is usually effective. Remember, haloperidol lowers the seizure threshold.

Seizures usually can be prevented, even in a patient with a history of withdrawal seizures, with liberal use of the benzodiazepine detoxifying agent and correction of magnesium deficit if one is present.

Antiseizure drugs, such as carbamazepine (Tegretol) or divalproex sodium (Depakote), may be useful for reducing the benzodiazepine dose. When used by themselves, however, they do not reduce seizures or delirium associated with withdrawal.

Diazepam (Valium) 5 to 20 mg can be administered by slow intravenous push in the rare patient who develops status epilepticus during withdrawal. Patients with no prior history of withdrawal seizures who develop them need full neurological workups.

Beta-blockers, such as propranolol (Inderal) and atenolol (Tenormin), are sometimes used in combination with benzodiazepines to slow heart rate and reduce tremors.

Many alcoholic patients are initially over hydrated and thus do not require parenteral hydration. Patients usually experience diuresis during the first 2 days of detoxification and may lose up to 2 kg (4.4 lb) of body weight. Patients with excessive vomiting, however, may be dehydrated and require fluid replacement, as well as acid-base balance monitoring [37].

Outpatient Versus Inpatient Detoxification

Patients receiving outpatient detoxification treatment usually are expected to travel to a hospital or other treatment facility daily, excluding weekends, for detoxification sessions. The sessions may be scheduled for daytime or evening hours, depending on the program.

For patients with mild to moderate alcohol withdrawal symptoms, characterized by hand tremor, perspiration, heart palpitation, restlessness, and loss of appetite, outpatient detoxification may be as safe and effective as inpatient detoxification but is much less expensive and less time-consuming.

Outpatients can maintain employment as well as family and social relationships. Compared with inpatients, outpatients retain greater freedom, maintaining day-to-day activities with fewer disruptions.

Among the drawbacks associated with outpatient detoxification is the increased risk of relapse resulting from the patient's easy access to alcoholic beverages. In addition, outpatients can choose not to keep their detoxification appointments and, consequently, fail to complete detoxification. Significantly more inpatients than outpatients completed detoxification.

Outpatient detoxification is not safe for alcoholics at risk for potentially life-threatening complications of withdrawal, such as delirium tremens, or those with medical conditions, such as pancreatitis, gastrointestinal bleeding, or cirrhosis. In addition, outpatient detoxification is not appropriate for suicidal or homicidal patients, those expected to have severe or medically complicated alcohol withdrawal, patients in adverse or disruptive family or job situations, or patients who would not be able to travel daily to the treatment facility.

The primary disadvantage of inpatient detoxification is its higher cost compared with outpatient alternatives. Overall treatment outcome may have more to do with patient characteristics than with detoxification setting [38, 39].

Ethanol Toxicity

Symptoms

The average blood alcohol concentration in fatal cases of ethanol overdose is above 0.4 g/dL; however, the lethal dose varies due to varying degrees of tolerance. Symptoms of ethanol toxicity include slow or irregular breathing; tachycardia; symptoms of myocardial depression; hypothermia, which may result in cardiac arrest; seizures from hypoglycemia; and changes in mental state, including sedation, confusion, or coma.

Treatment

The mainstay of medical treatment of patients with ethanol toxicity is supportive care. Hypoglycemia and respiratory depression are the two most immediate life-threatening complications that result from ethanol intoxication, especially in children. These should be corrected quickly. In children, 2–4 mL/kg of 25% dextrose solution is usually administered to correct hypoglycemia. A maintenance infusion of dextrose-containing intravenous fluids is often required. In adults, ketoacidosis may require the administration of glucose. Thiamine is given to protect against Wernicke-Korsakoff syndrome, especially if the patient is suspected of being an alcoholic.

If the patient is not maintaining good ventilation or if a significant risk of aspiration is observed, the airway should be secured with an endotracheal tube. Respiratory support and mechanical ventilation should be used if needed.

Intravenous access should be obtained and fluid deficit, if present, should be replaced. Electrolyte abnormalities should be corrected. Plasma expanders and vasopressors can be used to treat hypotension, if present. The patient's body temperature should be maintained.

If the ingestion occurred within 1 h of presentation, placing a nasogastric tube and evacuating the stomach contents can be helpful. The administration of activated charcoal is not recommended for isolated ethanol ingestions because it does not bind hydrocarbons or alcohols. If concomitant ingestion of other toxic products is suspected, activated charcoal may be effective in absorbing these toxins.

Because of the hemorrhagic gastritis that can follow ethanol ingestion, H_2 blockers or proton pump inhibitors should be given.

Forced diuresis is not helpful because 90% of ethanol metabolism occurs in the liver, and only 10% of the ethanol load is secreted in the urine. Hemodialysis can be used in patients whose clinical condition is deteriorating or in patients whose CNS depression, respiratory depression, or hypotension is refractory to standard therapy. Patients who have impaired hepatic function may require dialysis to clear the ethanol load [8, 40].

Recovery

General information about the recovery process and how to prevent relapse are discussed in Chaps. 16 and 17. A choice of three medications may be used to assist with recovery—disulfiram (Antabuse), acamprosate (Campral), and naltrexone (Vivitrol, Revia). These medications also are discussed in Chap. 16.

Other Alcohols

Other alcohols of medical interest include isopropyl alcohol, methyl alcohol, and propylene glycol.

Isopropyl Alcohol Toxicity

Isopropyl alcohol (isopropanol), also known as wood alcohol and rubbing alcohol, has a number of sources, including alcohol swabs, cleaning supplies, paint thinners, and perfumes.

Symptoms

Symptoms of an isopropanol overdose include:

Abdominal pain Ataxia Burns of cornea Coma Decreased reflexes Decreased urine output Dizziness	Flushing Headache Hypoglycemia Hypopnea Hypotension Hypothermia Nausea	Shock Slurred speech Tachycardia Throat pain Unconsciousness Vomiting (may contain blood)

Drinking large amounts of isopropyl alcohol can lead to internal bleeding, breathing difficulty, coma, and kidney failure. Children can absorb a large amount of isopropyl alcohol through the skin, so sponging with it to reduce fever is contraindicated.

Diagnosis

Isopropyl alcohol poisoning can occur from ingestion, inhalation, or cutaneous absorption. As little as 15 g of isopropyl alcohol can have a toxic effect on an average-sized adult. However, isopropyl alcohol is not nearly as toxic as methanol or ethylene glycol. An osmolar gap and ketonuria without metabolic acidosis, along with a fruity or sweet odor on the breath as the result of acetone metabolism, and CNS depression support the diagnosis.

Treatment

As with ethanol toxicity, treatment is primarily symptomatic. There is no role for fomepizole. Rarely, severe cases may require hemodialysis [8, 41, 42].

Methyl Alcohol Toxicity

Methyl alcohol (methanol), also known as wood alcohol, is used as an industrial solvent and in chemical manufacture. In the home, it is most likely to be found in the form of Canned Heat or in windshield-washing products. It is metabolized first to formaldehyde and then to formic acid, both of which are toxic to the central nervous system.

Symptoms

Symptoms of methanol toxicity include:

Bluish-colored lips and finger nails Bradycardia CNS depression Confusion Diarrhea Dizziness Dyspnea	Fatigue, leg cramps, weakness Headache Hypotension Liver damage Nausea and vomiting Odor of formaldehyde in breath and urine	Pancreatitis Prolonged coma Seizures Severe epigastric pain Unconsciousness Visual disturbance

The visual disturbance frequently is described as like being in a snowstorm. It can progress to blindness.

Diagnosis

Patients appear intoxicated but do not have the smell of alcohol on their breaths. Metabolic acidosis with an elevated anion gap and an osmolar gap occurs, and there is a decrease in serum bicarbonate.

The development of bradycardia, prolonged coma, seizures, and resistant acidosis implies a poor prognosis. Serum methanol concentrations higher than 20 mg/dL warrant treatment and concentrations higher than 50 mg/dl are considered serious enough to require dialysis. Serum formate levels are a better indication of clinical pathology, but are not widely available.

Treatment

A nasogastric tube should be inserted, and gastric lavage with sodium bicarbonate should be done if the patient is brought to the emergency department within 2 h of ingesting methanol. Supportive measures to maintain ventilation and blood pressure should be instituted. Activated charcoal may be used.

Acidosis should be treated by an intravenous sodium bicarbonate infusion to prevent retinal damage. Potassium chloride (KCl) infusion is needed only when hypokalemia occurs due to alkali therapy.

If methanol overdose is suspected, folinic acid should be administered at a dose of 1 mg/kg, with a maximal dose of 50 mg. It should be repeated every 4 h. If folinic acid is not immediately available, folic acid can be substituted at the same dose. Administration of folic or folinic acid enhances metabolism of formate.

The primary antidotal treatment of methanol involves blocking alcohol dehydrogenase. This enzyme can be inhibited by either ethanol or fomepizole. If ethanol is used as an antidote, the recommended target serum concentration is 100–150 mg/dL. Ethanol (10% in water) can be administered through the nasogastric tube (loading dose of 0.7 ml/kg) followed by 0.15 ml/kg/h infusion. Ethanol saturates alcohol dehydrogenase and retards methanol metabolism.

Methanol levels are frequently not immediately available. Thus, if methanol poisoning is suspected and the decision is made to use fomepizole, a loading dose of fomepizole can be given while the methanol level is being obtained.

Fomepizole should be administered as a loading dose of 15 mg/kg. Subsequent doses should be at 10 mg/kg every 12 h for four doses or until serum methanol falls below 20 mg/dl. Ethanol has been associated with more frequent adverse reactions than fomepizole, making fomepizole a better choice despite its expense. Fomepizole, like ethanol, inhibits alcohol dehydrogenase to slow methanol metabolism.

Hemodialysis, if needed, clears methanol as well as formate and hastens recovery. Indications for hemodialysis include an arterial pH < 7.10, a decline of >0 0.05 in the arterial pH despite bicarbonate infusion, a pH greater than 7.3 despite bicarbonate therapy, a rise in serum creatinine level by 90 mmol/L, or an initial plasma methanol concentration greater than or equal to 50 mg/dL [8, 42, 43].

Ethylene Glycol Toxicity

Symptoms

Young children are sometimes attracted to ethylene glycol by its sweet taste. It is sometimes ingested intentionally as an ethanol substitute or in a suicide attempt. It has been use to poison individuals in attempted or completed murders. Symptoms of ethylene glycol toxicity include:

Ataxia Bronchopneumonia Cardiac arrest Cardiac dysrhythmias Coma Congestive heart failure with cardiogenic pulmonary edema Convulsions	Death Disorientation Drowsiness Hypertension Hyperventilation Hypotension which may progress to circulatory collapse Kussmaul respirations	Irritation Myoclonic jerks Pulmonary edema with diffuse hemorrhagic exudates Restlessness Slurred speech Tachypnea

Other than its inebriating effects, ethylene glycol itself has relatively low toxicity. However, it is metabolized in the liver by successive oxidations to a variety of compounds that include glycolaldehyde, glycolic acid, glyoxylic acid, and oxalic acid. These compounds are more toxic than ethylene glycol itself.

Symptoms of ethylene glycol toxicity are most severe 6 to 12 h after ingestion when the acidic metabolites of ethylene glycol are at their maximal concentrations. Renal involvement may become apparent within 24 to 72 h after ingestion. Urinary crystal formation requires a sufficient amount of time for ethylene glycol to be metabolized into oxalate. Calcium oxalate formation depletes serum calcium levels and deposits in intestinal mucosa, liver, brain, heart, lung, and kidney.

Oliguric or anuric renal failure is the result in the most severe cases, and although permanent renal failure is rare, recovery of renal function may take up to 2 months. If untreated, severe ethylene glycol toxicity is usually fatal within 24 to 36 h.

Diagnosis

The absence of a strong odor of alcohol in a patient who appears intoxicated should raise the suspicion of ethylene glycol ingestion. Indicators of the presence of ethylene glycol poisoning include hyperventilation, laboratory data suggestive of an elevated anion gap metabolic acidosis, an osmolar gap, the presence of hypocalcemia, and urinary crystals.

Ethylene glycol or glycolic acid concentrations are definitive but may not be available. Urine microscopy to identify the presence of crystals should follow determination of the anion and osmolar gaps [39].

Three stages of ethylene glycol poisoning occur. Within the first few hours after ingestion, there is a transient excitation followed by CNS depression. After a delay of 4 to12 h, severe metabolic acidosis develops. Finally, deposition of oxalate crystals in the renal tubules occurs, followed by delayed renal insufficiency [8].

Treatment

Ethylene glycol is rapidly absorbed from the stomach, making treatment with gastric lavage less than optimum. Likewise, it requires large amounts of activated charcoal to bind relatively small amounts of ethylene glycol, and the therapeutic window for this action is less than an hour. Traditional treatment of ethylene glycol poisoning consists of sodium bicarbonate, ethanol or fomepizole, and hemodialysis as in methanol treatment. Hemodialysis, if needed, is effective in removing ethylene glycol and glycolic acid and correcting the metabolic acidosis. Dialysis indications include a pH less than 7.25, acute renal failure, ethylene glycol level greater than 50 mg/dL, or serum glycolic acid level less than 8 mmol/L [8, 44, 45].

Summary

The types of ethanol commonly consumed are divided into three major categories—beer, wine, and spirits. Alcohol use is the fourth leading preventable cause of death in the United States.

Alcohol is believed to mimic GABA's effect by binding to GABA receptors and thereby inhibiting neuronal signaling. Over 90% of consumed alcohol is metabolized in the liver; the rest is excreted unchanged by the lungs and the kidneys. The effects of various blood alcohol levels range from feeling warm and relaxed after one to two drinks to death from respiratory depression at much higher levels. Excessive drinking includes binge drinking, heavy drinking, and any drinking by pregnant women or people younger than age 21.

Several classifications of subtypes of alcoholism exist. The two most common ones are an observational classification and a genetic classification. Short-term health risks most often are the result of binge drinking, and include injuries, such as motor vehicle crashes, falls, drowning, and burns. Risks also include violence, homicide, suicide, sexual assault, and intimate partner violence. Over time, excessive alcohol use can lead to the development of chronic diseases and other serious problems involving virtually every organ system of the body. Low to moderate alcohol consumption may have beneficial effects on health. The acute phase of the alcohol abstinence syndrome has traditionally been divided into three stages. Drug treatment for detoxification involves two basic principles: (1) substituting another sedative-hypnotic agent for alcohol, usually a benzodiazepine, and (2) gradually tapering the dose. Overdose of ethanol, methanol, and ethylene glycol sometimes occurs.

References

1. Lovitz L. The alcohols: ethanol, methanol, isopropanol, ethylene glycol. Pediatr Clin N Am. 1986;33(2):311–23.
2. Alcoholic beverages. Encyclopedia.com website. http://www.encyclopedia.com/sports-and-everyday-life/food-and-drink/alcoholic-beverages/alcoholic-beverages. 2001.
3. What is a standard drink? National Institute of Alcohol Abuse and Alcoholism (NIAAA) website. https://niaaa.nih.gov/alcohol-health/overview-alcohol-consumption/what-standard-drink
4. Alcohol facts and statistics. National Institute of Alcohol Abuse and Alcoholism (NIAAA) website. https://pubs.niaaa.nih.gov/publications/AlcoholFacts&Stats/AlcoholFacts&Stats.pdf
5. Excessive drinking costs U.S. $223.5 billion. Center for Disease Control and Prevention (CDC). https://www.cdc.gov/features/alcoholconsumption/index.html. April 17, 2014.
6. Royce JE. Sociocultural aspects. In: Alcohol problems and alcoholism. New York: Free Press; 1981. p. 33–47.
7. Dubuc B. Neurotransmitters. The brain from top to bottom. McGill University website. http://thebrain.mcgill.ca. May 2012.
8. Masters SB. The alcohols. In: Katzung BG, Trevor AJ, editors. Basic and clinical pharmacology. 13th ed. New York: McGraw-Hill Education; 2015. p. 384–95.
9. Alcohol metabolism: an update. National Institute of Alcohol Abuse and Alcoholism (NIAAA) website.

https://pubs.niaaa.nih.gov/publications/AA72/AA72.htm. July 2007(72).
10. Zakhari S. Overview: how is alcohol metabolized by the body? Alcohol Res Health. 2006;29(4):245–255.
11. Blood alcohol concentration. Notre Dame University's student well-being/McDonald center website. http://mcwell.nd.edu/your-well-being/physical-well-being/alcohol/blood-alcohol-concentration. 2016.
12. Ritchie JM. The aliphatic alcohols. In: Gilman AG, Goodman LS, Rall TW, Murad F, editors. Goodman and Gilman's the pharmacological basis of therapeutics. New York: Macmillan; 1985. p. 372–84.
13. Alcohol use and cancer. American Cancer Society website. http://www.cancer.org/cancer/cancer-causes/diet-physical-activity/alcohol-use-and-cancer.html
14. Alcohol-related drug interactions. Pharmacist's letter/prescriber's letter. 2008;24(1):240106.
15. Fact sheets: alcohol use and your health. Center for Disease Control and Prevention (CDC) website. https://www.cdc.gov/alcohol/pdfs/alcoholyourhealth.pdf. July 25, 2016.
16. Researchers identify alcoholism subtypes. National Institute on Alcohol Abuse and Alcoholism (NIAAA) website. https://niaaa.nih.gov/news-events/news-releases/researchers-identify-alcoholism-subtypes. June 28, 2007.
17. Cloninger CR, Sigvardsson S, Bohman M. Type I and type II alcoholism: an update. Alcohol Health Res World. 1996;20(1):18–23.
18. Packard RC. The neurological consequences of alcoholism. Am Fam Physician. 1976;14:111–5.
19. Wernicke-Korsakoff Syndrome. New York Times. February 27, 2013.
20. Hesse K, Savitsky J. The elderly. In: Barnes HN, Aronson MD, Delbanco TL, editors. Alcoholism: a guide for the primary care physician. New York: Springer-Verlag; 1987. p. 167–75.
21. Budzikowski AS. Holiday heart syndrome treatment & management. Medscape website. http://emedicine.medscape.com/article/155050-treatment. December 21, 2016.
22. Ende J. Nutritional status, cardiovascular, hematologic, reproductive, and musculoskeletal systems. In: Alcoholism: a guide for the primary care physician. New York: Springer-Verlag; 1987. p. 134–44.
23. Milhorn HT. The diagnosis of alcoholism. Am Fam Physician. 1988;37(6):175–83.
24. Moulton AW, Cyr MG. The liver. In: Barnes HN, Aronson MD, Delbanco TL, editors. Alcoholism: a guide for the primary care physician. New York: Springer-Verlag; 1987. p. 167–75.
25. Saxe TG. Drug-alcohol interactions. Am Fam Physician. 1986;33(4):159–62.
26. Hodges DL, Kumar VN, Redford JB. Effects of alcohol on bone, muscle and nerve. Am Fam Physician. 1986;34(5):149–56.
27. Daley J, Harrington JT. Metabolic and renal effects of alcohol. In: Barnes HN, Aronson MD, Delbanco TL, editors. Alcoholism: a guide for the primary care physician. New York: Springer-Verlag; 1987. p. 145–50.
28. Poley W, Lea G, Vibe G. Alcohol and its effects on the individual. In: Alcoholism treatment manual. New York: Gardner Press; 1979. p. 17–31.
29. Danaei G, Ding EL, Mozaffarian D, Taylor B, Rehm J, Murray CJ, et al. The preventable causes of death in the United States: comparative risk assessment of dietary, lifestyle, and metabolic risk factors. PLoS Med. 2009;6(4):1–23.
30. Allen JP, Sillanaukee P, Strid N, Litten RZ. Biomarkers of heavy drinking. National Institute of Alcoholism and Alcohol Abuse (NIAAA) website. https://pubs.niaaa.nih.gov/publications/AssessingAlcohol/biomarkers.htm. August 2004.
31. Harm Reduction for Alcohol. What is reverse tolerance? Harm Reduction for Alcohol (HAMS) website. http://hams.cc/reverse
32. Benzer DG. Management of alcohol intoxication and withdrawal. In: ASAM principles of addiction medicine. Chevy Chase: The Society; 1994. 11(3).
33. Bayard M, Mcintyre J, Hill KR, Woodside J. Alcohol withdrawal syndrome. Am Fam Physician. 2004; 69(6):1443–50.
34. Sullivan JT, Sykora K, Schneiderman J, Naranjo CA, Sellers EM. Assessment of alcohol withdrawal: the revised clinical institute withdrawal assessment for alcohol scale (CIWA-Ar). Br J Addict. 1989;84:1353–7.
35. Prater CD, Miller KE, Zylstra RG. Outpatient detoxification of the addicted or alcoholic patient. Am Fam Physician. 1999;60(4):1175–82.
36. Miller NS, Gold MS. Management of withdrawal syndromes and relapse prevention in drug and alcohol dependence. Am Fam Physician. 1998;58(1):139–46.
37. Milhorn HT. Chemical dependence: diagnosis, treatment, and prevention. New York: Springer-Verlag; 1990.
38. Hayashida M. An overview of outpatient and inpatient detoxification. Alcohol Health Res World. 1998;22(1):44–46.
39. Muncie HL, Yasinian Y, Og L. Outpatient management of alcohol withdrawal syndrome. Am Fam Physician. 2013;88(9):589–95.
40. Fernandez E. Ethanol toxicity treatment & management. Medscape website. http://emedicine.medscape.com/article/820531-treatment. December 29, 2015.
41. Heller JL. Isopropanol overdose. MedlinePlus website. https://medlineplus.gov/ency/article/002660.htm. October 13, 2005.
42. Levine MD. Alcohol toxicity. Medscape website. http://emedicine.medscape.com/article/812411-overview. December 15, 2016.
43. Shrestha S. Methanol poisoning: symptoms, diagnosis and management. Medchrome website. http://medchrome.com/basic-science/pharmacology/methanol-poisoning. July 7, 2010.
44. Keyes DC. Ethylene glycol toxicity treatment & management. Medscape website. http://emedicine.medscape.com/article/814701-treatment. June 24, 2016.
45. Scalley RD, Ferguson DR, Piccaro JC, Scalley M, Archer TE. Treatment of ethylene glycol poisoning. Am Fam Physician. 2002;66(5):807–13.

5 Sedative-Hypnotic Dependence

Key Chapter Points

- Barbiturates were the earliest class of sedative-hypnotic agents to be developed. They largely have been replaced by benzodiazepines.
- Both dispositional and pharmacodynamic tolerance to barbiturates can develop, the latter being more important.
- Withdrawal symptoms are similar to those of alcohol dependence.
- Benzodiazepines are used for alcohol detoxification, along with treatment of a number of other disorders.
- Withdrawal symptoms from benzodiazepines, in some cases, can last for months.
- Flunitrazepam (Rohypnol) is a benzodiazepine that has a reputation as a date rape drug.
- Z drugs are a group of nonbenzodiazepine drugs used for the temporary treatment of insomnia. They have dependence risk and withdrawal symptoms similar to benzodiazepines.
- Gamma-hydroxybutyric acid (GHB) is a central nervous depressant that sometimes is used as a date rape drug.
- Carisoprodol (Soma) is a centrally acting skeletal muscle relaxant that has meprobamate as a metabolite.

In addition to alcohol, drugs that depress the central nervous system include barbiturates, benzodiazepines, insomnia medications collectively referred to as the Z drugs, GHB, a group of medications primarily of historical interest, meprobamate, and chloral hydrate.

These drugs are used mainly to calm and relax patients (sedatives or anxiolytics) or to induce sleep (hypnotics). Collectively, they are known as sedative-hypnotics.

Barbiturates

Barbiturates were the earliest class of sedative-hypnotic agents to be developed. They are central nervous system depressants derived from barbituric acid, a white, crystalline powder having no CNS depressant properties of its own.

The barbiturates largely have been replaced by benzodiazepines for treating medical and psychiatric problems because benzodiazepines proved to be significantly less dangerous in overdose. The barbiturate therapeutic dose is close to lethal dose, and there is no specific antidote for barbiturate overdose [1–3].

Prevalence of Use

In 1975, 17% of high school seniors reported having used barbiturates at some time in their lives. By 1972, the rate had fallen to 7%. However, the rate rose again to 12% in 2004 [4].

H.T. Milhorn, *Substance Use Disorders*, DOI 10.1007/978-3-319-63040-3_5

The Barbiturates

The major difference among the barbiturates is their length of action. They are divided into ultrashort-acting (thiopental, methohexital), short-acting (pentobarbital, secobarbital), intermediate-acting (amobarbital, butabarbital), and long-acting (barbital, phenobarbital) [5]. Barbiturates are listed in Table 5.1, as well as their onset of action and duration of action.

Barbiturates are usually abused in pill form. The long-acting barbiturates are usually not abused because of their slow onset of action. Secobarbital (Seconal) is a DEA Schedule II drug, Amobarbital (Amytal) and pentobarbital (Nembutal) are Schedule III drugs, and butabarbital (Butisol) is a Schedule IV drug [5].

Street Names

Street names for commonly abused barbiturates include

Amobarbital (Amytal)	Blue heavens, blue birds, blue devils, blues, blue tips, blue dolls, bull bullets
Butabarbital (Butisol)	Bute, stoppers
Pentobarbital (Nembutal)	Nembies, yellow jackets
Phenobarbital (Luminal)	Phennies, goofballs, phenos, purple hearts
Secobarbital (Seconal)	Red birds, seccies, red devils, reds, Mexican reds

Current Uses

Current barbiturate uses are:

Acute Convulsions

Acute onset convulsions, including status epilepticus and eclampsia during pregnancy, are indications for use of barbiturates.

Cluster and Migraine Headache Treatment

The combination of acetaminophen and caffeine with butalbital (Fioricet) is still used, as well as the combination of aspirin and caffeine with butalbital (Fiorinal).

Induction of General Anesthesia

Sodium pentothal (Thiopentone) routinely is used as an injectable induction agent in general anesthesia [6].

Lethal Injection

Most states use a three-drug combination for lethal injection—an anesthetic (sodium thiopental or pentobarbital), a paralytic agent (pancuronium bromide), and an agent to stop the heart (potassium chloride). Some states use a single drug—pentobarbital [7].

Preanesthetic Agent

Barbiturates are given prior to surgery to decrease anxiety and to ease the process of induction of general anesthesia. This also is an area where benzodiazepines have replaced barbiturates.

Reduction of Intracranial Pressure

Barbiturates are used to reduce intracranial pressure after a traumatic head injury.

Sedation

Barbiturates have been largely replaced by more modern and safer agents like benzodiazepines in this area.

Table 5.1 Barbiturate types based on onset of action and duration of action

Barbiturate type	Onset of action	Duration of action	Examples
Ultrashort-acting	Few seconds to 45 s	15 min to 3 h	Thiopental, methohexital
Short-acting	10–15 min	2–4 h	Pentobarbital, secobarbital
Intermediate-acting	15–30 min	4–6 h	Amobarbital, butabarbital
Long-acting	30–60 min	10–16 h	Barbital, phenobarbital

Sleep Induction (Hypnosis)

Barbiturates may be effective in short-term insomnia. They tend to lose their effectiveness after 2 weeks of use. They are seldom used for this anymore.

Treatment of Seizures

Prophylactic treatment of partial and generalized tonic-clonic and cortical focal seizures can be controlled with phenobarbital (Luminal) [6].

Pharmacology

Pharmacodynamics

Barbiturates increase the efficiency of synaptic transmission of the neurotransmitter gamma-aminobutyric acid (GABA) by acting on its receptors. A GABA receptor is a macromolecular complex that, in addition to containing sites for binding GABA, also contains sites for binding other molecules such as barbiturates that modulate GABA's activity. When barbiturates bind to a specific site on a GABA receptor, they increase the frequency with which the chlorine channel opens when GABA binds to its own site on this receptor. The resulting increase in the concentration of chloride ions in the postsynaptic neuron immediately hyperpolarizes it, making it less excitable [8].

Pharmacokinetics

Barbiturates are absorbed in the small intestine. Food in the stomach decreases absorption. Intramuscular injection is painful and causes necrosis at the injection site. Binding to plasma proteins varies from 80% for thiopental to 5% for barbital.

The highly lipid-soluble barbiturates, such as thiopental, rapidly cross the blood-brain barrier to induce sleep. The ultrashort duration of these drugs is due to rapid distribution in the body rather than elimination from it. The less lipid-soluble barbiturates equilibrate more slowly. Those with high partition coefficients are readily absorbed from the lumen of the renal tubules and therefore must be metabolized to metabolites with lower partition coefficients to be excreted. The barbiturates are metabolized in the liver by a variety of mechanisms, including oxidation to alcohols, phenols, ketones, and carboxylic acid [9].

With the exception of phenobarbital, only insignificant quantities of the barbiturates are excreted unchanged. The elimination half-lives of secobarbital and pentobarbital range from 18 to 48 h, depending on the individual. The elimination half-life of phenobarbital is 4–5 days. Multiple dosing of these agents can lead to cumulative effects [10].

The symptoms of barbiturate intoxication include altered level of consciousness, difficulty in thinking, drowsiness, faulty judgment, lack of coordination, shallow breathing, slow or slurred speech, sluggishness, and staggering [11].

Barbiturates may increase the patient's sensitivity to pain and thus leave him or her less responsive to narcotic pain medication. They also depress rapid eye movement (REM) sleep. In therapeutic doses, barbiturates have little effect on cardiac, skeletal, or smooth muscle [9].

Interaction with Other Drugs

Barbiturates act synergistically with other CNS depressant drugs, including alcohol and benzodiazepines, to cause cerebral and respiratory depression. Most other drug interactions result from induction of hepatic microenzymes, causing significant increase in clearance of corticosteroids, oral anticoagulants (warfarin), digitoxin, beta-adrenergic antagonists (propranolol, metoprolol), doxycycline, griseofulvin, quinidine, and phenytoin [9].

Health Risks

Drowsiness, dizziness, and decreased alertness may cause injuries from falls, automobile accidents, and other accidents. Barbiturates may cause elderly patients to develop low calcium concentrations because of a probable result of acceleration of vitamin D elimination. Hepatic enzyme induction lowers endogenous steroid hormone concentrations, which may cause endocrine disturbances. Barbiturates also competitively inhibit the metabolism of certain drugs, such as tricyclic antidepressants, to increase their serum concentrations.

Addicts who inject the drugs may get local necrosis, cellulitis, abscesses, bacterial endocarditis, hepatitis B, and acquired immune deficiency disorder (HIV/AIDS). Coma and death can occur [12, 13].

Tolerance

Both dispositional and pharmacodynamic tolerance to barbiturates can develop, the latter being more important. With chronic use, pharmacodynamic tolerance continues to develop over a period of weeks to months. Dispositional tolerance, on the other hand, reaches a peak in a few days. Despite the development of tolerance, the lethal dose of barbiturates essentially remains the same. Therefore, the dose necessary for an addict to get high may approach a lethal dose. Tolerance to barbiturates confers tolerance to other CNS depressant drugs because of the phenomenon of cross-tolerance [9].

Dependence

Barbiturate dependence is defined by the American Psychiatric Association's DSM-5 criteria given in Chap. 1.

Abstinence Syndrome

Symptoms

Barbiturates withdrawal symptoms can include restlessness, insomnia, weakness, dizziness, nausea, sweating, and anxiety. There may be tremors, seizures, hallucinations, and psychosis. Users may become hostile and violent. Without proper treatment, hyperthermia, circulatory failure, and death can result. Symptoms are less pronounced with longer-acting drugs, which in part may be due to self-detoxification [14].

Table 5.2 Barbiturate doses equivalent to 10 mg diazepam (Valium) (Based on Milhorn [5])

Barbiturate	10 mg diazepam equivalent (mg)
Butabarbital (Butisol)	100
Pentobarbital (Nembutal)	100
Secobarbital (Seconal)	100
Phenobarbital (Luminal)	30

Detoxification

Treatment of barbiturate abstinence syndrome involves estimating the usually daily barbiturate dose a patient has been taking, substituting diazepam in an equivalent dose, stabilizing the patient at the equivalent diazepam dose, and tapering the drug over 4–5 days for the shorter-acting barbiturates and up to a matter of weeks for the longer-acting ones. Barbiturate-diazepam equivalent doses are given in Table 5.2.

Overdose

Symptoms

In overdose, barbiturates can cause lack of coordination, ataxia, depressed respiration, slurred speech, nystagmus, stupor, coma, and death. The EEG may show periods of silence. Patients' pupils initially may be constricted and later dilated due to hypoxia. Pupillary and corneal reflexes may be diminished or absent.

Overdose has been associated with necrosis of sweat glands and bullous cutaneous lesions that heal slowly. Delayed gastric emptying may occur. Breathing may either be slow or rapid and shallow. Cheyne-Stokes breathing may occur. Eventually, hypothermia, shock, and death may occur.

Barbiturates cause a dose-dependent respiratory depression. At therapeutic sedative-hypnotic doses, respiratory depression is similar to that of normal physiologic sleep. As doses increase, the medullary respiratory center is progressively depressed with resultant decreases in respiratory rate and volume.

The barbiturates cause reduced tone and motility of the intestinal musculature, probably secondary to their central depressant action.

Table 5.3 Clinical manifestations of barbiturate toxicity (Based on Lafferty [12])

Neurologic manifestations			
Lethargy Coma Hypothermia	Decreased pupillary light reflex Nystagmus	Strabismus Vertigo Slurred speech	Ataxia Decreased deep tendon reflexes
Psychiatric manifestations			
Memory disturbances Poor judgment	Limited attention span Impaired thinking	Delirium Irritability	Combativeness Paranoia
Respiratory manifestations			
Respiratory depression	Acute respiratory distress	Hypoxia syndrome	Apnea
Cardiovascular manifestations			
Tachycardia Bradycardia	Diaphoresis	Hypotension	Shock
Skin manifestations			
Barbiturate blisters (i.e., bullous lesions typically found on the hands, buttocks, and knees)			
Other manifestations			
Severe electrolyte and endocrine disturbances	Renal dysfunction	Decreased bowel sounds	

There is no direct effect of barbiturates on the kidney, but severe renal impairment may occur secondary to hypotension [11, 12].

The patient with barbiturate toxicity may present with any or all of the signs and symptoms listed in Table 5.3.

Treatment

Treatment of the patient with barbiturate toxicity is predominantly supportive. The mainstay of treatment underscores the importance of preventing hypoxemia and hypotension. Management strategies generally fall into three major areas: supportive care, decontamination, and enhancement of elimination [12].

Supportive Care

The physician should provide supplemental oxygen and continue to monitor the airway status. Intubation can be done if necessary. Intravenous access should be obtained and an initial pulse oximeter reading should be done. The patient should be placed on a cardiac monitor. The physician should obtain a blood glucose and administer naloxone 2 mg IV to all patients with altered mental status. Fluid therapy should be done if the patient has a low blood pressure or appears to be in hypovolemic shock. Norepinephrine can be given if shock persists or worsens. A rectal temperature should be obtained to check for hypothermia. If the patient is hypothermic, careful rewarming should be initiated [12].

Gastrointestinal Decontamination

There is no evidence that the administration of activated charcoal improves clinical outcome. However, a single dose may be given within an hour of overdose if the clinician estimates that a clinically significant fraction of the ingested substance remains in the GI tract and the patient has an intact or protected airway [12].

Enhancement of Elimination

Enhanced urinary elimination has been well established as a treatment for phenobarbital and butalbital. This can be accomplished with an initial sodium bicarbonate bolus of 1 mEq/kg followed by a constant infusion. This infusion may be made by adding 100–150 mEq of sodium bicarbonate to 850 mL of D5W and titrating to maintain a urine pH of greater than 7.5 with an arterial pH of less than 7.50. The goal should be a urine output of 150–250 mL/h. Risks include hypokalemia, fluid overload, tetany, and the possibility of excessive elevations in arterial pH. Hemodialysis is effective but rarely required [12].

Benzodiazepines

Benzodiazepines are a class of psychoactive drugs whose core chemical structure is the fusion of a benzene ring and a diazepine ring. They, like alcohol and barbiturates, depress the central nervous system.

Clinically, benzodiazepines are used to treat various anxiety disorders, anxiety associated with medical illnesses, insomnia, convulsive disorders, acute status epilepticus, adjunct to other anticonvulsants, amnestic before surgery, spastic disorders, involuntary movement disorders, detoxification from alcohol and other substances, and agitation or anxiety associated with other psychiatric conditions. Other uses include adjunctive to surgery, dentistry, diagnostic studies (computed tomography [CT], magnetic resonance imaging [MRI]), cardioversion, and chemotherapy.

In 1988, the Committee of Safety of Medicines spelled out guidelines for the use of benzodiazepines. Benzodiazepines are DEA Schedule IV drugs [15–17].

The Benzodiazepines

The various benzodiazepines are listed in Table 5.4, along with their brand names, times to peak action, half-lives, and primary use [18].

Despite its long half-life (20–100 h), diazepam has a rapid onset of action—30–60 min orally and only a few minutes when given intravenously.

Street Names for Benzodiazepines

Street names for benzodiazepines include:

Candy Downers Sleeping pills Tranks Totem poles Chill pills	French fries Blues Z-bars Bricks Benzos Zannies	Bars Ladders Footballs Bennies, Goofballs Xs	Peanuts Phennies Christmas trees V Downers

Pharmacology

Pharmacodynamics

Like alcohol, benzodiazepines increase the efficiency of synaptic transmission of the neurotransmitter GABA by acting on its receptors. The GABA receptor is a macromolecular complex that, in addition to containing sites for binding GABA, also contains sites for binding other molecules such as benzodiazepines that modulate GABA's activity.

When benzodiazepines bind to a specific site on a GABA receptor, they do not stimulate it directly. Instead, they make it more efficient by increasing the frequency with which the chlorine channel opens when GABA binds to its own site on this receptor. The resulting increase in the concentration of chloride ions in the postsynaptic neuron hyperpolarizes this neuron, thus making it less excitable [19].

Pharmacokinetics

Benzodiazepines are completely absorbed after ingestion, except for clorazepate (Tranxene) which is converted to its active metabolite (nordazepam) by gastric juices in the stomach prior to absorption. With the exception of lorazepam (Ativan), the absorption of benzodiazepines tends to be erratic after intramuscular injection.

Benzodiazepines and their active metabolites bind to plasma proteins ranging from about 70% for alprazolam (Xanax) to nearly 99% for diazepam (Valium). Rapid uptake of benzodiazepines by the brain occurs after ingestion because of their high lipid solubilities (high partition coefficient) and the high perfusion rate of the brain.

The benzodiazepines are metabolized by several different microenzyme systems in the liver. All undergo glucuronidation by the liver prior to urinary excretion. Most have active metabolites, which, because they may have half-lives longer than the parent benzodiazepine, may have durations of action that bear little resemblance to the half-life of the original drug. Benzodiazepines do not produce enzyme induction [9].

Table 5.4 The benzodiazepines (Based on [18])

Drug name	Brand names	Time to peak (hours)	Half-life (hours)	Primary use
Alprazolam	Xanax	1–2	6–12	Anxiolytic
Chlordiazepoxide	Librium	1.5–4	5–30	Anxiolytic
Clonazepam	Klonopin	1–4	18–50	Anxiolytic, anticonvulsant
Clorazepate	Tranxene	Variable	36–100	Anxiolytic, anticonvulsant
Diazepam	Valium	1–2	20–100	Anxiolytic, anticonvulsant, muscle relaxant
Estazolam	Prosom	0.5–5	10–24	Hypnotic
Flunitrazepam	Rohypnol	0.5–3	18–26	Hypnotic
Flurazepam	Dalmane	1–1.5	40–250	Hypnotic
Halazepam	Paxipam	1–3	30–100	Anxiolytic
Lorazepam	Ativan,	2–4	10–20	Anxiolytic, anticonvulsant
Midazolam	Versed	0.5–1	3	Hypnotic
Oxazepam	Serax	3–4	4–15	Anxiolytic
Prazepam	Centrax	2–6	36–200	Anxiolytic
Quazepam	Doral	1–5	39–120	Hypnotic
Temazepam	Restoril	0.5–3	8–22	Hypnotic
Triazolam	Halcion	0.5–2	2	Hypnotic

The benzodiazepines act on the central nervous system to produce sedation, hypnosis, decreased anxiety, muscle relaxation, and anticonvulsant activity. They cause depressed REM sleep.

Alprazolam (Xanax), lorazepam (Ativan), oxazepam (Serax), chlordiazepoxide (Librium), clorazepate (Tranxene), diazepam (Valium), clonazepam (Klonopin), halazepam (Paxipam), and prazepam (Centrax) are mainly used as sedatives. Temazepam (Restoril), triazolam (Halcion), and flurazepam (Dalmane) are used as hypnotics. In addition, diazepam has muscle relaxant and anticonvulsant properties, and clonazepam is sometimes used to treat petit mal seizures.

In therapeutic doses, the drugs have little effect on the respiratory, cardiovascular, and gastrointestinal systems. They do not cause true anesthesia as do the barbiturates. Paradoxical excitement, although uncommon, does occur. When used for sedation, benzodiazepines are often referred to as "minor tranquilizers." Benzodiazepines, because of their dependence-producing properties, should not be prescribed for longer than 2–4 weeks [5].

Interactions with Other Drugs

Many drug interactions can occur with benzodiazepines. While it is rare that an overdose of benzodiazepines by itself would be fatal, when combined with other drugs that depress the central nervous system, the risk greatly increases. Other drugs that may be additive to the central nervous system depression if combined with a benzodiazepine include phenothiazines, opiates, barbiturates, MAO inhibitors, tricyclic antidepressants, alcohol, sedating antihistamines, and some illicit drugs.

Many benzodiazepines are broken down in the liver, and when combined with drugs that block this action, blood levels can rise. Lorazepam (Ativan), oxazepam (Serax), and temazepam (Restoril) are less likely to have this risk.

Rifampin may reduce the effectiveness of benzodiazepines, and the proton pump inhibitors omeprazole (Prilosec) and esomeprazole (Nexium) can elevate diazepam levels. Some herbal supplements (kava, St. John's wort) and grapefruit can have significant interactions with some benzodiazepines.

Kava may increase the central nervous system adverse effects of benzodiazepines. Combined use of St. John's wort with benzodiazepines may increase side effects, such as dizziness, drowsiness, impaired thinking, and difficulty concentrating. Grapefruit and grapefruit juice may interact with certain benzodiazepines, such as midazolam, triazolam, and alprazolam. Blood levels of these drugs may be increased, which may lead to potentially dangerous side effects.

Many drugs, including oral contraceptives, antifungal agents, and some antibiotics, inhibit cytochrome enzymes in the liver, thus reducing the rate of elimination of the benzodiazepines that are metabolized by CYP450 microenzymes. This can lead to excessive drug accumulation and increased side effects. In contrast, drugs that induce cytochrome P450 enzymes, such as St John's wort, rifampicin, carbamazepine, and phenytoin, accelerate elimination of many benzodiazepines and decrease their action [20].

Health Risks

Benzodiazepines may worsen or mask symptoms of depression. Consequently, this may deny the patient the opportunity of effective antidepressant medication. Moreover, they may result in disinhibition, which may lead to suicide attempts.

Benzodiazepines may cause cognitive impairment, mainly involving memory disturbance and subtle learning impairment. Cognitive impairment may not allow patients to make optimum responses to dangerous situations. Benzodiazepines may cause psychomotor impairment, which could affect activities such as driving an automobile and operating machinery [21]. Other health risks of long-term benzodiazepine use are given in Table 5.5.

Tolerance

Tolerance to all of the actions of benzodiazepines can develop, although at variable rates and to different degrees. Tolerance to the hypnotic effects tends to develop rapidly, which may be beneficial in daytime anxiolysis but makes long-term management of insomnia difficult. Patients typically notice relief of insomnia initially, followed by a gradual loss of efficacy. Tolerance to the anxiolytic effect seems to develop more slowly than does tolerance to the hypnotic effects [15].

Table 5.5 Health risks of long-term benzodiazepine use (Based on [22])

Decreased interest in doing normal things	Irritability	Skin rashes
Decreased energy	Loss of interest in sex or decreased sexual functioning	Slurred speech
Depression	Menstrual problems	Unpleasant dreams
Fatigue or drowsiness	Nausea	Unsteadiness
Headaches	Nervousness	Urinary retention or incontinence
Increased appetite and weight gain		Weakness

Dependence

Benzodiazepine therapy can give rise to physiologic and psychological dependence based on the drug's dosage, duration of therapy, and potency. Thus, dependence will develop sooner in a patient who is taking a high dosage of a high-potency agent such as alprazolam (Xanax) than in a patient who is receiving a relatively low dosage of a long-acting, low-potency agent such as chlordiazepoxide (Librium). As a result of physiologic dependence, withdrawal symptoms emerge with rapid dose reduction or abrupt discontinuation of the drug.

Psychologically, long-term use of benzodiazepines may lead to overreliance on the need for the agent and varying degrees of drug-seeking behavior. Patients may be reluctant to discontinue the drug because of misplaced fears or anticipatory anxiety. Some patients combine alcohol with benzodiazepines when they are not able to acquire the desired or "needed" effects [15].

Therapeutic dose dependence is the largest category of people dependent on benzodiazepines. These individuals typically do not escalate their doses to high levels or abuse their medication. Smaller groups who develop dependence include patients who escalate their dosage to higher levels and illicit drug users of benzodiazepines [6]. Benzodiazepine dependence is defined by the American Psychiatric Association's DSM-5 criteria discussed in Chap. 1.

Abstinence Syndrome

Symptoms

As a result of physiological dependence, withdrawal symptoms emerge after rapid dose reduction or abrupt discontinuation of a benzodiazepine. Figure 5.1 shows the withdrawal symptoms from different patterns of benzodiazepine use. One of five possibilities may occur:

1. *High dose, short half-life, short duration of use.* Symptoms include intense anxiety, insomnia, sensitivity to light and sound, and irritability. These symptoms may progress to tremulousness, diaphoresis, muscle twitching, tachycardia, elevated blood pressure, confusion, psychosis, hyperpyrexia, and seizures. Onset varies from a few hours to a few days depending on the half-life of the drug. Symptoms peak in 2–4 days for shorter half-life drugs (1). In (1a), instead of returning to baseline, the initial withdrawal symptoms are followed by a low-level continuation of anxiety and insomnia that lasts for weeks to months. In (1b) symptoms gradually decline and generally abate within a month.
2. *Long half-life, long duration of use.* Onset of withdrawal symptoms is delayed. Symptoms escalate over the next 3 weeks or so and then begin to decline. Overall they may last 6 weeks or more. The severity of the symptoms is not as severe as with the high-dose, short half-life benzodiazepines.
3. *Low dose, long duration of use (not shown).* The low-dose, long-duration abstinence syndrome consists of an initial response less intense than the one seen in (1), but instead of returning to baseline it continues at a low level of anxiety and insomnia that may wax and wane. Panic attacks and disturbing nightmares may occur, making it difficult for some patients to discontinue the benzodiazepine. The symptoms gradually decrease in intensity for up to 6 months or more.
4. *Rebound phenomenon (not shown).* A rebound phenomenon may occur after discontinuing a benzodiazepine taken in a therapeutic dose. It consists of anxiety and insomnia and may last only a few days. It's difficult to tell if the symptoms are withdrawal symptoms.
5. *Symptom reemergence (not shown).* The original symptoms may reoccur after cessation of the benzodiazepine. Unlike the rebound phenomenon, symptoms persist but do not fluctuate like the low-dose, long-duration abstinence syndrome [5, 22–24].

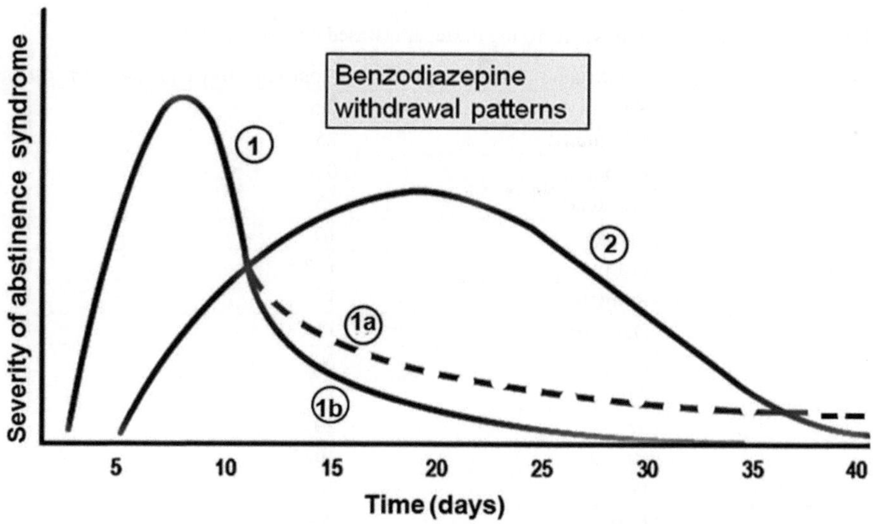

Fig. 5.1 Benzodiazepine abstinence syndromes (Based on [24])

In addition to anxiety, depression, and insomnia, withdrawal symptoms related to gastrointestinal, neurological, and musculoskeletal effects may occur.

Detoxification

Detoxification involves two steps: (1) substituting a benzodiazepine with a long half-life for the one the patient is taking and (2) tapering that medication over a period of time. Benzodiazepines with long half-lives are used for tapering because they allow smother detoxification. Diazepam is a time-proven choice.

The reduction schedule may be tailored to the individual patient as required. Four steps are involved as follow [25]:

Step 1: Transfer the patient to an equivalent daily dose of a long half-life benzodiazepine such as diazepam (Valium), taken as a single dose at night. Although simply tapering the patient's own medication is acceptable, other benzodiazepines don't always have a wide choice of doses available for tapering. Diazepam is supplied as 2, 5, and 10 mg scored tablets. Tablets can be combined with half tablets to improve the dose choices.

Step 2: Reduce the diazepam dose every 2–3 weeks in steps of 2 or 2.5 mg; if withdrawal symptoms occur, maintain this dose until symptoms improve.

Step 3: Continue to reduce the dose in smaller increments every 2–3 weeks until the lowest dose has been prescribed for the 2- to 3-week period.

Step 4: Stop completely.

The time needed to treat withdrawal may vary from 2 weeks to 6 months or more. Benzodiazepine equivalents are given in Table 5.6 [26]. Lorazepam in a dose of 1 mg, for instance, is equivalent to 10 mg of diazepam.

Overdose

Symptoms

Individuals who have overdosed on benzodiazepines have a depressed sensorium without the odor of alcohol on their breaths. They have slurred speech, an unsteady gait, and the absence of hypotension. Onset of symptoms is typically rapid, with most patients developing symptoms within 4 h. Paradoxical reactions such as anxiety, delirium, combativeness, hallucinations, and aggression can occur.

Severe consequences are rare following overdose of benzodiazepines alone, but the severity

Table 5.6 Benzodiazepine equivalent doses to 10 mg diazepam (Based on Ashton [26])

Benzodiazepine	Trade name	Approximately equivalent oral dosages (mg)
Alprazolam	Xanax	0.5
Chlordiazepoxide	Librium	25
Clonazepam	Klonopin	0.5
Clorazepate	Tranxene	15
Diazepam	Valium	10
Estazolam	Prosom	1–2
Flunitrazepam	Rohypnol	1
Flurazepam	Dalmane	15–30
Halazepam	Paxipam	20
Lorazepam	Ativan	1
Oxazepam	Serax	20
Prazepam	Centrax	10–20
Quazepam	Doral	20
Temazepam	Restoril	20s
Triazolam	Halcion	0.5

Table 5.7 Signs and symptoms of benzodiazepine overdose (Based on Gresham [27])

Signs			
Altered mental status Impairment of cognition Amnesia	Hallucinations Ataxia Coma Hypotension	Hypotonia Respiratory depression Nystagmus	Slurred speech Paradoxical agitation Weakness
Symptoms			
Agitation Anxiety	Blurred vision Confusion	Dizziness Drowsiness	Unresponsiveness

is increased considerably if benzodiazepines are used in overdose in combination with other sedating medications, such as barbiturates, alcohol, or opioids.

The duration of symptoms following benzodiazepine overdose alone is usually between 12 and 36 h. The signs and symptoms of benzodiazepine overdose are given in Table 5.7 [27].

Treatment

The cornerstone of treatment in benzodiazepine overdoses is supportive care and monitoring as with barbiturate overdose. Benzodiazepines are very rarely fatal in overdose. The altered mental status from benzodiazepine overdose greatly increases the risk of aspiration following oral charcoal dosing.

Flumazenil (Romazicon) is a specific antidote for benzodiazepine overdose, but its use is controversial. It should be used only when absolutely necessary. If used, the usual adult dose for benzodiazepine overdose initially is 0.2 mg IV one time over 30 s. Repeated doses of 0.5 mg may be given every minute. The maximum total dose is 3 mg. Patients responding partially at 3 mg may receive additional doses up to 5 mg. Most patients respond to 1–3 mg. In long-term benzodiazepine users, flumazenil may precipitate withdrawal and seizures [28].

Patients may be discharged from the emergency department if they remain asymptomatic at least 6 h post ingestion. Patients with hemodynamic instability, coma, or respiratory depression should be admitted to the intensive care unit. Respiratory depression, if present, may be treated with assisted ventilation. Patients with intentional overdoses require psychiatric evaluation before discharge.

In patients who have ingested benzodiazepines with tricyclic antidepressants, seizures and cardiac arrhythmias may follow flumazenil administration [10].

Flunitrazepam

Flunitrazepam (Rohypnol) is a benzodiazepine that deserves special attention. While commonly prescribed for anxiety and sleep disorders in Europe and Latin America, flunitrazepam was never approved for sale in the United States. In Mexico it is known as Rivotril.

Flunitrazepam pills are smuggled into the United States and sold on the street. The tablets contain 1 or 2 mg of flunitrazepam. They are odorless and tasteless, and the tablets readily dissolve in liquid.

In response to reports implicating flunitrazepam in sexual assaults (date rape), the manufacturer reformulated the tablets so that they are now green and include a dye that turns blue when they are dissolved in liquid.

The most common route of administration is oral; users swallow or chew the tablets or allow them to dissolve under the tongue. They may also crush the pills and snort the powder to feel the effects more quickly.

Users may take flunitrazepam with other drugs, including marijuana, ecstasy, LSD, or alcohol, to enhance the effects of the drug. The powder can be sprinkled on marijuana and smoked or dissolved in water and injected.

Heroin users use flunitrazepam to relieve withdrawal symptoms. Similarly, cocaine users take flunitrazepam to soften the effects of coming down from a binge. In the United States, flunitrazepam is a DEA Schedule II drug.

In response to the drug-facilitated sexual assaults, the United States Congress passed the Drug-Induced Rape Prevention Act in 1996. This act provided harsher penalties for the use of a controlled substance without an individual's consent and with the intent to commit a crime of violence, including sexual assault. Under this act, the punishment for the importation and distribution of flunitrazepam is up to 20 years in prison and a fine [29, 30].

Street Names

Street names for flunitrazepam include:

Ruffies	La Rocha	Poor man's Quaalude	Mind erasers
Roofies	Roape	Whiteys	Mexican
Rophies	Ropies		
Roches	Rib	Robutal	Valium
Roaches	Forget pill	Trip-and-fall	Circles

Pharmacology

Flunitrazepam depresses central nervous system activity. This manifests in reduced anxiety, sedation, muscle relaxation, and sleep. Rohypnol's sedative effects are approximately five to ten times stronger than diazepam. The effects of flunitrazepam appear 15–20 min after administration and last approximately 4–6 h. Some residual effects may be present 12 h or more after administration. The effects are much greater with the concurrent ingestion of alcohol or other sedating drugs [31].

Health Risks

Flunitrazepam causes anterograde amnesia, confusion, disinhibition, dizziness, drowsiness, headaches, nightmares, and tremors. It also can cause loss of muscle control, difficulty in talking, nausea, loss of consciousness, and hypotension [30]. Recreational users often combine it with other depressants, which intensify the impairment.

Dependence, Tolerance, and Abstinence Syndrome

Abuse of flunitrazepam may lead to physical dependence as it does with other benzodiazepines. Regular use results in increased tolerance to the drug. Withdrawal symptoms can range from restlessness and anxiety to more severe effects, such as tremors, hallucinations, and convulsions. Other symptoms may include headaches, muscle pain, tension, numbness, tingling of extremities, delirium, and shock.

Seizures caused by withdrawal from flunitrazepam may occur more than a week after the last use of the drug [29].

Overdose

Symptoms of flunitrazepam overdose may include Cheyne-Stokes respiration, seizures, coma, and death. Coma may be interrupted by agitation, with flailing activity described similar to a drowning swimmer fighting for air. Bradycardia and hypothermia are reported in about one-third of patients admitted to a hospital and appear to be correlated with the level of consciousness. Treatment is the same as benzodiazepine overdose described earlier. The flunitrazepam dose can be converted to a diazepam dose and tapered (1 mg flunitrazepam is equivalent to 10 mg diazepam) [31].

Z Drugs

The Z drugs are a group of nonbenzodiazepine drugs with effects similar to benzodiazepines. They include zolpidem (Ambien, Intermezzo), eszopiclone (Lunesta), and zaleplon (Sonata). Because of their short half-lives (2 h), they are prescribed for insomnia. The Z drugs are DEA Schedule IV, the same as the benzodiazepines.

In people more than 60 years of age, the benefits of these drugs may not justify the increased risk of falls, motor vehicle collisions, accidents, decreased mobility, and impaired cognitive functioning. Intoxication appears the same as alcohol, barbiturates, and benzodiazepines.

In March 2007, the FDA released a list of 13 drugs, including all three Z drugs, for which stronger labeling was required regarding potential risk from complex sleep-related behaviors, such as sleep-eating and sleep-driving [32, 33].

Pharmacology

Pharmacodynamics

The Z drugs modulate benzodiazepine-specific subunit sites, acting as specific agonists of the $GABA_A$ receptors. It is thought that the primary mode of action utilized by Z drugs is selective and carries a high affinity for the a1 hypnotic-inducing site on the benzodiazepine subunit within the $GABA_A$ receptor [33].

Pharmacokinetics

Most Z drugs causes sleep in less than an hour, and their effects last at least 4 h. Ambien, Ambien CR, and Lunesta can sustain sleep as long as 6–8 h [34].

Health Risks

Heath risks of the Z drugs are the same as for the benzodiazepines. The most common adverse effects include headache, gastrointestinal upset, and dizziness [33].

Dependence

The Z drugs, like benzodiazepines, should not be taken for more than 2–4 weeks. If taken longer, tolerance and dependence develop, and patients are incapable of sleeping without the medication [33]. Z drug dependence is defined within sedative-hypnotic criteria of the American Psychiatric Association's DSM-5 criteria discussed in Chap. 1.

Abstinence Syndrome

The Z drug abstinence syndrome resembles that from benzodiazepines, including insomnia, delirium, craving, anxiety, tremor, palpitations, and rarely, seizures and psychosis [33].

Detoxification

The Z drug dose should be gradually reduced or crossed over to an equivalent dose of diazepam, which has a much longer half-life. Z drug equivalents to 10 mg diazepam are zaleplon 20 mg, zolpidem 20 mg, and eszopiclone 3 mg. The diazepam dose is gradually tapered over a period of several weeks to months [26].

Gamma-Hydroxybutyric Acid

Gamma-hydroxybutyric acid (GHB) is a central nervous depressant that was initially sold and promoted in health food stores to improve physical performance, reduce stress, induce sleep, build muscle, and burn fat.

Most illicit GHB is sold in the form of a clear, odorless, nearly tasteless liquid. It is also available as a white powder. Acute use of GHB produces euphoria, progressing with higher doses to dizziness, hypersalivation, hypotonia, and amnesia.

GHB that is sold and used recreationally is obtained illegally from clandestine labs. It is easily manufactured from industrial chemicals. Internet websites offer instructions for home production and sell kits with the requisite materials. As a result, the chemical composition is highly variable.

GHB is used in social environments, such as parties, clubs, and raves, for its intoxicating, euphoric, and sedative effects. Because it can be mixed with almost any liquid and causes intoxication and amnesia, it has found a use as a date rape drug. It can be lethal when combined with alcohol or other depressants.

Gamma butyrolactone (GBL), a prodrug of GHB, is a clear liquid solvent. It is not approved for human consumption but has legitimate uses in cleaning and manufacturing chemicals. One of the hallmarks of GBL is the "gleeb" coma, which is a temporary unwakeable state. It also has a reputation as a date rape drug.

In 2000, GHB was classified as a DEA Schedule I drug. In 2002, sodium oxybate

(Xyrem), a formulation of GHB, was approved for the treatment of narcolepsy and classified as DEA Schedule III [35].

Street Names

Street names for GHB include:

Georgia home boy	Grievous bodily harm Jib	Liquid X	Vita G
Goop	Liquid E	Salty water	Growth hormone
Great hormones at bedtime	Liquid ecstasy	Soap	booster

Pharmacology

Pharmacodynamics

GHB acts at two receptor sites in the brain, the $GABA_B$ and specific GHB receptors. Action at these two receptor sites leads to the CNS depressant, stimulant, and psychomotor impairment effects of GHB [36]. Drugs.com

Pharmacokinetics

Roughly 95% of GHB is metabolized in the liver. Its half-life ranges from 30 to 60 min. Only 5% of the parent drug is excreted via the kidneys.

Effects are felt within 10–20 min of the initial ingestion; 45–90 min later, effects begin to peak. After effects, like grogginess and sleepiness, are felt for 2–12 h after use.

Consumption of less than 1 g of GHB acts as a relaxant, causing a loss of muscle tone and reduced inhibitions. Consumption of 1–2 g causes a strong feeling of relaxation and slows the heart rate and respiration. At this dosage level, GHB also interferes with blood circulation, motor coordination, and balance. In larger doses, 2–4 g, pronounced interference with motor and speech control occurs. A coma-like sleep may be induced [37].

GHB is easily manufactured from industrial chemicals. Internet websites offer instructions for home production and sell kits with the requisite materials [38].

Health Risks

GHB can cause nausea, vomiting, delusions, depression, vertigo, hallucinations, seizures, respiratory distress, loss of consciousness, slowed heart rate, lowered blood pressure, amnesia, and coma. GHB-related deaths have occurred.

When mixed with alcohol, the depressant effects of GHB are enhanced. This can lead to respiratory depression, unconsciousness, and coma.

GHB has surpassed Rohypnol (flunitrazepam) as the most common substance used in drug-facilitated sexual assaults (date rape) [38].

Tolerance, Dependence, and Abstinence Syndrome

Dependence on GHB can develop, and users develop tolerance. On cessation of use, users may experience physical and psychiatric withdrawal symptoms, including anxiety, tremor, insomnia, confusion, delirium, and hallucinations.

Abuse patterns of GBL are similar to GHB. So is tolerance, dependence, and abstinence syndrome [35].

Overdose

Symptoms

GHB overdose results in amnesia, headache, hallucinations, nausea and vomiting, respiratory depression, seizures, loss of consciousness, coma, and death. The sleep or deep sedation from which the person cannot be awakened by any means may last for about 3 h. Passing out while on GHB is sometimes called carpeting out, scooping out, or throwing down [39].

Treatment

Treatment of GHB overdose is primarily supportive. No specific antidote exists. The course of GHB overdose may be short lived, with rapid recovery. Therefore, many of these patients can be discharged from the emergency department without admission to the hospital [40].

Sedative-Hypnotics of Historical Interest

Sedative-hypnotics of historical interest include the barbiturate-like drugs, meprobamate, and chloral hydrate.

Barbiturate-Like Drugs

The barbiturate-like drugs include ethchlorvynol (Placidyl), ethinamate (Valmid), glutethimide (Doriden), methaqualone (Quaalude), and methyprylon (Noludar). These drugs were developed in an attempt to avoid some of the undesirable side effects of the barbiturates, including their potential for lethal overdose. However, they also were found to produce tolerance, dependence, and an abstinence syndrome [41].

Ethchlorvynol (Placidyl) was developed by Pfizer in the 1950s, and in the United States, it was sold by Abbott Laboratories under the trade name Placidyl. It was used to treat insomnia. During the late 1970s, ethchlorvynol was overprescribed, causing a minor epidemic of persons who became addicted to this drug. Some addicted persons tried to inject the drug directly into a vein, resulting in loss of limbs or death. Abbott discontinued production in 1999.

The drug had a rapid onset and short duration of action. It had anticonvulsant and muscle relaxant properties. Overdose was characterized by a prolonged coma, severe respiratory depression, hypotension, bradycardia, hypothermia, and cutaneous bullae. Intravenous injection was sometimes associated with pulmonary edema. It was especially dangerous in overdose because it was highly lipid soluble and resistant to excretion. Withdrawal symptoms in the severest form resembled delirium tremens [5].

Ethinamate (Valmid) was a short-acting hypnotic used to treat insomnia. It was said to be not effective for longer than 7 days. It had a rapid onset and a short duration of action. Overdose and withdrawal symptoms resembled those of barbiturates. Deaths from overdose occurred. It is no longer available in the United States [5].

Glutethimide (Doriden) was a hypnotic introduced by Ciba in 1954 as an alternative to barbiturates to treat insomnia. Before long, however, it became clear that glutethimide was just as likely to cause addiction and severe withdrawal symptoms. The drug community learned that when glutethimide was taken with codeine, it enabled the body to convert higher amounts of the codeine to morphine.

Because it produced pronounced anticholinergic activity, atony of the urinary bladder, mydriasis, and hyperpyrexia could occur. Bouts of tonic muscular contraction, twitching, and even convulsions were known to occur.

Patients with an overdose tended to show a cyclic level of consciousness because of rise and fall of the plasma concentration as the drug was absorbed from the gastrointestinal tract. It was exceptionally difficult to dialyze out of the body, making it exceptionally difficult to reverse overdoses.

Glutethimide was discontinued in the United States by manufacturers in 1993. It is a DEA Schedule II drug [5, 42].

Methaqualone (Quaalude) was synthesized in India in the 1951. It was introduced into the United States in 1965 as a treatment for insomnia and was believed to possess none of the abuse potential of the barbiturates. It did, however, become a very popular abused drug.

In prescribed doses, methaqualone promoted relaxation, sleepiness, and sometimes a feeling of euphoria. By the late 1960s, it had become a popular recreational drug. In 1972, methaqualone was one of the most prescribed sedatives in the United States. Its popularity, in part, was due to the belief that sex plus a Quaalude was better than sex alone.

Intoxication with methaqualone was similar to barbiturate intoxication. In addition, a prickling of the fingers, lips, and tongue sometimes occurred.

"Luding out" is a term designating Quaaludes taken with wine, which was a popular college pastime. In 1973, methaqualone was placed in DEA Schedule II and removed from the market in 1980 [5].

Methyprylon (Noludar) was developed by Hoffmann-La Roche to treat insomnia in1956. Intoxication and overdose were similar to barbiturates. Because of abuse of the drug, it was withdrawn from the United States market in 1989. It is a Schedule III drug [5, 43].

Meprobamate

Meprobamate (Miltown, Equanil) was synthesized in 1950 by Frank Berger and Bernard Ludwig working for Carter Products. The drug was used as an anxiolytic, and was the best-selling minor tranquilizer for a time.

The liver is the primary source of degradation, and the drug is capable of stimulating the hepatic microenzyme system.

The predominant manifestations of meprobamate overdose include stupor, vomiting, paresthesias, seizures, and coma. Profound and persistent hypotension may occur following large ingestions. Forced diuresis and dialysis are effective in removing the drug from the body. Repeated oral charcoal administration may be effective [5, 44].

The European Medicines Agency recommended suspension of marketing authorizations for meprobamate-containing medicines in the European Union in January 2012. In the United States, meprobamate is a Schedule IV drug.

Carisoprodol

Carisoprodol (Soma) is a centrally acting skeletal muscle relaxant. Its benefit is mostly due to its meprobamate metabolite. Carisoprodol, like meprobamate, has the potential to produce physical dependence of the barbiturate type following periods of prolonged use.

Withdrawal from the drug after extensive use may require hospitalization of medically compromised patients. In severe cases, the withdrawal can mimic the symptoms of alcohol withdrawal, including seizures. Because of abuse of the drug, it was placed in DEA Schedule IV in 2012 [45].

Chloral Hydrate

Chloral hydrate (Noctec) is supplied as gelatinous capsules that are taken orally. It is metabolized within 4 min into trichloroethanol by erythrocytes and plasma esterases and many hours later into trichloroacetic acid. In therapeutic doses for insomnia, chloral hydrate is effective within 60 min.

The irritant effects of chloral hydrate cause an unpleasant taste, epigastric distress, nausea, occasional vomiting, and flatulence. Persistent effects in the elderly are less pronounced than for other hypnotics. In addition, it interferes less with REM sleep. For these reasons, it was once widely prescribed to treat insomnia in the elderly. Today it is commonly used as an ingredient in the veterinary anesthetic Equithesin. Chloral hydrate is also still used as a sedative prior to Electroencephalogram (EEG) procedures, as it is one of the few available sedatives that does not suppress epileptiform activity.

Chloral hydrate is a DEA Schedule IV controlled substance in the United States and still available by prescription.

Mickey (Michael) Finn was an American saloon-keeper who allegedly drugged his customers in the 1920s. His name has been given to an alcohol drink to which chloral hydrate is added to make the drinker unconscious. It was called a "Mickey Finn."

Sudden withdrawal causes symptoms similar to those of the alcohol abstinence syndrome. Detoxification can be done using an equivalent dose of chlordiazepoxide (Librium) in a ratio of 25 mg Librium/200 mg chloral hydrate. Chloral hydrate overdose resembles barbiturate toxicity and is treated the same [5, 41, 46].

Summary

In addition to alcohol, drugs that depress the central nervous system include barbiturates, benzodiazepines, insomnia medication collectively referred to as the Z drugs, gamma-hydroxybutyric acid (GHB), a group of medications primarily of historical interest, meprobamate, and chloral hydrate.

Barbiturates were the earliest class of sedative-hypnotic agents to be developed. They largely have been replaced by benzodiazepines. Both dispositional and pharmacodynamic tolerance to barbiturates can develop, the latter being more important. Withdrawal symptoms are similar to those of alcohol dependence. Treatment of barbiturate abstinence syndrome involves estimating the usually daily barbiturate dose a patient has been taking, substituting diazepam in an equivalent dose, stabilizing the patient at the equivalent diazepam dose, and tapering the drug over 4–5 days for the shorter-acting barbiturates and up to a matter of weeks for the longer-acting ones. In overdose, barbiturates can cause lack of coordination, ataxia, depressed respiration, slurred speech, nystagmus, stupor, coma, and death.

Benzodiazepines are used for alcohol detoxification, along with treatment of a number of other disorders. Withdrawal symptoms from benzodiazepines, in some cases, can last for months.

Severe consequences are rare following overdose of benzodiazepines alone, but the severity is increased considerably if benzodiazepines are used in overdose in combination with other sedating medications, such as barbiturates, alcohol, or opioids.

Flunitrazepam (Rohypnol) is a benzodiazepine that has a reputation as a date rape drug.

Z drugs are a group of nonbenzodiazepine drugs used for the temporary treatment of insomnia. They have dependence risk and withdrawal symptoms similar to benzodiazepines.

Gamma-hydroxybutyric acid (GHB) is a central nervous depressant that sometimes is used as a date rape drug. Carisoprodol (Soma) is a centrally acting skeletal muscle relaxant that has meprobamate as a metabolite.

References

1. Barbiturate statistics. Erowid.org website. http://www.erowid.org/chemicals/barbiturates/barbiturates_stats.shtml
2. Cohen S. The barbiturates: has their time gone? In: The substance abuse problems: volume one. New York: Haworth Press; 1981. p. 119–24.
3. Mandal Ananya. Barbiturate history website. www.news-medical.net/health/Barbiturate-History.aspx. May 26, 2013.
4. O'Brien R, Barbiturates CS. The encyclopedia of drug abuse. New York: Facts on File; 1984. p. 35–8.
5. Milhorn HT. Chemical dependence: diagnosis, treatment, and prevention. New York: Springer; 1990.
6. Allgulander C. Barbiturates. In: Encyclopedia of psychopharmacology. Heidelberg/New York: Springer; 2014.
7. Denno DW. Gas chamber: execution device. Encycloepedia Britannica. February 9, 2012.
8. Olsen RW, Yang J, King RG, Dilber A, Stauber GB, Ransom RW. Barbiturate and benzodiazepine modulation of GABA receptor binding and function. Life Sci. 1986;39(21):1969–76.
9. Harvey S. Hypnotics and sedatives. In: Goodman LS, Gilman AG, Rall TW, Murad F, editors. Goodman and Gilman's the pharmacological basis of therapeutics. New York: Macmillan; 1985. p. 339–69.
10. Trevor AJ. Sedative-hypnotic drugs. In: Katzung BG, Trevor AJ, editors. Basic and clinical pharmacology. 13th ed. New York: McGraw-Hill Education; 2015. p. 369–83.
11. Heller JL. Barbiturate intoxication and overdose. MedlinePlus website. https://medlineplus.gov/ency/article/000951.htm. U.S. National Library of Medicine. October 9, 2015.
12. Lafferty KA. Barbiturate toxicity. Medscape website. http://emedicine.medscape.com/article/813155-overview. January 14, 2017.
13. Trevor AJ, Way WL. Sedative-hypnotics. In: Katzung BG, editor. Basic and clinical Pharmacology. Norwalk: Appleton and Lange; 1987. p. 241–53.
14. Barbiturates withdrawal symptoms & treatment. Pat Moore Foundation website. http://www.patmoorefoundation.com/barbiturates-withdrawal-symptoms-treatment
15. Longo LP, Brian J. Addiction: part I. Benzodiazepines – side effects, abuse risk and alternatives. Am Fam Physician. 2000;61(7):2121–8.
16. Lader M. History of benzodiazepine dependence. J Subst Abus Treat. 1991;8:53–9.
17. Laux G, Puryear DA. Benzodiazepines – misuse, abuse and dependency. Am Fam Physician. 1984;30(5):139–47.
18. Benzodiazepines: list of trade names, uses and dosage. UATests.com website. http://www.uatests.com/drug-information/benzodiazepines-list.php
19. Dubuc B. The brain from top to bottom. McGill University. http://thebrain.mcgill.ca. May 2012.
20. Benzodiazepines: overview and use. Drugs.com website. http://www.drugs.com/article/benzodiazepines.html. May 04, 2014.
21. West LM. Benzodiazepines: benefits versus risks. J Malta Coll Pharm Pract 2007;(Summer):13.
22. Benzodiazepines. NSW government, Health website. http://www.health.nsw.gov.au/mentalhealth/Factsheets/Pages/benzodiazepines.aspx. July 11, 2013.

23. Benzodiazepine abuse. WebMD website. http://www.webmd.com/mental-health/addiction/benzodiazepine-abuse#1
24. Smith DE, Wesson DR. Benzodiazepine withdrawal syndromes. J Psychoactive Drugs. 1983;15:85–95.
25. Benzodiazepine & 'z' drugs withdrawal protocol. NHS Northamptonshire website. http://www.neneccg.nhs.uk/resources/uploads/files/benzodiazepine_protocol.pdf
26. Ashton CBH. Comparison chart. Pharmer.org website. http://m.pharmer.org/forum/discussion-prescription-and-otc-meds/benzo-comparison-chart. April 2007.
27. Gresham C. Benzodiazepine toxicity. Medscape website. http://emedicine.medscape.com/article/813255-overview. April 29, 2016.
28. Flumazenil dosage. Drugs.com website. http://www.drugs.com/dosage/flumazenil.html
29. Flunitrazepam (Rohypnol). Center for Substance Abuse Research (CESAR) at the University of Maryland website. http://www.cesar.umd.edu/cesar/drugs/rohypnol.pdf
30. Date rape drugs fact sheet. Office on women's health in the office of the assistant secretary for health at the U.S. Department of health and human services website. http://www.womenshealth.gov/publications/our-publications/fact-sheet/date-rape-drugs.html. July 16, 2012.
31. Gahlinger PM. Club drugs: MDMA, Gamma-Hydroxybutyrate (GHB), Rohypnol, and Ketamine. Am Fam Physician. 2004;69(11):2619–27.
32. Insomnia treatment with non-benzodiazepines Ambien, Lunesta & Sonata. Drugs.com website. http://www.drugs.com/slideshow/insomnia-treatment-nonbenzodiazepines-1072. April 5, 2016.
33. Gunja N. The clinical and forensic toxicology of z-drugs. J Med Toxicol. 2013;9(2):155–62.
34. Tamura L. Z drugs keep sleep-aid market awake. Washington Post. February 15, 2011.
35. GHB. Center for Substance Abuse Research (CESAR) at the University of Maryland website. http://www.cesar.umd.edu/cesar/drugs/ghb.pdf
36. GHB or Gamma-Hydroxybutyrate. Drugs.com website. http://www.drugs.com/illicit/ghb.html
37. O'Connell T, Kaye L, Plosay JJ III. Gamma-Hydroxybutyrate (GHB): a newer drug of abuse. Am Fam Physician. 2000;62(11):2478–82.
38. Gamma Hydroxybutyrate (GHB). Office of National Drug Control Policy website. http://www.ncjrs.gov/pdffiles1/Digitization/194881NCJRS.pdf
39. What is GHB? Project GHB website. http://www.projectghb.org/content/what-ghb
40. Benzer T. Gamma-Hydroxybutyrate toxicity treatment & management. Medscape website. http://emedicine.medscape.com/article/820531-treatment. December 29, 2015.
41. Wilford BB. Sub-acute care. In: Review course syllabus. New York: American Medical Society on Alcohol and Other Drug Dependencies; 1987. p. 189–218.
42. Milhorn HT. Pharmacologic management of acute abstinence syndromes – withdrawal symptoms. Am Fam Physician. 1992;45(1):231–9.
43. Gwilt PR, Pankaskie MD, Zustiak R, Shoenthal DR. Pharmacokinetics of methyprylon following a single oral dose. J Pharm Sci. 1985;74:1001–3.
44. Hasson E. Treatment of meprobamate overdose with repeated oral doses of activated charcoal. Ann Emerg Med. 1986;15:73–6.
45. Carisoprodol. MedLibrary.org website. http://medlibrary.org/medwiki/Carisoprodol. June 22, 2001.
46. Mohammed MS, Aquino MF. The use of chloral hydrate in pediatric electroencephalography. Neurosciences. 2001;6(2):99–102.

6 Opioid Dependence

Key Chapter Points

- The opioid drugs reduce both the perception of pain and the reaction to it. They also produce euphoria, which leads to their abuse.
- Natural opiates (thebaine, opium, codeine, morphine) are obtained from the poppy plant (*Papaver somniferum*).
- Semisynthetic opioids are derived from opium but are chemically altered to make new substances. These drugs include heroin, oxycodone, hydrocodone, oxymorphone, and hydromorphone.
- Krokodil is a homemade drug, combining codeine, lighter fluid, gasoline, paint thinner, alcohol, and other ingredients.
- Synthetic opioids include meperidine, fentanyl, methadone, tramadol, and the antidiarrheal medications loperamide and diphenoxylate/atropine.
- Agonist-antagonist opioids include pentazocine, butorphanol, nalbuphine, and buprenorphine.
- Naltrexone and naloxone are opioid antagonists. They block the effects of opioids.
- Designer drugs are substances that are illegally developed in clandestine laboratories and which have structures and properties similar to those of DEA scheduled drugs.
- Buprenorphine, methadone, and clonidine can be used for opioid detoxification.
- Administration of naloxone can produce a dramatic reversal of respiratory depression from opioid overdose.

The term *opiate* is used to designate a group of drugs that are naturally occurring in the poppy plant *P. somniferum* (Fig. 6.1). They include thebaine, opium, codeine, and morphine. *Opioids* are substances that act on opioid receptors to produce morphine-like effects. They include the opiates.

The opioids are divided into three major groups—naturally occurring, semisynthetic, and synthetic. The naturally occurring opioids are the opiate drugs. Semisynthetic opioids are drugs that are made by minor alterations of the opiate drug molecules. Synthetic opioids are manufactured in the laboratory independent of the poppy plant. Opioids can further be divided into agonist, partial agonist, agonist-antagonist, and pure antagonist drugs [1].

Because of the tendency of opioid drugs to produce somnolence, they are often referred to as *narcotics*, a word that comes from *narcosis*, meaning sleep [2].

Prevalence of Use

Of the 21.5 million Americans 12 or older who had a substance use disorder in 2014, 1.9 million involved prescription pain relievers, and 586,000 involved heroin.

H.T. Milhorn, *Substance Use Disorders*, DOI 10.1007/978-3-319-63040-3_6

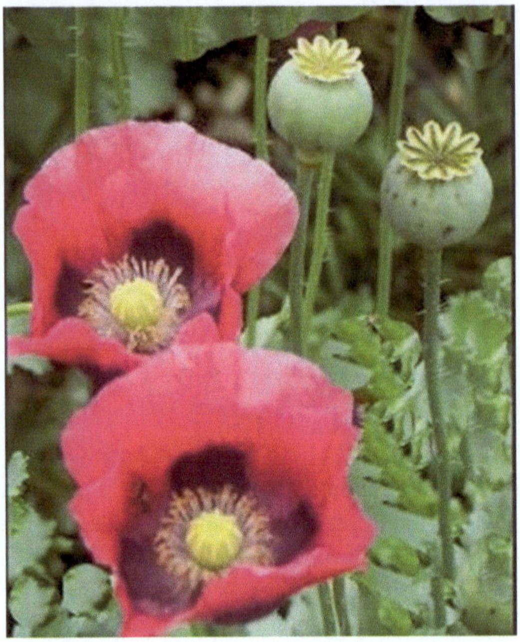

Fig. 6.1 The poppy plant

There were 18,893 overdose deaths related to prescription pain relievers and 10,574 overdose deaths related to heroin in 2014. Deaths from all opioids combined topped 33,000 in 2015. That means opioid deaths outnumbered firearm-related homicides nearly three to one [3–5].

The Opioid Drugs

Opioid drugs are classified as naturally occurring, semisynthetic, synthetic, partial agonists, agonist-antagonist, and antagonist (Table 6.1) [6].

Pharmacology

Pharmacodynamics

Three distinct families of endogenous opioid peptides have been identified—the enkephalins, the endorphins, and the dynorphins. By interacting with specific receptors, the endogenous opioids function as neurotransmitters, modulators of neurotransmission, or neurohormones. Endogenous opioids modulate reactions to painful stimuli.

There are three major categories of endogenous opioid receptors, designated as mu, kappa, and delta [7].

- *Mu receptors* are found primarily in the brain stem and medial thalamus. Mu receptors are responsible for supraspinal analgesia, respiratory depression, euphoria, sedation, decreased gastrointestinal motility, and physical dependence.
- *Kappa receptors* are found in the limbic and other diencephalic areas, brain stem, and spinal cord and are responsible for spinal analgesia, sedation, dyspnea, dependence, dysphoria, and respiratory depression.
- *Delta receptors* are located largely in the brain, and their effects are not well studied. They may be responsible for psychomimetic and dysphoric effects.

The receptors influence the likelihood that ion channels will open, which reduces the excitability of neurons. This reduced excitability is the source of the euphoric effect of opioids and appears to be mediated by the mu and delta receptors. The euphoric effect also appears to involve another mechanism in which the GABA-inhibitory interneurons of the ventral tegmental area are involved. By attaching to mu receptors, exogenous opioids reduce the amount of GABA released. Normally, GABA reduces the amount of dopamine released in the nucleus accumbens. By inhibiting this inhibitor, the opioids increase the amount of dopamine produced and the amount of pleasure felt. Exogenous opioids, such as morphine and heroin, bind to the same receptors as the endogenous opioids [8].

Pharmacokinetics

Most opioid drugs are well absorbed from subcutaneous and intramuscular sites, as well as from the nose and gastrointestinal tract. Despite rapid absorption from the gastrointestinal tract, some opioid drugs (morphine, hydromorphone, oxymorphone)

Table 6.1 The opioid drugs(Based on Milhorn [6])

Generic names	Trade names
Naturally occurring opioids	
Opium	Paregoric, Parepectolin, Pantopon, B & O Supprettes, Donnagel-PG
Morphine	Morphine Sulfate, Duramorph, Roxanol
Codeine	Empirin with Codeine, Tylenol with Codeine, Phenergan with Codeine, Robitussin and other cough compounds
Semisynthetic opioids	
Heroin (diacetylmorphine)	None
Oxymorphone	Numorphone, Opana, Opana ER
Hydrocodone	Hycodan, Hycomine, Vicodin, Norco
Oxycodone	Percodan, Percocet, Tylox, OxyContin, OxyContin CR
Synthetic opioids	
Hydromorphone	Dilaudid
Fentanyl	Actiq, FentoraTM, Duragesic
Methadone	Methadose, Dolophine
Tramadol	Ultram
Meperidine	Demerol
Dextromethorphan	Benylin, Delsym, Sucrets, Bromfed-DM, Robitussin, Vicks Formula 44
Partial agonists	
Buprenorphine	Buprenex, Probuphine
Buprenorphine-naloxone	Suboxone
Agonist-antagonists	
Pentazocine	Talwin
Butorphanol	Stadol
Nalbuphine	Nubain
Antagonists	
Naltrexone	Vivitrol, Revia
Naloxone	Narcan
Others	
Loperamide	Imodium
Diphenoxylate/atropine	Lomotil

are far less potent when absorbed that way than when administered parenterally because of a significant first-pass effect by the liver. Therefore, the oral dose of these compounds must be greater than the parenteral dose. On the other hand, some opioids (methadone, codeine) do not undergo significant first-pass effect so that their oral dose is close to their parenteral dose. Yet others are intermediary in oral to parenteral potency.

Opioids bind to plasma proteins with varying degrees of affinity. However, they rapidly leave the blood and localize in parenchymatous tissues, such as the lungs, liver, kidneys, and spleen. Although these drugs maintain low concentrations in skeletal muscles, this tissue serves as the main reservoir for the drugs because of its bulk. Brain concentrations are usually relatively low compared to concentrations in other tissues.

The opioids are converted in large part by the liver to metabolites that are readily excreted by the kidneys. Compounds that have a free hydroxyl group, such as morphine, are conjugated with glucuronic acid. Esters, such as meperidine and heroin, are hydrolyzed by esterases [1, 7, 9].

The opioid drugs cause central nervous system and peripheral (cardiovascular, respiratory, gastrointestinal, genitourinary, endocrine, skin) effects.

Central Nervous System Effects

The opioid drugs reduce both the perception of pain and the reaction to it. They also produce euphoria, which leads to their abuse. In addition, they reduce anxiety and stress and produce sleep. Respiratory depression can occur because the drugs inhibit the respiratory brain stem mechanism, in particular the responsiveness to carbon dioxide. Suppression of the cough reflex is a well-known effect of the opioids. All opioid agonists constrict the pupils except meperidine, which in large doses may dilate them. Opioids also activate the brain stem chemoreceptor trigger zone to produce nausea and vomiting. Truncal rigidity may occur with some opioids, thus reducing thoracic compliance and interfering with ventilation. The effect is most apparent with high doses of highly lipid-soluble opioids like fentanyl (Sublimaze) [9, 10].

Peripheral Effects

Peripheral effects occur with the cardiovascular, gastrointestinal, genitourinary, endocrine, immune, and integumentary systems.

Cardiovascular System

Most opioid drugs in therapeutic doses do not have significant effects on the heart, cardiac rate and rhythm, or blood pressure in the supine position. Meperidine (Demerol) is an exception because its antimuscarinic action can result in tachycardia.

Opioids do produce peripheral vasodilation, reduce peripheral resistance, and inhibit the baroreceptor reflex. Therefore, when patients in the supine position raise their upper torsos, they may suffer orthostatic hypotension and may have syncope. Therefore, precautions should be taken with patients who have decreased blood volumes [9, 10].

Gastrointestinal System

The opioids constrict biliary smooth muscle, which may cause biliary colic. Constriction of the sphincter of Oddi may result in reflux of biliary secretions and elevated plasma amylase and lipase levels. In addition, the drugs decrease large intestine motility, leading to constipation. In the stomach, motility is decreased, and tone is increased. Gastric acid secretion is decreased.

Genitourinary System

The opioids depress renal function, probably because they decrease renal plasma flow. Ureteral and bladder tone are increased, and increased urethral sphincter tone may lead to urinary retention. In addition, mu receptor agonists have an antidiuretic effect.

Opioids also enhance renal tubular sodium reabsorption. Occasionally uterine colic caused by a renal stone is made worse by opioid-induced increase in ureteral tone. Opioid-induced uterine tone may prolong labor [9, 10].

Endocrine System

The opioid analgesics stimulate the release of antidiuretic hormone, prolactin, and somatropin but may inhibit the release of luteinizing hormone. Patients receiving chronic opioid therapy may have low testosterone levels resulting in decreased libido, energy, and mood. Women may experience dysmenorrhea or amenorrhea [9, 10].

Immune System

Opioids modulate the immune system by effects on lymphocyte proliferation, antibody production, and chemotaxis. In addition, leukocytes migrate to the site of tissue injury and release opioid peptides, which help counter inflammatory pain. However, natural killer cell cytolytic activity and lymphocyte proliferation are usually inhibited by opioids, which may play a role in tumor progression [9, 10].

Integumentary System

Opioids produce flushing and warming of the skin, sometimes accompanied by sweating, urticaria, and pruritus. Although peripheral histamine release is an important contributor, all opioids can cause pruritus via a central (spinal cord and medulla) action on pruritoceptive neural circuits. When opioids are administered by the epidural or spinal routes, their usefulness may be limited because of intense pruritus of the lips and torso [9, 10].

Clinical Uses of Opioids

Clinical uses of opioids include analgesia and treatment of acute pulmonary edema, cough, and diarrhea. Opioids are frequently used as premedication drugs before anesthesia and surgery because of their sedative, anxiolytic, and analgesic properties [1].

Opioid Conversion

Opioid doses can be converted from one opioid drug to another. For example, when switching a patient from oxycodone to oral morphine, the conversion ratio is two, that is, 5 mg of oxycodone is equivalent to 10 mg of morphine. Some examples are given in Table 6.2 [11].

Interactions with Other Drugs

Opioids act synergistically with CNS depressants, including antipsychotic agents, to depress the sensorium and respiration. Hyperpyrexia, hypertension, and coma have been reported when opioids are used with monoamine oxidase (MAO) inhibitors.

Erythromycin increases and rifampicin (Rifadin) decreases the effects of opioids. Cimetidine (Tagamet) may increase the effects of opioids by increasing their duration of action. Carbamazepine (Tegretol), phenytoin (Dilantin), and the barbiturates can enhance the metabolism of opioids that rely on hepatic metabolism. Other pharmacokinetic interactions include those with benzodiazepines, tricyclic antidepressants, and metoclopramide (Reglan) [1, 12].

Table 6.2 Opioid dose equivalents(Based on [11])

	Potency ratio with oral morphine	Equivalent dose to 10 mg oral morphine (mg)
Codeine	0.1	100
Hydromorphone	7.5	1.3
Morphine	1	10
Oxycodone	2	5
Tramadol	0.15	67

Opioid Agonists

Natural Opiates

Natural opiates are obtained from the poppy plant (*P. somniferum*), a plant indigenous to the Middle East and Southeast Asia. Extraction only is required to get the drugs—thebaine, opium, codeine, and morphine [6].

Thebaine

Thebaine, an opiate alkaloid of opium, was isolated in 1835. Because of its toxicity, it is not used therapeutically. It is converted into several medications, including oxycodone, oxymorphone, nalbuphine, naloxone, naltrexone, buprenorphine, and etorphine. It is a Schedule II controlled substance [2].

Opium

Opium is made by air-drying the juice of the unripe seed pods of the Oriental poppy. Farmers cut open the pod and collect the gum with a scraping knife, bundling it into bricks, cakes, or balls. Opium can be smoked or ingested orally. One of the most common oral methods of opium use involves making tea infused with opium alkaloids. It also is used by vaporizing it in an opium pipe [2].

Opium is sometimes abused in combination with other drugs. For example, “Black” is a combination of marijuana, opium, and methamphetamine, and “Buddha” is potent marijuana spiked with opium.

During the 1870s, patent medicines containing opium proliferated in Europe and the United States. The most important of these was paregoric, a tincture of opium combined with camphor, for diarrhea. It is still used today. Paregoric is a DEA schedule III drug. Heroin addicts sometimes use it when they cannot get heroin, giving it the name *blue velvet*.

The Harrison Narcotic Act of 1914 placed opium under strict federal control, and the

Controlled Substances Act of 1970 made it a DEA Schedule II drug [1, 13–16].

Codeine

Codeine (3-methylmorphine) is found in concentrations of 1–3% in opium from the poppy pods. Today, most codeine is produced from morphine. It comes in two forms: Codeine phosphate is an odorless, white crystalline powder soluble in water. Codeine sulfate consists of white crystals that are soluble in alcohol. Therefore, codeine phosphate is used in elixirs and in injectable form, and codeine sulfate is used in tablet form.

Codeine can be used orally, intramuscularly, or subcutaneously. About 10% of codeine is converted to morphine in the liver. Taken orally, its half-life is 2.5–3 h with a peak effect in about 30–60 min. Its effect lasts 3–4 h.

Codeine's analgesic potency is less than that of morphine, so it is used for mild pain. It is considered moderately addictive, and withdrawal symptoms are relatively mild.

Codeine is metabolized by CYP2D6 and therefore is susceptible to drug-drug interactions.

The FDA has issued a Public Health Advisory regarding a very rare but serious side effect in nursing infants whose mothers are taking codeine and are apparent ultrarapid metabolizers of codeine, resulting in rapid and higher levels of morphine in the breast milk. This can cause potentially fatal neonatal respiratory depression [2, 7].

Its most common medical use is as an antitussive in cough syrups (10–15 mg per dose). For pain, codeine is usually combined with acetaminophen (Tylenol #3 or #4) or ibuprofen (Nurofen Plus). It may be combined with promethazine (Phenergan) for cough and colds. Individuals wishing to obtain a high drink codeine-containing cough syrup straight or take pills whole or crushed and mixed with water to allow faster absorption into the body. When codeine is used recreationally, the dose is between 60 and 400 mg.

Codeine may be combined with butalbital, caffeine, and aspirin (Fiorinal with codeine) or butalbital, caffeine, and acetaminophen (Fioricet with codeine) for migraine headache treatment, and it is combined with *carisoprodol* and aspirin for painful muscle spasm (Soma Compound with Codeine).

Codeine in its pure form is a Schedule II substance, whereas in combination with other analgesics, it is Schedule III.

Dihydrocodeine is a semisynthetic opioid that is very similar in structure to codeine. Its analgesic properties are generally considered equipotent to codeine. It is indicated for moderate to moderately severe pain as well as coughing and shortness of breath. It comes in tablet and injectable forms. Synalgos-DC tablets contain dihydrocodeine, aspirin, and caffeine [7].

Morphine

Morphine is the principal alkaloid of opium. It is named for Morpheus, the god of sleep and dreams. It constitutes about 10% of opium.

For moderate to severe pain, morphine can be administered orally, parenterally, or rectally. It also is used as an adjunct to anesthesia and as a treatment of pulmonary edema caused by left ventricular failure. When taken orally, it is less effective than when given intravenously.

Morphine, like other prescription opioids, can quickly lead to dependence, even when the user begins taking it for legitimate medical reasons.

Opioid addicts prefer the shorter-acting heroin to morphine. Morphine is a DEA Schedule II drug [2, 7, 15].

Semisynthetic Opioids

Semisynthetic opioids are derived from opium but are chemically altered to make new substances. These drugs include heroin, oxycodone, hydrocodone, oxymorphone, and hydromorphone.

Heroin

Diacetylmorphine (heroin) is usually injected (*mainlined*) or smoked. Purer forms of heroin are inhaled. Suppository or vaginal insertions are known as *plugging*. Heroin also can be injected subcutaneously (*skin-popping*). It is rapidly converted to morphine by the liver.

Pure heroin is a white, crystalline, water-soluble powder with a bitter taste. It may vary in color from white to dark brown because of impurities. Mexican heroin, known as "black tar," may be sticky like roofing tar or hard like coal.

The dose of heroin is difficult to estimate because it is cut a number of times as it passes down the line from the large distributer to the street pusher. Adulterants include quinine, sugar, starch, and powdered milk. Talcum powder is sometimes used to cut heroin and can be dangerous because it does not dissolve in the bloodstream.

To prepare heroin for injection, addicts dilute the powder in a little water, put it in a spoon, and boil it over a flame from a match or cigarette lighter for a few seconds. They then filter the liquid through a piece of cloth and draw it up in a syringe for injection.

Intramuscular injection of heroin produces the euphoric high within 5–8 min, and when the drug is sniffed or smoked, the effects are felt within 10–15 min. After using heroin the user feels a surge of euphoria (*rush*) accompanied by a warm flushing of the skin, a dry mouth, and heavy extremities. Following this initial euphoria, the user goes *on the nod* for several hours—a period of alternating between a wakeful and drowsy state [2, 16]. Heroin is a DEA Schedule I drug.

Heroin use increased 63% between 2002 and 2013, and heroin-related overdose deaths nearly quadrupled over the same time period. In 2013, an estimated 517,000 people reported that they had used heroin in the last year or had a heroin-related dependence, a 150% increase from 2007. More than 10,500 people died of heroin overdose in 2014. In 2015, heroin deaths surpassed firearm-related homicides for the first time ever. The number of heroin deaths was 12,989, and the number of firearm-related homicides was 12,979 [5]. The prevalence of heroin use by age range is given in Table 6.3 [17].

Table 6.3 Prevalence of use of heroin in 2015 by age range (%)(From [17])

	Ages 12-17	Ages 18–25	Ages 26 or older
Lifetime	0.10	1.80	2.10
Past year	0.10	0.60	0.30
Past month	0.00	0.30	0.10

People who use heroin over the long term may develop collapsed veins, endocarditis, skin abscesses, constipation and stomach cramping, liver or kidney disease, and lung complications, including various types of pneumonia. In addition to the effects of the drug itself, street heroin often contains dangerous chemicals that can clog blood vessels leading to the lungs, liver, kidneys, or brain, causing permanent damage. Also, sharing drug injection equipment and having impaired judgment from drug use can increase the risk of contracting infectious diseases such as HIV and hepatitis B and C. It also can cause miscarriages, coma, and death [18].

Oxycodone

The chemical structure of oxycodone is similar to codeine and is almost as potent as morphine. Oxycodone products can be administered intramuscularly, intravenously, subcutaneously, rectally, and orally through pills and tablets.

Extended release oxycodone (OxyContin) taken orally can remain effective for up to 12 h, making it the longest-acting oxycodone product available. OxyContin, sold as tablets, is typically crushed by addicts into a powder to be snorted or mixed with liquid to be injected. Others heat a tablet that has been placed on a piece of foil and then inhale the vapors.

An abuse-deterrent combination of oxycodone with naloxone (Targin) is available in managed-release tablets. If crushed and injected, the naloxone precipitates opioid withdrawal symptoms and blocks the effect of oxycodone. All oxycodone products are in DEA Schedule II.

Under pressure from the federal government, the manufacturer reformulated OxyContin pills so they can't be crushed, making it impossible to inject or snort the drug [2, 7, 19].

Hydrocodone

Hydrocodone products have been among the most popular pharmaceutical drugs associated with drug diversion, trafficking, and addiction. Therapeutically, it usually is combined with acetaminophen (Norco) or ibuprofen (Vicoprofen). Hydrocodone also is an ingredient in several cough and cold preparations, including Tussionex (hydrocodone bitartrate plus chlorpheniramine maleate).

In 2014, the DEA moved all hydrocodone-containing products to DEA Schedule II [7, 16, 20].

Oxymorphone

Many people who became addicted to OxyContin have switched to other forms of opioids, including oxymorphone (Opana), which is almost twice as potent as OxyContin. This has resulted in drug overdoses in some who switched from OxyContin to oxymorphone.

People using oxymorphone to get high crush the drug and either snort or inject it. Because it is an extended-release pill, crushing it releases the drug all at once.

In 2011, the FDA approved a formulation designed to prevent abuse by making the drug tough to crush or dissolve for injection [7, 16].

Hydromorphone

Hydromorphone (Dilaudid) is about eight times as potent as morphine. It is available for oral use (tablet and liquid), injection, and rectal suppository. It is highly water-soluble, which allows for very concentrated formulations. In patients with renal failure, it may be preferred over morphine.

Hydromorphone's abuse potential is high and at one time was a popular street drug. Many of its side effects such as nausea and vomiting are not as severe as those produced by morphine.

For orally administered immediate-release preparations, the onset of action is approximately 30 min with a duration of action of 4 h. All hydromorphone products are in DEA Schedule II [7, 16].

Krokodil

Krokodil is a homemade drug, combining codeine, lighter fluid, gasoline, paint thinner, alcohol, and other ingredients. It was first used in Russia in 2003. One of the street names for krokodil is "Russian Magic," referring to its short but intense production of euphoria. The euphoric effects may last less than 2 h.

Due to the short high, many users find themselves in a rapid repetition of drug injection to avoid withdrawal symptoms, which are similar of those of heroin. Users tend to inject the drug because it delivers a faster high than when taken in tablet form. The onset of effects is an hour or 2 for pill form and 5–10 min if used intravenously. Although the drug can be ten times cheaper than heroin, it gives a heroin-like effect.

Those who inject the drug into their veins can develop extreme skin ulcerations, infections, and gangrene (a discolored green-black scale-like skin that resembles a crocodile, hence the street name "krokodil").

A common reason for death is the loss of skin and the resulting infection. The drug also destroys the blood vessels it is injected into, causing vascular blockage. Pneumonia and meningitis have been reported. There have been multiple news reports of users in the United States who have had extreme skin ulcerations, infections, and the development of scale-like skin lesions due to the use of krokodil. There also have been news reports of amputations due to the drug.

Frequent administration may lead to binge patterns that can last for days. Users suffer risk for exhaustion due to sleep deprivation, memory loss, and problems with speech. Addiction is an obvious problem with krokodil use due to its high potency and short duration of effect [21, 22].

Synthetic Opioids

Synthetic opioids have a similar effect as opiates, although they have no structural resemblance. They include meperidine, fentanyl, methadone, tramadol, and the antidiarrheal medications loperamide and diphenoxylate/atropine.

Meperidine

Meperidine (Demerol) is supplied as tablet, liquid for injection, or syrup and is for moderate to severe pain. Mepergan Fortis is a narcotic pain reliever that is combined with promethazine (Phenergan) to prevent and treat nausea and vomiting from meperidine. The brand name Mepergan Fortis has been discontinued, but generic versions are available.

Meperidine can produce effects that can be felt 10–15 min after it is ingested and has a half-life of approximately 3 h. It is metabolized in the liver to normeperidine, which has a half-life of 15–30 h and has significant neurotoxic properties. It sometimes produces seizures. If the tablets are crushed, snorted, or injected, this can lead to serious side effects and/or death.

Although all opioids have some propensity to reduce shivering, meperidine is reported to have the most pronounced anti-shivering properties, mainly thorough action on subtypes of the α_2 adrenoceptor [1].

Once a first-line analgesic for acute pain, its use has dramatically fallen over the years due to its side effects. It is a DEA Schedule II controlled substance [2, 7, 23].

Fentanyl

Fentanyl is up to 100 times more powerful than morphine and 30–50 times more powerful than heroin. It began being abused recreationally by the 1970s. Initially, it was stolen from pharmacies. It has since been synthesized in clandestine laboratories and is frequently cut with heroin or cocaine. Manufacture of the drug requires relatively little technical knowledge. Theft has also been identified at nursing homes and other long-term care facilities.

Fentanyl is supplied in several forms—nasal spray, injectable, sublingual tablets, buccal tablets, and transdermal patches. Fentanyl patches are abused by removing the gel contents from the patches and then injecting or ingesting the material. Patches have also been frozen, cut into pieces, and placed under the tongue or in the cheek cavity for drug absorption through the oral mucosa. Fentanyl oral transmucosal lozenges and fentanyl injectable are also diverted and abused.

Fentanyl injection is used as premedication prior to surgery, for anesthesia induction, as an adjunct to regional anesthesia, or for pain control in the postoperative setting.

Two other legal forms of fentanyl are available. Sufentanil (Sufenta) is approximately five to ten times more potent than fentanyl and 500 times as potent as morphine. Alfentanil (Alfenta) is a short-acting opioid used for anesthesia in surgery. It has one-fourth to one-tenth potency of fentanyl and has about one-third the duration of action but with an onset of effects four times faster than fentanyl [1, 2, 7, 16].

Fentanyl, which is often used in anesthesia to prevent pain after surgery or other procedures, is commonly laced in heroin, causing significant problems across the country, particularly because heroin abuse has increased. The DEA has issued warnings to law enforcement agencies, about the fact that fentanyl can be absorbed through the skin, and accidental inhalation of airborne powder can occur [24].

Carfentanil (Wildnil), an analogue of fentanyl, is used as a tranquilizing agent for elephants and other large mammals. It is 100 times more potent than fentanyl and 1000 times more potent than morphine. Carfentanil is not approved for use in humans. Drug dealers, in an attempt to stretch their supply and deliver a stronger, longer high, sometimes cut heroin with carfentanil to save money. In recent years, a number of overdose deaths have been attributed to carfentanil. In 2016, heroin cut with carfentanil caused 255 overdoses across four states in 1 week. Carfentanil is a DEA Schedule II drug [25].

Lofentanil is very similar to carfentanil in effects but has a longer duration of action. This makes it unsuitable for most practical applications, with carfentanil being the preferred agent for tranquilizing large animals [26].

Methadone

Although the main use of methadone (Dolophine) is the long-term maintenance of opioid addicts, there are addicts who use methadone as their primary drug of choice.

Supplies of the drug for these users are illegal and are diverted from legitimate methadone programs by enrolled methadone patients.

In 2000, there were an estimated 1200 methadone treatment facilities in the United States. Methadone is available in oral solutions, tablets, and injectable solution.

Methadone can be prescribed by any physician for pain management just like other prescription opioid. Its analgesic action lasts 4–8 h. It has the potential to initiate torsades de pointes, a potentially fatal arrhythmia caused by a lengthening of the QT interval. It is a DEA Schedule II drug.

In 2001, regulations over methadone were modified to allow physicians and other healthcare professionals to provide methadone more effectively and consistently for opioid maintenance. However, methadone's main use continues to be in methadone maintenance programs where it is administered over a prolonged period of time as treatment for opioid dependence, such as one that occurs with heroin opioids [7, 27, 28].

Tramadol

Tramadol (Ultram) is an analogue of codeine. In therapeutic doses it does not cause the untoward effects of other opioids, such as sedation and constipation. It is used to treat moderate to moderately severe pain. Available dosage forms include liquids, syrups, drops, elixirs, effervescent tablets, powders for mixing with water, capsules, tablets, suppositories, and liquid for injection. Serious side effects may include seizures, increased risk of serotonin syndrome, decreased alertness, and drug addiction.

Opioid addicts take tablets orally or crush them for snorting to get a euphoric high. Long-term use of high doses of tramadol will cause physical dependence and a withdrawal syndrome. In most cases, tramadol withdrawal begins 12–20 h after the last dose. Tramadol withdrawal tends to last longer than that of other opioid drugs. Seven days or more of acute withdrawal symptoms can occur as opposed to typically 3 or 4 days for other codeine analogues.

On July 2, 2014, the DEA placed tramadol into Schedule IV of the Controlled Substances Act [7, 29].

Antidiarrheal Medications

People who are addicted to illegal narcotics or narcotic prescription pain killers, when they cannot get their drugs of choice, sometimes use antidiarrheal drugs. Other addicts use them just as a new experience.

Loperamide

Loperamide (Imodium) is an over-the-counter medication. It acts on the opioid receptors in the large intestine to decrease its activity and thereby increase the amount of time substances stay in the intestine, allowing for water absorption. It is supplied in 2 mg caplets.

Loperamide is increasingly being abused by people attempting to self-treat their opioid addiction, with sometime fatal results due to cardiac dysrhythmias [30, 31].

Diphenoxylate HCl/Atropine

Diphenoxylate HCl/atropine (Lomotil) is a prescription medication. It is supplied as an oral solution and a tablet that contains diphenoxylate HCl 2.5 mg and atropine sulfate 0.025 mg. A dose of 40–120 tablets per day taken for a prolonged period of time produces opioid dependence. Suddenly stopping the medication after this dose produces opioid withdrawal symptoms. Diphenoxylate/atropine is a DEA Schedule V medication [32].

Opioid Agonist-Antagonists

Agonist-antagonist opioids include pentazocine (Talwin), butorphanol (Stadol), nalbuphine (Nubain), and buprenorphine (Buprenex). All of these drugs have a lower abuse potential than the pure agonist opioid analgesics, such as morphine. All have been abused; however, pentazocine has been the most abused.

Pentazocine

Pentazocine (Talwin) is supplied as Talwin NX (pentazocine HCl 50 mg/naloxone HCl 0.5 mg) tablets and pentazocine injectable (pentazocine HCl 30 mg/mL). It is about one-fourth as potent as morphine and is approved to treat moderate pain. Side effects are similar to those of morphine, but withdrawal symptoms are milder. Given subcutaneously or intravenously, the duration of action is 2–3 h.

If the tablets are crushed and injected, the naloxone negates the narcotic effect of pentazocine. Taken orally the naloxone is inactivated by the stomach acid.

Severe injection site necrosis and sepsis have occurred, sometime requiring amputation of a limb. I had a patient whose physician prescribed him pentazocine for self-home injection for chronic pain. When I saw the patient for admission to a treatment center, he had pockmarks covering his buttocks and upper posterior extremities from local infections resulting from the injections.

The combination of pentazocine and the antihistamine tripelennamine is known as T's and Blues. Tripelennamine is added to increase the effect of the pentazocine. Pentazocine is a DEA Schedule IV drug.

It was approved by the FDA in June 1967. Pentazocine was originally classified in Schedule V but was changed to Schedule IV in 1979 [7, 16].

Nalbuphine

Nalbuphine (brand name formerly Nubain) injection is used to relieve moderate to severe pain. It also is used with other medications and anesthetic agents before, during, and after surgery and other medical procedures. Nalbuphine is ten times more potent than pentazocine as an antagonist and will precipitate withdrawal in an opiate-tolerant individual. It successfully has been used off-label to treat opioid-induced itching.

It has an FDA boxed warning for "Asthma, chronic obstructive pulmonary disease (COPD), co-administration with other CNS depressants, infection, pulmonary disease, respiratory depression, respiratory insufficiency, uremia."

Nalbuphine abuse is rarely encountered by law enforcement personnel. A limited number of anecdotal reports suggest that nalbuphine is abused by health-care professionals and by body builders (anabolic steroid users). It is a DEA Schedule IV drug [7, 33, 34].

Butorphanol

Butorphanol produces analgesia equivalent to nalbuphine and buprenorphine but appears to produce more sedation. The trade name Stadol has been discontinued by the manufacturer, but the drug is available in generic form. The duration of action is 3–4 h.

The most common indication for butorphanol is management of migraine using the intranasal spray formulation. It also may be used parenterally for management of moderate-to-severe pain, as a supplement for balanced general anesthesia, and management of pain during labor. Butorphanol is also quite effective at reducing postoperative shivering due to its kappa agonist activity.

Butorphanol injection, and the nasal spray, exposes patients and other users to the risks of opioid addiction, abuse, and misuse. It is a DEA Schedule IV medication [7, 10, 16, 35].

Buprenorphine

Buprenorphine (Buprenex) is an opioid analgesic used to treat moderate to severe pain. It is supplied as an injectable solution (0.3 mg/mL) and sublingual tablets (2 mg and 8 mg). It is a DEA Schedule III drug.

Buprenorphine is the first partial opioid available for maintenance of opioid-dependent patients by certified physicians outside the traditional opioid treatment delivery system.

The DEA will issue qualified physicians a second DEA number beginning with an "X" after the physician has notified the Center for Substance Abuse Treatment that they have met specified criteria.

For opioid maintenance, buprenorphine is supplied as Subutex (2 mg and 8 mg sublingual tablets) and buprenorphine/naloxone (Suboxone) sublingual films containing buprenorphine/naloxone (2/0.5 mg, 4/1 mg, 8/2 mg, and 12/3 mg). Naloxone is added to block the effects of opioid drugs (euphoria and pain reduction) and prevent people from injecting Suboxone. Suboxone also must be prescribed by a certified physician.

In 2016, the FDA approved the first buprenorphine implant (Probuphine) for treatment of opioid dependence. The device is designed to provide a constant, low-level dose of buprenorphine for 6 months in patients who are already stable on low-to-moderate doses of other forms of buprenorphine as part of a complete treatment program.

Buprenorphine produces the euphoric effects sought by opioid abusers; therefore, it is susceptible to abuse in both of the forms approved for treating opiate addiction [7, 10, 36, 37].

Suboxone has a high street value because opioid addicts use it to prevent withdrawal when their opioid of choice is unavailable. They barter or exchange it for money, heroin, or other illegal drugs [38].

Opioid Antagonists

Opioid antagonists include naltrexone and naloxone.

Naltrexone

Naltrexone blocks the effects of opioids. It competes with these drugs for opioid receptors in the brain. Light alcohol consumption stimulates the release of opioid peptides in brain regions that are associated with reward and reinforcement and that mediate, at least in part, the reinforcing effects of alcohol. However, chronic heavy alcohol consumption induces a central opioid deficiency, which may be perceived as opioid withdrawal, promoting alcohol consumption.

In 1984, the FDA approved naltrexone as a treatment for heroin addiction. In 1995, the FDA approved naltrexone as a treatment for alcohol dependence [7, 39].

Naltrexone is supplied as Revia and Vivitrol, both for the maintenance of opioid- or alcohol-dependent patients.

Revia comes in 50 mg scored tablets. It tightly binds to mu opiate receptors to block opioid attachment, thereby blocking the high normally obtained from opioid drugs. The treatment settings are the physician's office, opioid treatment programs, and other health-care settings.

Naltrexone can precipitate withdrawal in patients who have not been abstinent from short-acting opioids for at least 7 days or who have not been abstinent from long-acting ones, such as methadone, for at least 10 days. It is not a scheduled medication [40, 41].

Vivitrol is given by intramuscular injection into alternating buttocks every 4 weeks. It is supplied as vials containing 380 mg of naltrexone extended-release suspension. The FDA approved Vivitrol for the treatment of alcohol dependence in 2006 and opioid dependence in 2010 [42].

Naloxone

Naloxone (Narcan) blocks the effects of opioid medication, including extreme drowsiness, slowed breathing, or loss of consciousness. It is used to treat a narcotic overdose in an emergency situation. Naloxone is also used to help diagnose whether a person has overdosed on an opioid drug [43].

Designer Drugs

Designer drugs are substances that are illegally developed in clandestine laboratories and which have structures and properties similar to those of scheduled drugs. The purpose of developing designer drugs is to circumvent the countries' narcotic laws. Because the government was powerless to prosecute people for these drugs until after they had been marketed successfully, laws were passed to give the DEA power to emergency schedule chemicals for a year.

There have been at least two designer opioid groups—fentanyl analogues and meperidine analogues. Designer cannabinoids, hallucinogens, and stimulants have all been developed over the years [44, 45].

Street Names

Street names for opioid drugs are given in Table 6.4.

Health Risks

The adverse health effects of chronic opioid use are related not only to the pharmacological action of the drugs but also to methods used to administer them and to the lifestyles of the users. Addicts get serious infections because of lack of aseptic techniques when they share needles and syringes. Cellulitis, skin abscesses, thrombophlebitis, bac-

Table 6.4 Street names for opioid drugs

Opium	Aunti Aunti Emma Big O Midnight Oil Mira	Pen Yan Gee God's Medicine Dream Gun Dover's Powder	Guma Zero Skee Chinese Molasses Chinese Tobacco
Codeine	Cody Captain Cody	Loads Schoolboy	Syrup Doors & Fours (Tylenol #4)
Morphine	White Stuff Miss Emma M	Morph Drone Monkey	Goodfellow TNT
Heroin	Horse Skag Smack Junk	Black tar White China white Boy	Brown White lady White Horse Sugar
Heroin and marijuana	Atom bomb Canade	Woola Woolie	Woo-woo
Heroin and cold medicine	Cheese		
Heroin and ecstasy	Chocolate chip cookies	H bomb	
Heroin and alprazolam	Bars		
Heroin and LSD	Beast	LBJ	
Heroin and cocaine	Belushi Boy-girl He-she	Dynamite Goofball H&C	Primo Snowball
Heroin and crack	Chocolate rock Dragon rock	Moonrock	Speedball
Heroin and Ritalin	Pineapple		
Oxycodone	Hillbilly heroin Percs Roxy	Oxy Ox OC	Kicker Oxycotton Oxycet
Hydrocodone	Hydro Norco Vikes Perks	Hydros Tabs Watsons 357 s	Loris Vic Vicos Watson-387
Oxymorphone	Blues Blue heaven New blues Octagons Stop signs	Pink Pink heaven biscuits Pink lady O bomb	Mrs. O OM Pink O The O bomb Biscuit

(continued)

Table 6.4 (continued)

Hydromorphone	Juice Footballs Dust D Big	Dill D Hydro Super 8 M-2 M-80s	Dillies Hospital heroin Moose White triangles
Meperidine	Monkey White stuff	Demmies	Pain killer
Fentanyl	China white China girl Apache	Goodfella Friend Dance fever	Murder 8 Tango and cash
Methadone	Amidone Fizzies Jungle juice Juice	Green machine Dose Done Dolls	Chocolate Chip cookies (Methadone plus MDMA)

terial endocarditis, intracranial and pulmonary abscesses, hepatitis B, and HIV/AIDS are common among them. In addition, cardiac dysrhythmias, collapsed veins, constipation, pneumonia, itching, malnutrition, and sexually transmitted diseases may occur [16, 46, 47].

Tolerance

Chronic opioid users develop tolerance to the drug's analgesic, euphoric, and mental clouding, sedation, respiratory depression, antidiuresis, nausea and vomiting, and cough suppressive effects. They develop moderate tolerance to bradycardia but minimal tolerance to miosis, constipation, and seizures.

Tolerance to the euphoriant and respiratory effects dissipates within a few days after patients stop taking the drugs. However, tolerance to the emetic effect may persist for several months.

Addicts develop tolerance to the agonist-antagonist opioids to a much lesser extent than to the agonist drugs. They do not develop tolerance to the antagonist actions of agonist-antagonist drugs or to the pure antagonists [48].

Opioid-induced hyperalgesia is a condition manifested clinically as hyperesthesia and/or allodynia (pain elicited by a normally nonpainful stimulus). It occurs in some patients receiving chronic opioid therapy. The abnormal pain often arises from an anatomically distinct region and is of a different quality than the original pain problem. Treatment is to reduce the opioid dose and hence tolerance [49].

Dependence

With chronic use of opioid drugs, dependence develops. The addict has to have the drugs to prevent unpleasant withdrawal symptoms. Opioid dependence is defined by the American Psychiatric Association's DSM-5 criteria discussed in Chap. 1.

Principles for Prescribing to Prevent Opioid Dependence

Because of the current opioid epidemic in this country, the CDC in 2016 published prescribing guidelines for chronic pain. The primary care physician can use these principles to minimize problems involving tolerance and dependence when prescribing opioid analgesics [50].

Determining When to Initiate or Continue Opioids for Chronic Pain

1. Nonopioid analgesics, especially in chronic pain management, should be considered. These include acetaminophen (Tylenol)

and nonsteroidal anti-inflammatory drugs (NSAIDS). Physicians should consider opioid therapy only if expected benefits for both pain and function are anticipated to outweigh risks to the patient. If opioids are used, they should be combined with nonpharmacologic therapy and nonopioid pharmacologic therapy as appropriate.

2. Before starting opioid therapy for chronic pain, physicians should establish treatment goals and should consider how opioid therapy will be discontinued if benefits do not outweigh risks. Physicians should continue opioid therapy only if there is clinically meaningful improvement in pain and function that outweighs risks to patient safety.
3. Before starting and periodically during opioid therapy, physicians should discuss with patients known risks and realistic benefits of opioid therapy and patient and clinician responsibilities for managing therapy.

Opioid Selection, Dosage, Duration, Follow-up, and Discontinuation

4. When starting opioid therapy for chronic pain, physicians should prescribe immediate-release opioids instead of extended-release/long-acting opioids.
5. When opioids are started, physicians should prescribe the lowest effective dosage. Physicians should use caution when prescribing opioids at any dosage, should carefully reassess evidence of individual benefits and risks when considering increasing dosage to ≥50 morphine milligram equivalents (MME)/day, and should avoid increasing dosage to ≥90 MME/day or carefully justify a decision to titrate dosage to ≥90 MME/day.
6. Long-term opioid use often begins with treatment of acute pain. When opioids are used for acute pain, physicians should prescribe the lowest effective dose of immediate-release opioids and should prescribe no greater quantity than needed for the expected duration of pain severe enough to require opioids. Three days or less will often be sufficient; more than 7 days will rarely be needed.
7. Physicians should evaluate benefits and harms with patients within 1–4 weeks of starting opioid therapy for chronic pain or of dose escalation. Physicians should evaluate benefits and harms of continued therapy with patients every 3 months or more frequently. If benefits do not outweigh harms of continued opioid therapy, physicians should optimize other therapies and work with patients to taper opioids to lower dosages or to taper and discontinue opioids.

Assessing Risk and Addressing Harms of Opioid Use

8. Before starting and periodically during continuation of opioid therapy, physicians should evaluate risk factors for opioid-related harms. Physicians should incorporate into the management plan strategies to mitigate risk, including considering offering naloxone when factors that increase risk for opioid overdose, such as history of overdose, history of substance use disorder, higher opioid dosages (≥50 MME/day), or concurrent benzodiazepine use, are present.
9. Physicians should review the patient's history of controlled substance prescriptions using state prescription drug monitoring program (PDMP) data to determine whether the patient is receiving opioid dosages or dangerous combinations that put him at high risk for overdose. Physicians should review PDMP data when starting opioid therapy for chronic pain and periodically during opioid therapy for chronic pain, ranging from every prescription to every 3 months.
10. When prescribing opioids for chronic pain, physicians should use urine drug testing before starting opioid therapy and consider urine drug testing at least annually to assess for prescribed medications as well as other controlled prescription drugs and illicit drugs.

11. Physicians should avoid prescribing opioid pain medication and benzodiazepines concurrently whenever possible.
12. Physicians should offer or arrange evidence-based treatment (usually medication-assisted treatment with buprenorphine or methadone in combination with behavioral therapies) for patients with opioid use disorder.

Table 6.5 Opioid withdrawal symptoms(Based on Heller [51])

Abdominal cramping Agitation Anxiety Confusion Diarrhea Dilated pupils Dysphoric mood	Fatigue Fever Hot/cold flashes Insomnia Lacrimation Muscle aches Muscle spasm	Nausea/vomiting piloerection (gooseflesh) Restless legs Rhinorrhea Skin-crawling sensation Sweating Yawning

Abstinence Syndrome

Opioid withdrawal refers to a wide range of symptoms that can occur once opioid intake is interrupted or reduced. The amount, length, and intensity of the symptoms vary from person to person. For some individuals it can be an easy process, and for others it can be moderate to severe. As a rule, deaths do not occur with opioid withdrawal as they sometimes do with alcohol withdrawal.

The onset, intensity, and duration of withdrawal symptoms are related to the half-life of the abused drug. With morphine and heroin, withdrawal signs and symptoms start within 6–10 h after the last dose, peak in 36–48 h, and then gradually subside. By 5 days, most of the effects have disappeared. With long-acting drugs, such as methadone, the abstinence syndrome usually starts within 30 h of last methadone exposure, may not peak for several days, and may last as long as 2 weeks. Because the methadone abstinence syndrome has a longer course, the symptoms may be less severe [50].

Symptoms

Opioid withdrawal symptoms include anxiety, muscle aches, rhinorrhea, sweating, abdominal pain, goose bumps, and nausea and vomiting. Withdrawal symptoms are very uncomfortable but are not life threatening. Opioid withdrawal symptoms are given in Table 6.5 [51].

A transient, explosive abstinence syndrome can inadvertently be precipitated by the administration of naloxone (Narcan) or other antagonist. Within 5 min of injection of the antagonist, withdrawal signs and symptoms appear. They peak in 10–20 min and subside in about 1 h.

The expression "kicking the habit" probably comes from the leg movements that result from muscle spasms [52].

Detoxification

The FDA has approved buprenorphine (Subutex) and methadone (Dolophine) for opioid detoxification. Clonidine (Catapres), which has not been approved by the FDA, is often used.

Buprenorphine

Buprenorphine (Subutex) 0.6–1.2 mg sublingually is given every day or three times a week. It has been shown to work better than other medications for treating withdrawal from opioids, and it can shorten the length of detoxification. It may also be used for long-term maintenance after detoxification. Adverse effects include respiratory depression, headache, and constipation.

A combination dose of buprenorphine and naloxone (Suboxone) is a widely used method of opioid withdrawal treatment that works to prevent the user from feeling the effects of opioids while also reducing cravings. This method of treatment requires the user to have first entered the early stages of opioid withdrawal before Suboxone is given.

An initial 4/1 mg dose of buprenorphine/naloxone is recommended. This dose can be followed in 24 h with a second dose of 4/1 mg if indicated. Over the following 2 days, the dose of buprenorphine/naloxone should be increased to

12/3 mg–16/4 mg per day. The medication can be given over a longer period of time if) needed [53, 54].

Methadone

To detoxify an opioid addict with methadone, the dose of the abused drug is converted to a daily methadone equivalent; 1 mg of methadone is equivalent to 1–2 mg of heroin, 3–4 mg of morphine, and 0.5 mg of meperidine (Demerol).

Methadone is given orally in divided doses twice a day and tapered over 4–5 days. Alternatively, the dose of the abused drug itself can be tapered. Detoxification from methadone, because of its long half-life, is probably best done by tapering the methadone itself over 3 weeks.

When the daily opioid dose is uncertain, a 10-mg dose of methadone is given orally and its effects assessed over 30–60 min. If withdrawal symptoms are not suppressed, an additional 10-mg dose is given, and the patient is again observed. This process is repeated until withdrawal symptoms are suppressed. A similar dose is administered 12 h later. Methadone is then given twice daily and tapered over 5–14 days, depending on the half-life of the abused drug.

For patients addicted to methadone, the following detoxification schedule can be used [55]:

- Decrease dose by 20–50% per day until you reach 30 mg/day
- Then decrease by 5 mg/day every 3–5 days to 10 mg/day
- Then decrease by 2.5 mg/day every 3–5 days

Since it is against federal law to prescribe an opioid to a known narcotic addict, detoxification using methadone must be done in an inpatient facility.

Clonidine

Clonidine is not approved by the FDA for opioid detoxification; however, it is commonly used. For detoxification from most opioid agents, clonidine is initially given in a dose of 0.1–0.3 mg orally every 4–6 h for 4–5 days. With long-acting opioids such as methadone, clonidine may have to be continued for 2 weeks or more, and tapering may be required to prevent rebound hypertension.

Clonidine primarily reduces anxiety, agitation, muscle aches, sweating, rhinorrhea, and muscle cramping. Adverse effects include bradycardia, hypotension, dry mouth, and drowsiness.

Transdermal clonidine patches promote a smoother withdrawal. Patches are available in three sizes that deliver doses equivalent to the twice-daily oral doses of 0.1, 0.2, and 0.3 mg. Because of the time required to reach a therapeutic blood level with transdermal administration, a 0.2 mg loading dose should be given, and then oral clonidine, 0.1–0.2 mg every 6 h, should then be given for the first 24 h. The patches can be left in place up to 7 days.

The use of clonidine in opioid withdrawal is limited because of its hypotensive and sedative adverse effects. It also does not manage withdrawal symptoms such as cravings and general malaise. Treatment should be modified as required to keep the systolic blood pressure above 90 mm Hg [56].

Nausea and vomiting additionally can be controlled by giving the patient ice chips followed by small amounts of juice. When this is not effective, promethazine (Phenergan) 25–50 mg orally, intramuscularly, or by suppository can be given every 6 h as needed. Loperamide (Imodium), two capsules initially followed by one capsule every 6 h as needed (not to exceed eight in 24 h), can be given for diarrhea. Ibuprofen (Motrin), 400 mg every 4 h as needed, can be given for pain.

Buprenorphine has been found superior to clonidine in alleviating most of the subjective and objective opioid withdrawal symptoms [57].

Rapid Detoxification

The rapid detoxification technique, developed about 25 years ago by physicians who hoped to mitigate the discomfort of withdrawal, relies on a general anesthetic to sedate the patient for several hours while an opioid blocker precipitates withdrawal. The method is not covered by insurance and is not readily available in most locations.

Although some advertise anesthesia-assisted detoxification as a fast and painless method to kick opioid addiction, the evidence does not support those statements [58].

Opioid Overdose

Symptoms

The classic triad of coma, pinpoint pupils, and depressed respiration strongly suggests opioid toxicity. Body temperature tends to fall, and the skin becomes cold and clammy. Skeletal muscles may become flaccid, and the tongue may fall back and block the airway. Needle tracts may be present. The patient may be somnolent or comatose. A toxicology screen can be helpful [59].

Treatment

The first step in managing on opioid overdose is to establish an adequate airway to ventilate the patient. Pulmonary edema, when present, must be treated vigorously. Administration of naloxone (Narcan) (0.4–0.8 mg) can produce a dramatic reversal of respiratory depression. The dose is repeated every 2–3 min until the patient responds or until 10 mg has been given. The dose has to be repeated periodically because the duration of action is much shorter than those of the opioid drugs. Usually it is possible to titrate the naloxone dose to restore respiration without producing severe opioid withdrawal symptoms. Grand mal seizures produced by meperidine overdose are relieved by the administration of naloxone [60].

Summary

The opioids are divided into three major groups—naturally occurring, semisynthetic, and synthetic. Natural opiates (thebaine, opium, codeine, morphine) are obtained from the poppy plant (*P. somniferum*). Semisynthetic opioids are derived from opium but are chemically altered to make new substances. These drugs include heroin, oxycodone, hydrocodone, oxymorphone, and hydromorphone. In 2014, opioid deaths outnumbered firearm-related homicides nearly three to one. The opioid drugs reduce both the perception of pain and the reaction to it. They also produce euphoria, which leads to their abuse.

Krokodil is a homemade drug, combining codeine, lighter fluid, gasoline, paint thinner, alcohol, and other ingredients. There have been multiple news reports of users in the United States who have had extreme skin ulcerations, infections, and the development of scale-like skin lesions due to the use of krokodil. There also have been news reports of amputations due to the drug.

Synthetic opioids include meperidine, fentanyl, methadone, tramadol, and the antidiarrheal medications loperamide and diphenoxylate/atropine.

Agonist-antagonist opioids include pentazocine, butorphanol, nalbuphine, and buprenorphine.

Naltrexone and naloxone are opioid antagonists. They block the effects of opioids.

Designer drugs are substances that are illegally developed in clandestine laboratories and which have structures and properties similar to those of DEA scheduled drugs. Buprenorphine, methadone, and clonidine can be used for opioid detoxification.

Buprenorphine is the first partial opioid available for maintenance of opioid-dependent patients by certified physicians outside the traditional opioid treatment delivery system. The DEA will issue qualified physicians a second DEA number beginning with an "X" after the physician has notified the Center for Substances Abuse Treatment that they have met the specified criteria. Because of the current opioid epidemic in this country, the CDC in 2016 published prescribing guidelines for chronic pain. Administration of naloxone can produce a dramatic reversal of respiratory depression from opioid overdose.

References

1. Schumacher MA, Basbaum AI, Ramana K, Naidu RK. Opioid agonist and antagonist. In: Katzung BG, Trevor AJ, editors. Basic and clinical pharmacology. 13th ed. New York: McGraw-Hill Education; 2015. p. 531–51.
2. O'Brien R, Cohen S. The encyclopedia of drug abuse. New York: Facts on File; 1984.
3. Substance use disorders. Substance Abuse and Mental Health Services Administration (SAMHSA). https://www.drugabuse.gov/publications/drugfacts/treatment-statistics. October 27, 2015.
4. Pew M. The ethics of an antidote. Worker's Compensation. http://workerscomp.theclm.org/home/article/The-Ethics-of-an-Antidote-Naloxone?tick=1272438492875420000
5. Ingraham C. Heroin deaths surpass gun homicides for the first time, CDC data shows. Washington Post. December 8, 2016.
6. Milhorn HT. Chemical dependence: diagnosis, treatment, and prevention. New York: Springer; 1990.
7. Trescot AM, Datta S, Lee M, Hansen H. Opioid pharmacology. Pain Physician J. http://www.painphysicianjournal.com/current/pdf?article=OTg3&journal=42
8. Dubuc B. The brain from top to bottom. McGill University. http://thebrain.mcgill.ca/flash/i/i_03/i_03_m/i_03_m_par/i_03_m_par_heroine.html#drogues. 2012.
9. Jaffe JH, Martin WR. Opioid analgesics and antagonists. In: Gilman AG, Goodman LS, Rall TW, Murad F, editors. Goodman and Gilman's pharmacological basis of therapeutics. New York: Macmillan; 1985. p. 491–531.
10. Way WL, Way EL. Opioid analgesics and antagonists. In: Katzung BG, editor. Basic and clinical pharmacology. Norwalk: Appleton and Lange; 1987. p. 336–49.
11. Dose equivalent and changing opioids. The Royal College of Anaesthetists. Faculty of Pain Management. https://www.rcoa.ac.uk/faculty-of-pain-medicine/opioids-aware/structured-approach-to-prescribing/dose-equivalents-and-changing-opioids. 2016.
12. Maurer PM, Bartkowski RR. Drug interactions of clinical significance with opioid analgesics. Drug Saf. 1993;8(1):30–48.
13. Drug fact sheet. Drug Enforcement Administration (DEA). http://www.dea.gov/druginfo/drug_data_sheets/Opium.pdf
14. History of opium, morphine, and heroin. In the Known Zone. http://www.intheknowzone.com/substance-abuse-topics/heroin/history.html
15. Opium throughout history. PBS Frontline. http://www.pbs.org/wgbh/pages/frontline/shows/heroin/etc/history.html
16. Wilford BB, editor. Major drugs of abuse. In: Drug abuse: a guide for primary care physicians. Chicago: American Medical Association; 1981. p. 21–84.
17. National survey on drug use and health: trends in prevalence of various drugs for ages 12 or older, ages 12 to 17, ages 18 to 25, and ages 26 or older. National Institute on Drug Abuse (NIDA). https://www.drugabuse.gov/national-survey-drug-use-health. 2015.
18. Heroin. National Institute on Drug Abuse (NIDA). https://www.drugabuse.gov/drugs-abuse/heroin. January 2017.
19. Oxycodone. Center for Drug Abuse Research (CESAR). University of Maryland. http://www.cesar.umd.edu/cesar/drugs/oxycodone.asp. 2013.
20. Little known facts about the history of hydrocodone. About Addiction. http://www.about-addiction.com/little-known-facts-about-the-history-of-hydrocodone
21. Krokodil drug facts. Drugs.com. https://www.drugs.com/illicit/krokodil.html. October 21, 2014.
22. Doheny K. Krokodil. Drug FAQ, WebMD. http://www.webmd.com/mental-health/addiction/news/20130930/krokodil-drug-faq#1. September 30, 2013.
23. Shlafer M, Marieb E. Narcotic analgesics and their antagonists. In: The nurse, pharmacology, and drug therapy. Redwood City: Addison-Wesley; 1989. p. 332–55.
24. Cassels C. Fentanyl: DEA sounds nationwide alarm on drug's dangers, Medscape. http://www.medscape.com/viewarticle/841683. March 18, 2015.
25. Mettler K. Heroin cut with elephant tranquilizer may have caused 60 overdoses across two states in just 48 hours. The Washington Post. August 25, 2015.
26. Laduron PM, Janssen PF. Axoplasmic transport and possible recycling of opiate receptors labelled with 3H-lofentanil. Life Sci. 1982;31(5):457–62.
27. Toombs JD, Kral LA. Methadone treatment for pain states. Am Fam Physician. 2005;71(7):1353–8.
28. Methadone. Center for Drug Abuse Research (CESAR). University of Maryland. http://www.cesar.umd.edu/cesar/drugs/methadone.pdf. 2013.
29. Tramadol. Drug Enforcement Administration (DEA). http://www.deadiversion.usdoj.gov/drug_chem_info/tramadol.pdf. July 2014.
30. Imodium abuse: anti-diarrhea medication containing loperamide dangerous for self-treatment of opioid addiction. American College of Emergency Physicians. May 3, 2016.
31. Eggleston W, Clark KH, Marraffa JM. Loperamide abuse associated with cardiac dysrhythmia and death. Ann Emerg Med. 2017;69:83–6.
32. Lomotil abuse and dependence. MedicationDaily.com. http://www.medicationdaily.com/lomotil/info/abuse-and-dependence
33. Usman E. Nubain reduces opioid-related itching. Medpage Today. http://www.medpagetoday.com/MeetingCoverage/APS/39031. May 10, 2013.
34. Nalbuphine hydrochloride. Drug Enforcement Administration (DEA). https://www.deadiversion.usdoj.gov/drug_chem_info/nalbuphine.pdf. August 2013.
35. Aukerman G, Knutson D, Miser WF. Management of the acute migraine headache. Am Fam Physician. 2002;66(11):2123–31.
36. DEA requirements for DATA Waived Physicians (DWPs). Drug Enforcement Administration (DEA). www.deadiversion.usdoj.gov/pubs/docs/dwp_buprenorphine.htm

37. FDA approves first buprenorphine implant for treatment of opioid dependence. U. S. Food and Drug Administration (FDA). News & Events, May 26, 2016.
38. Suboxone: the new drug epidemic? National Pain Report. http://nationalpainreport.com/suboxone-new-drug-epidemic-8821747.html. September 23, 2013.
39. Gonzole JP, Brogden RN. Naltrexone: a review of its pharmacodynamic and pharmacokinetic properties and therapeutic efficacy in the management of opioid dependence. Drugs. 1988;35:192–213.
40. Revia (naltrexone HCl) tablets, U.S. Food and Drug Administration (FDA). https://www.fda.gov/Safety/MedWatch/SafetyInformation/ucm374896.htm. October 2013.
41. Revia. Office of Alcoholism and Substance Abuse Services (OASAS). https://www.oasas.ny.gov/AdMed/FYI/FYI-ReVia.cfm. September, 2011.
42. Vivitrol. Drugs.com. www.drugs.com/vivitrol.html
43. Naloxone. Drugs.com. https://www.drugs.com/naloxone.html
44. The new street drug to watch: acetyl fentanyl. Fox News. August 22, 2014.
45. Semour RD, Inaba D, Landsy M. Analogs of sedative-hypnotics, and treatment issues. In: The new drugs: look-alike, drugs and deception, and designer drugs. Center City: Hazelden; 1989. p. 39–44.
46. Schonberg SK, editor. Specific drugs. In: Substance abuse: a guide for health professionals. Elk Grove Village: American Academy of Pediatrics; 1988. p. 115–182.
47. Gabbey AE. Opioid (opiates) abuse and addiction. HealthLine. http://www.healthline.com/health/opioids-and-related-disorders. October 25, 2016.
48. Tolerance to opioid pain medications. Institute for Chronic Pain. http://www.instituteforchronicpain.org/treating-common-pain/tolerance-to-opioid-pain-medications. July 10, 2014.
49. DuPen A, Shen D, Ersek M. Mechanisms of opioid-induced tolerance and hyperalgesia. Pain Manag Nurs. 2007;8(3):113–21.
50. CDC guideline for prescribing opioids for chronic pain. Agency for Healthcare and Quality. U. S. Department of Health and Human Services. https://www.guideline.gov/summaries/summary/50153/cdc-guideline-for-prescribing-opioids-for-chronic-pain---united-states-2016?q=pain+management. March 18, 2016.
51. Heller JL. Opiate and opioid withdrawal. MedlinePlus. https://medlineplus.gov/ency/article/000949.htm. April 20, 2016.
52. Heroin in the brain: its chemistry and effects. PBS Frontline. http://www.pbs.org/wgbh/pages/frontline/shows/heroin/brain
53. Donaher PA, Welsh C. Managing opioid addiction with buprenorphine. Am Fam Physician. 2006;73(9):1573–8.
54. Opioid detoxification with buprenorphine, SuboxoneAssistedTreatment. http://www.suboxone-assistedtreatment.org/44.html. April 14, 2007.
55. Tapering and discontinuing opioids. Department of Defense. http://www.healthquality.va.gov/guidelines/Pain/cot/OpioidTaperingFactSheet23May2013v1.pdf. May 2013.
56. Nicholls L, Bragaw L, Ruetsch C. Opioid dependence treatment and guidelines. J Manag Care Pharm. 2010;16(1-b):14–21.
57. Digregorio GJ, Bukovinsky MA. Clonidine for narcotic withdrawal. Am Fam Physician. 1981;24(3):203–4.
58. Nigam AK, Tripathi Ray R. Buprenorphine in opiate withdrawal: a comparison with clonidine. J Subst Abus Treat. 1993;10(4):391–4.
59. Whitten, L. Study finds withdrawal no easier with ultrarapid opiate detox. National Institute on Drug Abuse. https://www.drugabuse.gov/news-events/nida-notes/2006/10/study-finds-withdrawal-no-easier-ultrarapid-opiate-detox. October 1, 2006.
60. Everett, S. Opioid toxicity treatment & management. Medscape. http://emedicine.medscape.com/article/815784-overview. December 19, 2016.

Stimulant Dependence

7

Key Chapter Points

- Central nervous system stimulants include the amphetamines, cocaine, methylphenidate, phentermine, modafinil, bath salts, flakka, and caffeine.
- Amphetamines are drugs that have a stimulant effect on the central nervous system (CNS) that can be both physically and psychologically addictive. They include methamphetamine.
- Cocaine is a bitter, crystalline alkaloid obtained from coca leaves and widely used as an illicit drug for its stimulant and euphorigenic properties.
- Methylphenidate is used to treat attention-deficit disorder (ADD), attention-deficit hyperactivity disorder (ADHD), and narcolepsy. It often is abused.
- Phentermine is a stimulant similar to amphetamine. It acts as an appetite suppressant by affecting the central nervous system. It also is sometimes abused.
- Modafinil (Provigil) is used to improve wakefulness in patients with excessive sleepiness associated with narcolepsy or other sleep disorders. It has the potential to produce euphoria.
- The chemicals in bath salts belong to a family of designer recreational drugs that are related to cathinone, a stimulant found in the khat plant.
- Bulk bags or bottles of pure caffeine powder are readily available online. These products are attractive to young people looking for added caffeine stimulation or for help in losing weight.

Central nervous system stimulants are a class of drugs that speed up physical and mental processes. They include the amphetamines, cocaine, methylphenidate, phentermine, modafinil, bath salts, flakka, and caffeine.

Prevalence of Use

The prevalence of use of central nervous system stimulants by age range for 2015 is given in Table 7.1 [1].

The Amphetamines

Amphetamines are drugs that have a stimulant effect on the central nervous system (CNS) that can be both physically and psychologically addictive. Amphetamines have been much abused recreationally. The street term “speed” refers to its stimulant effects.

Disorders medically treated with amphetamines include obesity, Parkinson’s disease, attention-deficit hyperactivity disorder, and narcolepsy.

H.T. Milhorn, *Substance Use Disorders*, DOI 10.1007/978-3-319-63040-3_7

In the 1970s and 1980s, illicit cocaine abuse replaced much of the illicit amphetamine use. Production and trafficking soared again in the 1990s as the result of organized crime in the Southwestern United States and Mexico. The 1970 Comprehensive Drug Abuse Prevention and Control Act classified amphetamines as DEA Schedule II drugs [2].

Prevalence of Use

Illicit amphetamine use reached its recent peak in the mid-1990s and has been declining ever since. In the United States, prevalence of use for ages 12 years and older in 2006 was 1.5%, in 2007 it was 1.2%, and in 2008 it was 1.1%. It has been decreasing ever since [3].

The Drugs

Current amphetamines on the market include amphetamine sulfate (Dexedrine), methamphetamine HCl (Desoxyn), dextroamphetamine (Dexedrine), lisdexamfetamine (Vyvanse), benzphetamine (Didrex), and amphetamine plus dextroamphetamine (Adderall). These drugs and their indications are given in Table 7.2.

Table 7.1 Prevalence of use of central nervous system stimulants in 2015 by age range (%) (From [1])

	Ages 12–17	Ages 18–25	Ages 26 or older
Past year	2.00	7.30	1.10
Past month	0.50	2.20	0.40

Street Names

Street names for amphetamines include:

Amphetamine	Goey, louee, speed, uppers, whiz, bennies, peaches, splash, whites
Dextroamphetamine	Dexies, kidi-speed, pep pills, uppers, oranges, footballs
Biphetamine	Black beauty, black birds, black mollies, copilots

Pharmacology

Pharmacodynamics

Amphetamines are similar in structure to dopamine, so they can enter the presynaptic neuron terminal via its dopamine transporters as well as by diffusing through the neural membrane directly. Once inside the presynaptic neuron, amphetamines force the dopamine molecules out of their storage vesicles into the synaptic cleft, thus increasing the postsynaptic neuron firing rate.

Amphetamines also seem to reduce the reuptake of dopamine and, in high concentrations, to inhibit monoamine oxidase A. Amphetamines may also excite dopaminergic neurons via glutamate neurons, thus removing the inhibiting effect due to glutamate receptors. By releasing this natural brake, amphetamines make the dopaminergic neurons more readily excitable [4].

Pharmacokinetics

Amphetamines are absorbed well from the gastrointestinal tract, which is the only legal route of

Table 7.2 The amphetamines and their trade names and indications

Drug	Trade name	Indications
Amphetamine sulfate	Dexedrine	ADHD, narcolepsy, obesity
Methamphetamine HCl	Desoxyn	ADHD
Dextroamphetamine	Dexedrine	ADHD, narcolepsy, obesity
Lisdexamfetamine	Vyvanse	ADHD
Benzphetamine	Didrex	Obesity
Amphetamine *plus* dextroamphetamine	Adderall, Adderall XR, Biphetamine	ADHD

administration. They are distributed throughout the body and easily enter the CNS. Both central and peripheral effects occur in 30–60 min when taken orally. However, they can be smoked and injected. Heavy users often progress rapidly to intravenous administration.

Amphetamines are excreted in the urine unchanged. Excretion is significantly increased in the presence of acidic urine.

Centrally, amphetamines stimulate the cerebral cortex, the brain stem, and the reticular activating system. Major responses include elevated mood, mydriasis, increased ability to concentrate, hyperalertness, increased motor activity, decreased fatigue, and suppressed appetite. These drugs produce a calming effect in hyperactive children.

Peripherally, amphetamines produce increased respiratory rate and a rise in blood pressure and pulse rate.

Injection of amphetamines produces an almost instant "rush" or "flash." Users compare this to the sensation of orgasm. After shooting up the drug, users feel energetic and self-confident. They become more sociable, and they have feelings of enhanced sexuality. Orgasm is delayed in both men and women, prolonging and intensifying sexual intercourse.

Because users are eager to reexperience the initial sensation, they develop a pattern of use called a "run." They inject the drug over and over again, each injection separated from the preceding one by a few hours. A run may last several days. During this time, users do not eat or sleep and may experience frightening visions or feel that bugs are crawling on their skin. They may develop paranoid symptoms, sometimes leading to violence. At the end of the run, users sink into an exhausted sleep ("crash"), which may last for several days.

Within hours after oral ingestion, amphetamines increase alertness and cause euphoria, agitation, and confusion. Bruxism and skin flushing may occur. With increasing dosage, tachycardia and dysrhythmias may occur. Hypertensive crisis and vasoconstriction may lead to stroke. HIV and hepatitis infection in inner cities have been closely associated with needle sharing by intravenous users [5–7].

Interactions with Other Drugs

Whereas acidifying agents, such as ascorbic acid, increase urinary excretion of amphetamines, alkalizing agents, such as sodium bicarbonate, decrease urinary excretion, thus increasing their effects. Amphetamines increase tricyclic antidepressant blood levels and decrease the effects of antihypertensive agents. They alter the blood sugar levels in patients on hypoglycemic agents and make diabetes more difficult to control.

Amphetamines decrease the effect of lithium, causing poor control of bipolar disorder. When used with MAO inhibitors, they increase the risk of a severe hypertensive episode and stroke.

Foods that contain tyramine (Chianti wines, aged cheeses, liver) in combination with the amphetamines increase blood pressure, central nervous system stimulation, and cardiac activity. Finally, amphetamines, when used with other sympathomimetic preparations, including over-the-counter ones, increase potentially serious cardiovascular and central nervous system risks [8].

Methamphetamine

Methamphetamine is a synthetic drug with more rapid and lasting effects than the amphetamines. It is used illegally as a stimulant and legally as a prescription drug to treat narcolepsy and maintain blood pressure.

Prevalence of Use

Prevalence of methamphetamine use by age range in 2015 is given in Table 7.3. It is estimated that 4.7 million Americans have tried methamphetamine at some point in their lives [9].

Street Names

Street names for methamphetamine include:

Methamphetamine	
Crystal form	Base, crystal, d-meth, fast, glass, ice, meth, speed, whiz, pure, wax, crank, quartz, speed
Liquid form	Leopard's blood, liquid red, ox blood

Table 7.3 Prevalence of use of methamphetamine in 2015 by age range (%) (From [1])

	Ages 12–17	Ages 18–25	Age 26 and older
Lifetime	0.30	3.30	6.40
Past year	0.20	0.90	0.60
Past month	0.10	0.40	0.40

Methamphetamine and other drugs:

Methamphetamine and coffee	Biker coffee
Methamphetamine and cocaine	Croak, shabby
Methamphetamine and MDMA	Hugs and kisses, P and P, party and play
Methamphetamine and crack	Mexican speed balls, twisters, tire
Methamphetamine, heroin, cocaine, flunitrazepam, and alcohol	The five-way

Table 7.4 Time course of methamphetamine effects based on route of use

Route of use	Intensity of effect	Onset	Lasts
Smoking or injection intravenously	Intense	A few seconds	A few minutes
Snorting	Less intense than smoking or injecting	3–5 min	15–30 min
Orally	Less intense than snorting	15–20 min	Lasts longer than snorting

Pharmacology

Methamphetamine is an extremely addictive stimulant drug that is chemically similar to amphetamine. It takes the form of a white, odorless, bitter-tasting crystalline powder.

Methamphetamine in its powder form ("Crystal") is ingested orally, smoked, snorted, or dissolved in water or alcohol and injected. "Glass" or "ice" (pure methamphetamine) is most often smoked in a glass pipe, allowing for quick absorption into the bloodstream without the risks of injecting the drug.

Smoking methamphetamine or injecting the drug delivers it very quickly to the brain where it produces an immediate, intense euphoria. Because the pleasure fades quickly, users often use repeated doses in a "binge and crash" pattern.

Users of methamphetamine are at three times more risk for getting Parkinson's disease than people who do not use the drug.

Most of the methamphetamine abused in the United States is manufactured in "super labs" here or, more often, in Mexico. However, the drug is also easily made in small clandestine laboratories, with relatively inexpensive over-the-counter ingredients, such as pseudoephedrine.

Methamphetamine production also involves a number of other, very hazardous chemicals. Toxicity from these chemicals can remain in the environment around a methamphetamine production lab long after the lab has been shut down, causing a wide range of health problems for people living in the area.

To curb production of methamphetamine, pharmacies and other retail stores are required by law to keep logs of purchases of products containing pseudoephedrine. Individuals may only purchase a limited amount of those products on a single day. Some states have made pseudoephedrine a prescription drug [10–12].

The time course of methamphetamine effects based on route of use is given in Table 7.4.

The most dangerous stage of methamphetamine abuse occurs when an abuser has not slept in several days and is irritable and paranoid. This behavior is referred to as "tweaking," and the user is known as the "tweaker." The tweaker craves for more methamphetamine but finds it difficult to achieve the original high.

"Meth mouth" is severe tooth decay and loss of teeth, as well as tooth fracture, acid erosion, and other oral problems that occur in chronic methamphetamine users [13].

Table 7.5 Short-term and long-term health effects of the amphetamines (Based on [2])

Short-term effects of amphetamines	
Increased body temperature Failure of the cardiovascular system Paranoia Hostility or agitation Irregular heart rate Tachycardia Elevated blood pressure Decreased appetite	Dry mouth or dehydration Dilated pupils Increased activity Increased talkativeness Nausea and vomiting An increase or decrease in sexual activity Twitching Increased feelings of power, greatness, or great competence
Long-term effects of amphetamines	
Toxic psychosis Behavioral disorders Rapid and pounding heartbeat Trouble breathing Mood swings Mental instability Convulsions Coma	Malnutrition due to decreased appetite Loss of coordination Pale skin Rotting teeth (meth mouth) Ulcers Weakness Unusual tiredness after a binge Death

Health Risks

Short-term and long-term health risks of the amphetamines are given in Table 7.5.

Tolerance

Tolerance to the amphetamines develops as neurons become desensitized to the amphetamine effects and neurotransmitters become depleted, resulting in the need to use more amphetamine to get the desired response. Increased tolerance leads to more drug exposure, which increases the risk of dependence.

Tolerance develops rapidly, often after only a few doses. Tolerance to the lethal dose also occurs, so that individuals addicted to amphetamines may only experience moderate effects after using hundreds of times more than the therapeutic dose.

Tolerance does not develop to the ability of the amphetamines to produce psychosis. Because the amphetamines cause anorexia, ketone bodies may be found in the urine. These acidify the urine, causing increased secretion of amphetamines. This contributes to tolerance [6–8].

Dependence

Amphetamine dependence is defined by the American Psychiatric Association's DSM-5 criteria discussed in Chap. 1.

Abstinence Syndrome

Amphetamine abstinence syndrome consists of sleepiness, hunger, irritability, depression, and amphetamine craving. The depression may last for months, often leading to relapse and sometimes to suicide. Protracted depression may respond to antidepressants, which should be prescribed for 2–3 months [8].

Amphetamine Overdose

Symptoms

The diagnosis of amphetamine overdose is made based on the greatly exaggerated CNS and peripheral nervous system signs. An empty prescription bottle or drug screen may be helpful.

Central nervous system manifestations include change in mental status, disorientation, headache, dyskinesias, agitation, formication, and symptoms of stroke. Cardiovascular manifestations include chest pain and palpitations.

Gastrointestinal manifestations include dry mouth, nausea and vomiting, and diarrhea. Skin manifestations include diaphoresis, erythematous painful rashes, needle marks, and infected deep ulcerations [13].

Treatment

Standard procedures to reduce drug absorption (activated charcoal, magnesium citrate) may be instituted.

Patients presenting with psychomotor agitation should be checked for hypoxia, hypoglycemia, and hyperthermia. Hyperthermia is associated with a poor prognosis, and when it occurs it should be managed with aggressive cooling measures, such as ice packs and fanning. Violent activity should be immediately controlled with benzodiazepines. Dopamine antagonists, such as haloperidol (Haldol), are generally contraindicated because they impair heat dissipation, although they can be used for psychosis if necessary.

Benzodiazepines decrease the centrally mediated and peripheral sympathomimetic outflow that contributes to the symptoms of stimulant-associated chest pain. They decrease the myocardial workload by controlling the psychomotor hyperactivity, lowering the systemic arterial blood pressure, and reducing the heart rate. Seizures may require intravenous diazepam (Valium) or lorazepam (Ativan). Nitroglycerin, a standard treatment for myocardial ischemia, decreases myocardial workload by lowering mean arterial pressure and maintaining myocardial perfusion, thereby relieving chest pain.

Patients who demonstrate myocardial ischemia by ECG or serum markers or who have hemodynamic instability should be considered for cardiac catheterization or thrombolysis when cauterization is not available. They should be admitted to a cardiac care unit [13].

Cocaine

Cocaine is derived from the leaves of the *Erythroxylum coca* plant (Fig. 7.1). It is a bitter, crystalline alkaloid obtained from coca leaves and widely used as an illicit drug for its stimulant and euphorigenic properties. Because cocaine blocks nerve transmission and constricts blood vessels, cocaine in the hydrochloride form is useful for topical application in otolaryngology surgery. This is its only medical use. It is a DEA Schedule II drug [14].

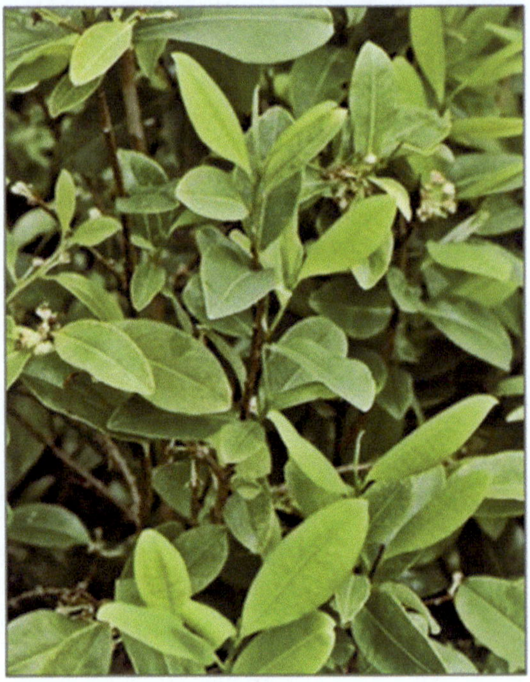

Fig. 7.1 *Erythroxylum coca* plant

Prevalence of Use

Prevalence of use of cocaine HCl and crack use in 2015 by age range is given in Table 7.6.

Table 7.6 Prevalence of use of cocaine HCl and crack use in 2015 by age range (%) (From [1])

		Ages 12–17	Ages 18–25	Ages 26 or older
Cocaine HCl	Lifetime	0.80	11.70	16.60
	Past year	0.60	5.40	1.30
	Past month	0.20	1.70	0.60
Crack	Lifetime	0.10	1.50	4.10
	Past year	0.00	0.30	0.30
	Past month	0.00	0.10	0.20

The Drugs

Cocaine is illicitly used in a variety of forms—coca leaves, coca paste, cocaine HCl, freebase cocaine, and crack or rock cocaine (Fig. 7.2 [15]).

Coca Leaves

The Indians of the Andes toast coca leaves and chew them along with an alkaline substance or mix powdered leaves with alkaline ash from

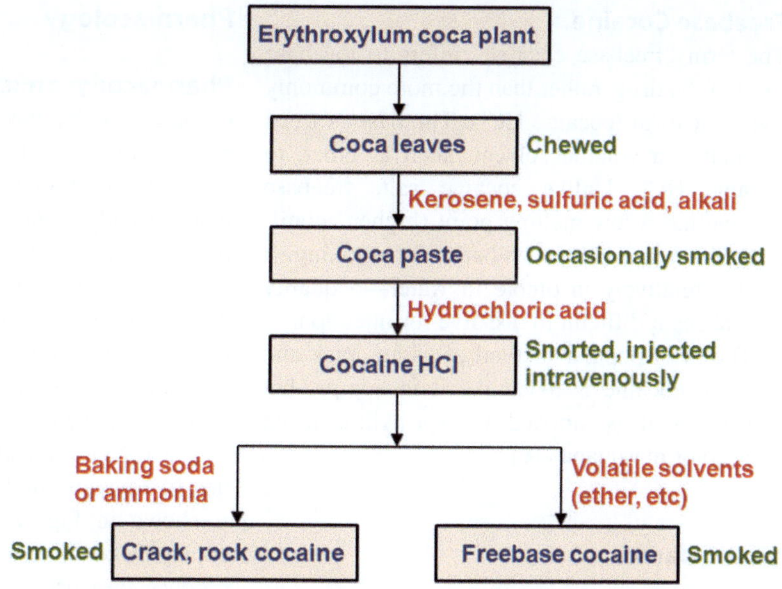

Fig. 7.2 Forms of cocaine (Based on Milhorn [15])

other burned leaves and chew the material. The alkaline substance improves buccal absorption. The practice is limited to the Indians of the Andes Mountains [16].

Coca Paste

Coca paste is made by mixing coca leaves with gasoline, kerosene, or sulfuric acid to extract a crude paste containing 40–80% cocaine. It is smoked in the form of a brown cigarette and can be dangerous because of the impurities it contains. It has not become a popular form of cocaine use in the United States [16].

Cocaine Hydrochloride

Cocaine HCl is the purified form of cocaine. It is extracted from coca paste with hydrochloric acid. It is smuggled into the United States in this pure form, which is then cut with adulterants, such as glucose, inositol, mannitol, lactose, lidocaine, tetracaine, procaine, caffeine, or flour.

This form of cocaine is snorted or injected intravenously. It is not effective when smoked because it does not volatilize sufficiently due to its high melting point. When snorted, cocaine HCl is first placed on a hard, flat surface, such as a mirror and chopped into lines with a razor blade to remove lumps. The lines are inhaled up the nose through a straw or a rolled up bill. When used intravenously, it sometimes is combined with CNS depressant drugs to decrease its irritability effects [16]. The combination of cocaine and heroin is known as a "speedball," and the act of snorting the combination is known as "speed balling."

Rock/Crack Cocaine

Crack is the name given to cocaine HCl that has been processed with baking soda or ammonia and heated to transform it to a more potent, smokable form. Because the end result is small pieces of material that resemble rocks, it is called rock cocaine. Because it makes a crackling sound when smoked, it is also referred to as crack cocaine.

Crack cocaine was first developed during the cocaine boom of the 1970s, and its use became enormously popular in the mid-1980s. It is generally smoked through a glass hand pipe or water pipe. Users report combining crack cocaine with heroin, marijuana, or other types of drugs to create more intense effects. Crack cocaine is highly addicting [16].

Freebase Cocaine

The term "freebase cocaine" refers to the base form of the drug, rather than the more commonly used salt form (cocaine HCl). The base is freed by adding a volatile solvent, such as ether, to cocaine HCl. Unlike cocaine salt, freebase cocaine has a low melting point (higher volatility), which makes it much better for smoking. It is also relatively insoluble in water—a quality that makes it difficult to dissolve for injection.

The most popular method of using crack and freebase cocaine is to smoke it in a pipe, but sometimes it is smoked by sprinkling it on tobacco or marijuana [16].

Street Names

Street names for the various forms of cocaine and for cocaine combined with other drugs include:

Cocaine in general	All-American drug, Aunt Nora, barbs, blow, coke, dream, foo-foo dust, her, king's habit, Peruvian lady, snow, stardust, witch and zip
Crack cocaine	Beam, bopper, candy, CDs, electric kool-aid, girl, mighty white, pop, real tops, rock, seven up, space, twinkie, yam
Powder cocaine	Aspirin, aunt, candy sugar, devil's dandruff, fast white lady, flave, pariba, shake, shrile, soft, sugar boogers, uptown, white dragon, Yao
Inhaled cocaine	Blow blue, blow coke, booster, cork the air, do a line, geeze, hitch up the reindeers, horning, one and one, pop, sniff, snort, toke
Cocaine mixed with marijuana	51, bazooka, blunt, candy sticks, cocktail, dirties, Greek, gremmies, lace, premos, primo turbo, splitting, tio, woolie
Cocaine mixed with heroin	Belushi, boy-girl, crisscrossing, dynamite, flamethrowers, goofball, H & C, he-she, murder one, primos, smoking gun, snowball, speedball, whiz bang
Cocaine mixed with other drugs and chemicals	Beam me up Scottie, bumping up, C & M, candy flipping on a string, cigamos, cotton brothers, croak, draf, five-way, handlebars, pseudocaine, shabu, snow seals

Pharmacology

Pharmacodynamics

Cocaine acts by blocking the reuptake of neurotransmitters, such as dopamine, norepinephrine, and serotonin. By binding to the transporters that normally remove the excess of these neurotransmitters from the synaptic gap, this prevents cocaine from being reabsorbed by the presynaptic neurons that released them and thus increases their concentration in the synapses. As a result, the natural effect of dopamine on the postsynaptic neurons is amplified [4].

The effect of cocaine on dopamine concentration in a synapse in the reward center of the brain is shown in Fig. 7.3. Anything that increases dopamine concentration in the synaptic cleft will produce euphoria, and anything that decreases the concentration will produce dysphoria. The normal situation is depicted in Fig. 7.3a. The nerve signal traveling down the presynaptic neuron causes release of dopamine from the storage vesicles. The dopamine is released into the synaptic cleft, diffuses across the space, and interacts with postsynaptic receptors, which cause the creation of postsynaptic nerve signals equal in magnitude to the presynaptic nerve signals.

As depicted in Fig. 7.3b, acute cocaine use blocks the reuptake of dopamine into the presynaptic storage vesicle, which increases the dopamine concentration in the synaptic cleft. The increased concentration causes an increased stimulation of postsynaptic receptors and a greater than normal postsynaptic nerve signal, resulting in euphoria.

With chronic cocaine use (Fig. 7.3c), the dopamine concentration in the synaptic cleft falls to a lower level because of partially depleted dopamine in the presynaptic storage vessels. However, because of continued cocaine use, the dopamine concentration remains high enough to prevent dysphoria despite the partially depleted storage vesicles.

When the addict can no longer obtain and use cocaine (Fig. 7.3d), the dopamine concentration in the synaptic cleft falls even lower, causing the postsynaptic nerve signal to be less than normal.

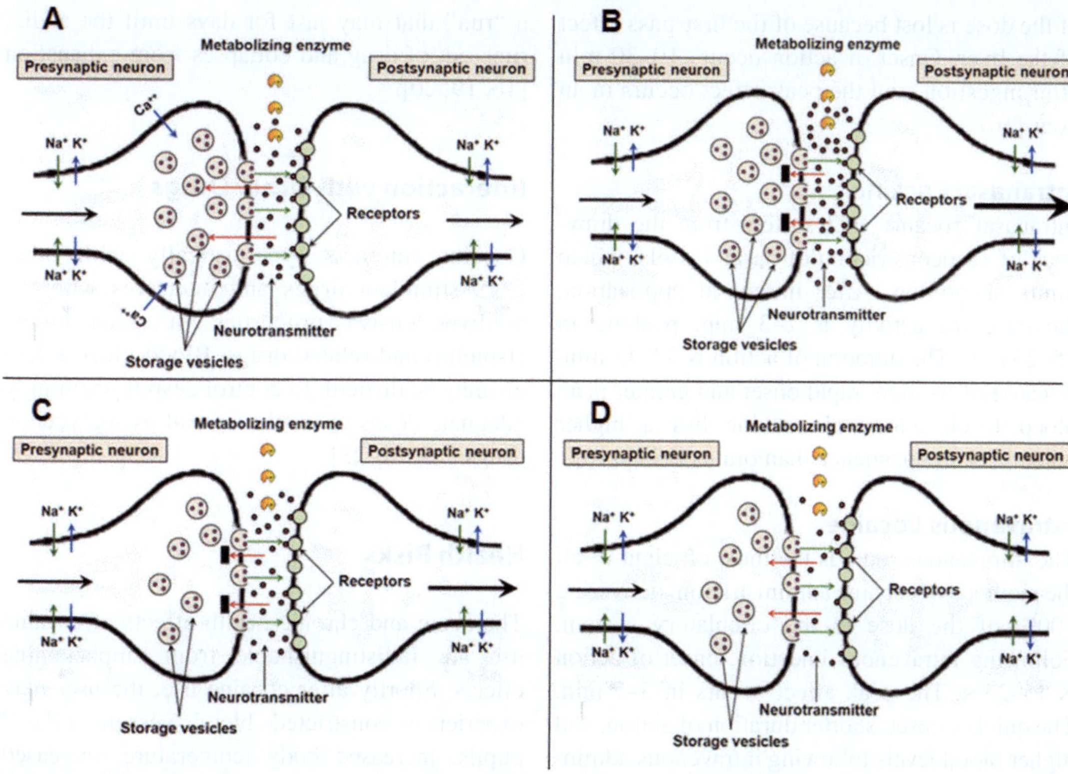

Fig. 7.3 Effect of acute and chronic cocaine use on dopamine concentration in the synaptic cleft. (**a**) Normal situation, (**b**) acute cocaine use, (**c**) chronic cocaine use, and (**d**) the absence of cocaine after prolonged use

The result is constant dysphoria. And what will relieve the discomfort? More cocaine of course [16, 17].

Pharmacokinetics

Cocaine is metabolized by plasma and liver esterases to the metabolites benzoylecgonine and ecgonine methyl ester, which are excreted in the urine.

A potentially dangerous interaction between cocaine and alcohol takes place. Taken in combination, the two drugs are converted by the body to *cocaethylene*, which has a longer duration of action in the brain and is more toxic than either drug alone. The mixture of cocaine and alcohol is the most common two-drug combination that results in drug-related deaths [18].

The rapidity of onset and the duration of action of cocaine depend on both the form of cocaine and its route of administration [15].

Coca Leaf Chewing

Chewing coca leaves is a relatively safe practice because they contain only 0.5–1% cocaine. Although buccal absorption is initially effective, the local vasoconstrictive effect of cocaine greatly slows absorption. As a result, the peak blood level reached is relatively low.

The time of onset with chewing coca leaves is 5–10 min, with a duration of effects of 45–90 min [16].

Coca Paste Smoking

Coca paste smoking causes a rapid and intense high, which is short in duration. Effects begin in 8–10 min. Its peak effect is in 1–5 min. The dependence potential for coca paste is high [15].

Oral Cocaine

Oral intake of cocaine HCl also results in relatively low blood level. Between 80% and 90%

of the dose is lost because of the first-pass effect of the liver. Onset of action occurs 10–30 min after ingestion, and the peak effect occurs in an hour [16].

Intranasal Cocaine

Intranasal cocaine HCl suffers from the drawback of vasoconstriction of nasal vessels, which limits absorption. After intranasal application, the onset of activity is 2–3 min, peaking in 15–20 min. The duration of action is 30–45 min. Because of its more rapid onset and greater peak blood level, intranasal cocaine has a higher potential for dependence than oral cocaine [16].

Intravenous Cocaine

The intravenous route is the most efficient of all the methods of cocaine administration, delivering 100% of the dose to the circulatory system. Following intravenous injection, onset of action is 15–25 s. The peak effect occurs in 3–5 min. The quicker onset, shorter duration of action, and higher blood levels following intravenous administration make this mode of administration more addictive than the intranasal route [16].

Crack/Freebase Cocaine

Crack is not pharmacologically different from freebase cocaine. Both are smoked. The effect occurs rapidly and intensely because of four factors: (1) crack/freebase cocaine has a lower temperature of volatilization than the HCl form, and as a result a larger percentage of it enters the lungs; (2) the large surface area of the pulmonary membrane allows rapid access of crack/freebase cocaine to the bloodstream; (3) the shorter distance to the brain the crack/freebase cocaine has to traverse when compared to the longer distance for intravenous injection contributes to the rapidity of response; and (4) crack/freebase cocaine is much more lipid soluble than the HCl form, allowing quick passage into the central nervous system.

The duration of action of crack/freebase cocaine is 5–10 min, with the peak effect occurring in 1–5 min. Administration of the drug must be repeated about every 20 min to maintain the euphoria and avoid the crash. This often leads to a "run" that may last for days until the addict runs out of drug and collapses from exhaustion [16, 19, 20].

Interaction with Other Drugs

Cocaine interacts synergistically with other CNS stimulant drugs and interferes with the antihypertensive properties of guanethidine (Ismelin) and related drugs. Blood glucose levels may be difficult to control despite seemingly adequate doses of insulin or oral hypoglycemic drugs [15, 21–23].

Health Risks

The acute and chronic health effects of cocaine use are indistinguishable from amphetamine effects. Shortly after cocaine use, the user may experience constricted blood vessels, dilated pupils, increased body temperature, increased heart rate, and higher blood pressure (short-term effects).

During the euphoric period after cocaine use, which can last up to 30 min, the user may experience hyperstimulation, reduced fatigue, and mental alertness. However, some users may have unpleasant experiences such as restlessness, irritability, and anxiety.

During a cocaine binge, when cocaine is used repeatedly, the user may experience increasing restlessness, irritability, and paranoia. For some users, binging on cocaine can lead to a period of paranoid psychosis, auditory hallucinations, and a disconnection with reality.

Repeated cocaine use, rather than occasional recreational use, can cause irregular heartbeat, heart attack, chest pain, respiratory failure, headaches, stroke, and seizures. It also may cause abdominal pain, nausea, and malnourishment due to the drug's ability to decrease appetite.

Snorting or injecting cocaine can produce specific health effects. Snorting cocaine can cause chronically runny nose, nosebleeds, loss of smell, hoarseness, and swallowing problems. Nasal septum perforation may occur. Injecting cocaine can cause allergic reactions and increased risk for contracting HIV, hepatitis, and other blood-borne diseases [24–27].

Tolerance

Tolerance develops from continuous cocaine use much as it does with amphetamines but probably more quickly. Tolerance does not appear to develop to the ability to produce psychosis [15, 24].

Dependence

Cocaine dependence is defined by the American Psychiatric Association's DSM-5 criteria discussed in Chap. 1. Its ability to produce dependence depends on the form of the drug used and the route of administration. Chewing coca leaves and ingesting cocaine produces mild stimulation and thus has little risk of dependence. Snorting cocaine HCl has a much higher risk of dependence: however, because it constricts blood vessels in the nose, absorption is limited. Intravenous cocaine and inhalation of crack cocaine have the highest risk for dependence [15, 28].

Abstinence Syndrome

The cocaine abstinence syndrome consists of negativism, pessimism, lack of patience, irritability, sleepiness, hunger, fatigue, depression, and intense craving. The depression is described as *anhedonia*, which is defined as the inability to experience pleasure from activities usually found enjoyable (exercise, hobbies, music, sexual activities, social interactions) [14, 25, 29].

Overdose

Overdose symptoms and treatment are similar to those of the amphetamines [30, 31].

Methylphenidate

Methylphenidate (Ritalin) is used to treat attention-deficit disorder (ADD), attention-deficit hyperactivity disorder (ADHD), and narcolepsy. Other trade names are Ritalin SR, Ritalin LA, Metadate ER, Metadate CD, Methylin ER, and Concerta. In the past, methylphenidate was used off label as an adjunct to antidepressants for difficult-to-control depression. It is a Schedule II drug.

Methylphenidate is a mild central nervous system stimulant. In the United States, for abuse, it typically is diverted from legitimate sources. In some cases abusers obtain the drug from peers, friends, or family members. Often individuals who have legitimate prescriptions will sell or give away their supply. Methylphenidate also is acquired through theft from individuals with legitimate prescriptions or from school medicine dispensaries.

Most individuals who abuse methylphenidate either swallow the tablets or crush them to produce a powder, which is snorted. Some abusers dissolve the tablets in water and then inject the mixture.

Abuse of methylphenidate typically is associated with preadolescents, teenagers, and young adults. Although less common, methylphenidate is abused by older adults as well. The increased use of the drug to treat attention-deficit hyperactivity disorder (ADHD) has resulted in a corresponding increase in abuse. Abusers who inject the drug are at risk because insoluble fillers in methylphenidate tablets can block small blood vessels, leading to gangrene.

"Pharming" is the term used by abusers of the drug who mix methylphenidate with other controlled substances or alcohol. Users try these combinations in an effort to sustain the high for longer periods of time [32, 33].

Street Names

Street names for methylphenidate and methylphenidate plus pentazocine include [33]:

Methyl-phenidate	Jif Kiddy-cocaine Pineapple R-ball Rids Uppers Vitamin R	Diet coke Kibbles and bits Kiddy coke Skippy Smart drug Smarties West coast	Coke junior Poor man's cocaine R pop Skittles Study buddies
Methylphenidate plus pentazocine	Crackers One and ones	Ritz and Ts Set	Ts and ritz Ts and Rs

Pharmacology

Pharmacodynamics

Methylphenidate primarily acts as a norepinephrine-dopamine reuptake inhibitor. It shares part of its basic structure with catecholamines. It is most active at modulating levels of dopamine and, to a lesser extent, norepinephrine. Methylphenidate binds to and blocks dopamine and norepinephrine transporters.

Pharmacokinetics

Methylphenidate taken orally has a duration of action of 2–4 h for the instant-release form (Ritalin), 3–8 h for sustained release (Ritalin SR), and 8–12 h for extended release (Concerta). When taken orally, methylphenidate slowly raises dopamine levels over the course of an hour or so. By contrast, when inhaled or injected, Ritalin reaches the brain in seconds, producing a high.

Methylphenidate is completely metabolized in the liver to inactive products that are excreted in the urine. The main urinary metabolite is ritalinic acid. Taking methylphenidate with a meal speeds absorption [32, 33].

Health Risks

Some of the most common health risks associated with methylphenidate include insomnia, anorexia, nausea, dizziness, headache, and growth retardation. Elevated blood pressure and heart rate can occur, although the magnitudes of these are usually small. For people who already have hypertension, methylphenidate increases the risk for congestive heart failure and arrhythmias. In addition, taking an overdose of methylphenidate can cause hyperactivity, confusion, and seizures. Other effects are the same as for the amphetamines and cocaine [34].

Tolerance, Dependence, and Abstinence Syndrome

Children and adults prescribed methylphenidate to treat ADHD or narcolepsy do not appear to develop tolerance to its therapeutic effects, but abusers develop tolerance to the euphoric effects they seek from the drug.

Chronic heavy use can lead to physical dependence. Withdrawal symptoms include exhaustion and severe emotional depression. Methylphenidate abusers may experience cravings for the drug and feelings of panic if the drug becomes temporarily unavailable [32].

Phentermine

Phentermine is a stimulant similar to amphetamine. It acts as an appetite suppressant by affecting the central nervous system. It is indicated as a short-term adjunct in a regimen of weight reduction based on exercise, behavioral modification, and caloric restriction in the management of obesity. It is not meant to be used for more than a few weeks. It is bound to a resin to make it last longer and to help prevent abuse.

Phentermine is for those with an initial body mass index ≥ 30 kg/m^2 or ≥ 27 kg/m^2 in the presence of other risk factors. Phentermine is a DEA Schedule IV drug [35].

Health Risks

Common phentermine side effects may include feeling restless or hyperactive, headache, dizziness, tremors, insomnia, dry mouth or an unpleasant taste, diarrhea or constipation, upset stomach, increased or decreased interest in sex, and impotence [35].

Tolerance, Dependence, and Abstinence Syndrome

Tolerance is said to develop to phentermine, but the occurrence of dependence and abstinence syndrome is uncertain. There have been reports of phentermine abuse for its stimulant properties [35].

Modafinil

Modafinil (Provigil) is used to improve wakefulness in patients with excessive sleepiness associated with narcolepsy or other sleep disorders. It is often prescribed "off label" for ailments like severe jet lag and ADHD. It blocks norepinephrine and dopamine transporters and increases dopamine in the nucleus accumbens, actions that suggest the potential for dependence. Although it is supposed to be a nonaddictive stimulant because it doesn't cause a high, it does have the potential for producing euphoria [36].

Bath Salts

In addition to methylenedioxypyrovalerone (MDPV), bath salts sometimes consist of other synthetic stimulants, such as mephedrone or methylone. These chemicals refer to a family of designer recreational drugs that are related to cathinone, a stimulant found in the khat plant. Effects are similar to those of amphetamine.

Khat is a shrub grown in East Africa and southern Arabia. People in these countries sometimes chew its leaves for their mild stimulant effects. Synthetic variants of cathinone are much more potent than the natural product.

The names given to this drug are intentionally misleading, and the warning that these products are "not for human consumption" is an effort by the manufacturers to sidestep drug laws.

Bath salts are marketed as cheap substitutes for other stimulants, such as methamphetamine, cocaine, and MDMA (ecstasy).

Synthetic cathinones usually take the form of a white or brown crystal-like powder and are sold in small plastic or foil packages. In addition to the name bath salts, it is sold as jewelry cleaner, plant food, and phone screen cleaner.

Brand names for bath salt drugs include:

Blue silk	Wave	Ocean	White
Cloud	Meow	burst	lightning
nine	meow	Stardust	White knight
Drone	Pure ivory	Vanilla sky	
Ivory	Red dove		

The drug can be purchased on the street, online, and in drug paraphernalia shops. It can be injected, snorted, or taken as tablets. The speed of onset is 15 min, while the length of the high from these drugs is 4–6 h. These synthetic stimulants are designated as DEA Schedule I substances under the Controlled Substances Act [37].

Health Risks

Short-term and long-term health risks of bath salts are very similar to those of amphetamines and cocaine. Excited delirium, resulting in extreme agitation and violent behavior, can occur. This may lead to dehydration, breakdown of skeletal muscle tissue, and kidney failure. Deaths have occurred [37].

Tolerance, Dependence, and Abstinence Syndrome

Tolerance almost certainly develops to synthetic cathinones. They can be addictive. Human users have reported that cessation of the drugs can trigger intense cravings. Withdrawal symptoms can occur and consist of anxiety, depression, insomnia, tremors, and paranoia [37].

Flakka

Alpha-pyrrolidinovalerophenone (alpha-PVP) has the popular name *flakka*. It is a synthetic drug similar to bath salts. It is also known by the name *gravel* because of the way it looks. It is a mix of one or more chemicals that mimic the effects of an amphetamine-like stimulant.

Flakka is typically white or pink in color and is found in crystal form. The drug may be smoked, eaten, snorted, injected, or vaporized in e-cigarettes.

The duration of the effects of the drug can last as few as 3–4 h but can also linger for several days.

Flakka, like other psychostimulants, can cause a condition known as excited delirium that involves hyperstimulation, paranoia, and hallucinations. During this state, body temperature can rapidly elevate to as high as 105–106°F. This can trigger a cascade of events, which can lead to kidney damage and failure as a result of rhabdomyolysis.

Flakka cases are significantly increasing from no reported cases in 2010 to 85 cases in 2012 and greater than 670 in 2014. The drug has been linked to deaths by suicide as well as heart attacks. It also can dangerously raise body temperature and lead to kidney damage or kidney failure. In 2014, the DEA listed it as DEA Schedule I [38].

Intoxication and Overdose

Intoxication and stimulant effects of flakka are similar to those of other CNS stimulants [38].

Caffeine

Caffeine is the most commonly used mood-altering drug in the world. It is found in many plants, including coffee, tea, kola nut, and cocoa pod. Coffee is the leading dietary source of caffeine among adults in the United States, while soft drinks represent the largest source of caffeine for children.

Many over-the-counter medications contain caffeine. In recommended doses, Excedrin Extra Strength tablets (2) have 130 mg, Anacin Maximum Strength tablets (2) have 64 mg, and a Midol Maximum Strength tablet has 60 mg. One NoDoz tablet has 200 mg of caffeine [39].

In the United States, the average per capita daily intake among adult caffeine consumers is 280 mg (the equivalent of 17 oz of brewed coffee or 84 oz of soft drink) [40].

Typical amounts of caffeine found in food and drink products include tea (50 mg), coffee (90 mg), cola (40 mg), and ginger ale and sprite (0 mg). Hershey's dark chocolate (1.8 oz) has 31 mg of caffeine, and Hershey's milk chocolate (1.55 oz) has 9 mg [40].

In caffeine nonusers or intermittent users, low dietary doses of caffeine (20–200 mg) generally produce positive mood effects, such as increased well-being, happiness, increased energy, alertness, and sociability [39].

Caffeine Powder

Bulk bags or bottles of pure caffeine powder are readily available online. These products may be attractive to young people looking for added caffeine stimulation or for help in losing weight.

These products are essentially 100% caffeine. A single teaspoon of pure caffeine is roughly equivalent to the amount in 28 cups of coffee.

Severe caffeine overdose can cause fast and erratic heartbeat, seizures, vomiting, diarrhea, and disorientation.

It is difficult to measure accurately pure powdered caffeine with common kitchen measuring tools, which makes it easier to consume a lethal amount.

The FDA is aware of at least two deaths of young men who used caffeine powder. The FDA advises consumers to avoid pure powdered caffeine [40].

Caffeine Intoxication

Caffeine intoxication usually requires at least 250 mg of caffeine—equivalent to what is found in two-and-a-half cups of coffee.

Symptoms of caffeine intoxication given in DSM-5 include restlessness, nervousness, excitement, insomnia, flushed face, dieresis, gastrointestinal disturbance, muscle twitching, rambling flow of thought and speech, tachycardia or cardiac arrhythmia, periods of inexhaustibility, and psychomotor agitation. Individuals with panic and anxiety disorders are especially sensitive to the effects of caffeine [41].

Caffeine Tolerance and Dependence

Regular use of high doses of caffeine (750–1200 mg/day) produces complete tolerance to some but not all of the effects of caffeine. Caffeine tolerance can be seen within a week of steady use. During that short period, the receptors that caffeine interacts with change in number and function so that the effects of small caffeine doses are no longer felt. The rush and nervous energy seen with the first few uses of the drug goes away with continued use.

Regular use of as little as two to three cups of coffee per day can trigger a withdrawal effect marked by tiredness or sleepiness. Despite this, caffeine dependence is not included in DSM-5. This is because it does not meet the American Psychiatric Association's criteria for dependence [42].

Caffeine Abstinence Syndrome

Caffeine abstinence syndrome from DSM-5 consists of headache; marked fatigue or drowsiness; dysphoric mood, depressed mood, or irritability; difficulty in concentrating; and flu-like symptoms (nausea, vomiting, or muscle pain/stiffness).

Withdrawal symptoms have an onset of 12–24 h after terminating caffeine intake, peak in 20–48 h, and have a duration of 2–7 days [43].

Caffeine Overdose

Symptoms

Caffeine overdose most commonly occurs when caffeine amounts greater than 500 mg are consumed. Caffeine can be lethal at very high doses, that is, 3–20 g.

Symptoms of caffeine overdose can include breathing trouble, changes in alertness, confusion, convulsions, diarrhea, dizziness, fever, and hallucinations. Increased thirst, increased urination, irregular heartbeat, muscle twitching, tachycardia, insomnia, and vomiting can also occur. Complete cardiovascular collapse has occurred, and a number of deaths have occurred from caffeine overdose [44].

Treatment

Mild caffeine overdose does not usually require special treatment. A serious overdose, however, may require hospitalization and initial treatment with activated charcoal.

Benzodiazepines (lorazepam, diazepam) may be required to treat severe anxiety, as well as seizures. Additional medications may be needed to control the heart rate or treat an abnormal heart rhythm (beta-blockers, calcium channel blockers). In the hemodynamically stable patient, amiodarone can be used to treat ventricular tachycardia (VT). If the patient is hemodynamically unstable, electrical cardioversion is indicated.

Those who do not respond to initial treatment may require medication to support the blood pressure (dopamine, phenylephrine) if hypotension is refractory to intravenous fluid boluses. In severe cases, dialysis may be required to remove the caffeine from the bloodstream [44].

Summary

Central nervous system stimulants include the amphetamines, cocaine, methylphenidate, phentermine, modafinil, bath salts, flakka, and caffeine.

Amphetamines are drugs that have a stimulant effect on the central nervous system (CNS) that can be both physically and psychologically addictive. They include methamphetamine. The most dangerous stage of methamphetamine abuse occurs when an abuser has not slept in several days and is irritable and paranoid.

Cocaine is a bitter, crystalline alkaloid obtained from coca leaves and widely used as an illicit drug for its stimulant and euphorigenic properties. Because cocaine blocks nerve transmission and constricts blood vessels, cocaine in the hydrochloride form is useful for topical application in otolaryngology surgery.

Methylphenidate is used to treat attention-deficit disorder (ADD), attention-deficit hyperactivity disorder (ADHD), and narcolepsy. Abuse of methylphenidate typically is associated with preadolescents, teenagers, and young adults. Phentermine is a stimulant similar to amphetamine. It acts as an appetite suppressant by affecting the central nervous system. It also is sometimes abused. Modafinil (Provigil) is used to improve wakefulness in patients with excessive sleepiness associated with narcolepsy or other sleep disorders. It has the potential to produce euphoria.

The chemicals in bath salts belong to a family of designer recreational drugs that are related to cathinone, a stimulant found in the khat plant. Bulk bags or bottles of pure caffeine powder are readily available online. These products are attractive to young people looking for added caffeine stimulation or for help in losing weight. Caffeine dependence is not included in DSM-5. This is because it does not meet the American Psychiatric Association's criteria for dependence.

References

1. National survey on drug use and health: trends in prevalence of various drugs for ages 12 or older, ages 12 to 17, ages 18 to 25, and ages 26 or older. National Institute on Drug Abuse (NIDA). https://www.drugabuse.gov/national-survey-drug-use-health. 2015.
2. Amphetamines. Center for Substance Abuse Research (CESAR)/University of Maryland. http://www.cesar.umd.edu/cesar/drugs/amphetamines.asp
3. Various stimulant drugs show continuing gradual declines among teens in 2008, most illicit drugs hold steady. Michigan News/University of Michigan. http://ns.umich.edu/new/releases/6882-various-stimulant-drugs-show-continuing-gradual-declines-among-teens-in-2008-most-illicit-drugs-hold-steady. December 15, 2008.
4. Dubuc B. The brain from top to bottom. McGill University. http://thebrain.mcgill.ca/flash/i/i_03/i_03_m/i_03_m_par/i_03_m_par_heroine.html#drogues. May 2012.
5. Christian L. Drugs of abuse. In: Katzung BG, Trevor AJ, editors. Basic and clinical pharmacology. 13th ed. New York: McGraw-Hill Education; 2014. p. 552–6.
6. O'Brien RC. The encyclopedia of drug abuse. Facts on File: New York; 1984.
7. Wilford BB, editor. Major drugs of abuse. In: Drug abuse: a guide for the primary care physician. Chicago: American Medical Association; 1981. p. 21–84.
8. Shlafer M, Marieb EN. Substance use and misuse. In: The nurse, pharmacology and drug therapy. Redwood City: Addison-Wesley; 1989. p. 509–28.
9. Anglin MD, Perrochet B, Burke C, Stamper E, Dawud-Noursi S. History of the methamphetamine problem. J Psychoact Drugs. 2011:137–41.
10. Methamphetamine. Center for Substance Abuse Research (CESAR)/University of Maryland. http://www.cesar.umd.edu/cesar/drugs/meth.asp
11. Methamphetamine. National Institute on Drug Abuse (NIDA). https://www.drugabuse.gov/drugs-abuse/methamphetamine. February 2017.
12. Winslow BT, Voorhees KI, Pehl KA. Methamphetamine abuse. Am Fam Physician. 2007;76(8):1169–74.
13. Handly N. Amphetamine toxicity. Medscape. December 16, 2016.
14. Tennant FS. Cocaine withdrawal step by step. Emergency Medicine. 1987;65–68.
15. Milhorn HT. Chemical dependence: diagnosis, treatment, and prevention. New York: Springer; 1990.
16. Vereby K, Gold MS. From coca leaves to crack: the effects of dose and routes of administration on abuse liability. Psychiatr Ann. 1988;18:513–20.
17. Wyatt RJ, Karourn F, Suddath R, Hitri A. The role of dopamine in cocaine use and abuse. Psychiatr Ann. 1988;18:531–4.
18. Golan DE, Tashjian AH, Armstrong EJ, Armstrong AW, editors. Principles of pharmacology: the pathophysiological basis of drug therapy. 3rd ed. Philadelphia: Lippincott Williams & Wilkins, Wolters Kluwer; 2011.
19. Gold M. Crack abuse: its implications and outcomes. Resid Staff Physician. 1987;33:45–53.
20. Bouknight LG. Cocaine – a particularly addicting drug. Postgrad Med. 1988;83:115–31.

21. Gottheil E, Weinstein SP. Cocaine risks: a review. Fam Pract Recertification. 1983;5:78–90.
22. Garvin FH. Chronic neuropharmacology of cocaine: progress in pharmacotherapy. J Clin Psychiatry. 1988;49:11–6.
23. Dackis CA, Gold MS. Psychopharmacology of cocaine. Psychiatr Ann. 1988;18:528–30.
24. The health effects of cocaine use and abuse: short-term and long-term effects. VeryWell. https://www.verywell.com/the-health-effects-of-cocaine-abuse-66706. November 16, 2016.
25. DrugFacts: cocaine. National Institute on Drug Abuse (NIDA). https://www.drugabuse.gov/publications/drugfacts/cocaine. June 2016.
26. Cregler LL, Mark H. Medical complications of cocaine abuse. N Engl J Med. 1986;345:1495–500.
27. Miller GW. The cocaine habit. Am Fam Physician. 1985;31:173–6.
28. Bouknight LG. Cocaine – a particularly addicting drug. Postgrad Med. 1988;83:115–31.
29. Brower KJ, Paredes A. Cocaine withdrawal. Arch Gen Psychiatry. 1987;44(3):297–8.
30. Dittmar PK, Olmedo R. An evidence-based approach to cocaine-associated emergencies. Emerg Med. 2008;10(1):1–20.
31. Dwyer BJ, editor. Cocaine: helping patients avoid the end of the line. Emerg Med Rep. 1985;6:17–26.
32. Ritalin. Center for Substance Abuse Research (CESAR). University of Maryland. http://www.cesar.umd.edu/cesar/drugs/ritalin.asp. 2013.
33. Ritalin Fast Facts. National Drug Intelligence Center (NDIC). http://www.justice.gov/archive/ndic/pubs6/6444. September 2003.
34. Methylphenidate. MedlinePlus. https://medlineplus.gov/druginfo/meds/a682188.html. February 15, 2016.
35. Phentermine. Drugs.com. http://www.drugs.com/pro/phentermine.html. 2015.
36. Biaggioni I, Roberson D. Adrenoceptor agonists and sympathomimetic drugs. In: Bertram GK, Trevor AJ, editors. Basic and clinical pharmacology. 13th ed. New York: McGraw-Hill; 2015.
37. The effects of bath salts use. Drug Abuse. http://drugabuse.com/library/the-effects-of-bath-salts-use
38. Glatter R. Flakka: the new designer drug you need to know about. Forbes. http://www.forbes.com/sites/robertglatter/2015/04/04/flakka-the-new-drug-you-need-to-know-about/#209ed1ba20bf. April 4, 2015.
39. Caffeine content for coffee, tea, soda and more. Mayo Clinic. http://www.mayoclinic.org/healthy-lifestyle/nutrition-and-healthy-eating/in-depth/caffeine/art-20049372. May 13, 2014.
40. Kotz D. FDA warns against dangers of caffeine powder. Boston Globe. July 23, 2014.
41. Gilbert SG. Caffeine. Toxipedia. http://www.toxipedia.org/display/toxipedia/Caffeine. June 13, 2012.
42. DSM-5. Diagnostic and statistical manual of mental disorder. In: American Psychiatric Association. 5th ed. Arlington: American Psychiatric Publishing; 2013.
43. Caffeine: how much is too much? Mayo Clinic. http://www.mayoclinic.org/healthy-lifestyle/nutrition-and-healthy-eating/in-depth/caffeine/art-20045678. April 14, 2014.
44. Schueler SJ, Beckett JH, Gettings DS. Caffeine overdose. Treatment. FreeMD. http://www.freemd.com/caffeine-overdose/treatment.htm. May 23, 2011.

8 Nicotine Dependence

Key Chapter Points

- In 1964, the Surgeon General of the United States published a report about the dangers of cigarette smoking.
- Cigarette smoking kills more than 480,000 Americans each year, with an estimated 49,000 of these deaths from exposure to secondhand smoke.
- The smoke itself consists of mainstream smoke, which smokers inhale directly from cigarettes, and sidestream smoke, which enters the atmosphere from the lit ends of cigarettes.
- Smoking causes about 90% of all lung cancer deaths in men and women. About 80% of all deaths from chronic obstructive pulmonary disease (COPD) are caused by smoking.
- The use of e-cigarettes could lead to a 21% drop in deaths from smoking-related diseases when cigarette smokers are switched to them.
- In 1986, the US Surgeon General declared that the use of smokeless tobacco is not a safe substitute for smoking cigarettes.
- Patients can follow five steps to conduct a brief smoking intervention.
- To overcome dependence on tobacco, patients need to become aware of their triggers, so they can develop plans to deal with them.
- Nicotine dependence medications include nicotine replacement therapy, bupropion (Zyban), and varenicline (Chantix).
- Because it occurs so often in those attempting to quit smoking, relapse must be considered part of a program to stop smoking.
- Nicotine is a potentially lethal poison at high exposure levels.

Tobacco is the dried prepared leaves of *Nicotiana tabacum*, an annual plant widely cultivated in the United States (Fig. 8.1). It is the source of various alkaloids, the principal one being nicotine. Nicotine is a psychoactive agent whose continued use usually leads to dependence.

Tobacco can be smoked in cigarettes, pipes, or cigars, chewed as chewing tobacco, placed between the lower lip and the gum, or sniffed through the nose as snuff. Nicotine also can be inhaled from vaporized liquid nicotine in e-cigarettes.

In 1964, the Surgeon General of the United States published a report about the dangers of cigarette smoking. The report said that the nicotine and tar in cigarettes cause lung cancer [1]. In 1965, the Congress of the United States passed the Federal Cigarette Labeling and Advertising Act. The bill said that every cigarette pack must have a warning label on its side stating, "Cigarettes may be hazardous to your health." This law later was expanded to require that the specific dangers of smoking be labeled on each cigarette pack.

The Congress passed a law in 1971 that made it illegal for tobacco companies to advertise cigarettes on television or radio [2].

H.T. Milhorn, *Substance Use Disorders*, DOI 10.1007/978-3-319-63040-3_8

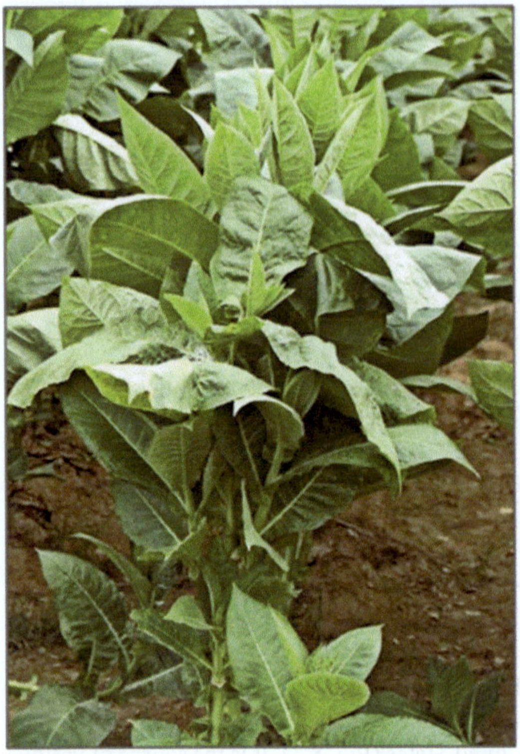

Fig. 8.1 Tobacco plant

Table 8.1 Prevalence of use of cigarette smoking in 2015 for various age ranges (%) (From [3])

	Ages 12–17	Ages 18–25	Ages 26 or older
Lifetime	14.20	56.10	67.50
Past year	8.90	37.70	24.60
Past month	4.90	28.40	21.50

Cigarettes

Nicotine is one of the more than 4000 chemicals in cigarettes and their smoke. Cigarette smoking kills more than 480,000 Americans each year, with an estimated 49,000 of these deaths from exposure to secondhand smoke. Table 8.1 [3] gives the prevalence of use of cigarette smoking in 2015 for various age ranges.

Table 8.2 Trends in cigarette smoking 1965–2014 (From [4])

	Adults	Males	Females
1965	42.4	52.0	34.0
1988	26.5	29.5	23.8
2014	16.8	18.8	14.8

Table 8.3 Percentage of smokers in 2015 by group (Based on [5])

Group	Percentage
Age range	
Aged 25–44	20.0
≥ 65 years old	8.5
Education	
GED certificate	43.0
Undergraduate college degree	7.9
Economic status	
Below the poverty level	26.3
Above the poverty level	15.2
Sexual orientation	
Lesbian/gay/bisexual adults	23.9
Straight adults	16.6

Trends in Cigarette Smoking

Over the last 40 years or so, there has been a rather dramatic decline in cigarette smoking, from 42.4% in 1965, to 26.5% in 1988, and to 18.8% in 2014 (Table 8.2 [4]). The decline has occurred with both males and females.

Percentage of Smokers by Group

In addition to sex, the percentage of adults who smoke cigarettes varies by age range, education, economic status, and sexual orientation (Table 8.3 [5]).

Despite the fact that cigarette smoking is the largest single preventable causes of death and disability in the United States, many patients report that they have not been counseled by their primary care physician to quit. This failure is, in part, due to the fact that physicians need to be trained in helping patients quit smoking [6].

Pharmacology

Pharmacodynamics

Nicotine imitates the action of the neurotransmitter acetylcholine by binding to nicotinic receptors. Tobacco dependence arises because nicotinic receptors are present on the neurons of the ventral tegmental area that project their terminations into the nucleus accumbens. In smokers, repeated nicotine stimulation increases the amount of dopamine released in the nucleus accumbens. Between cigarettes, chronic smokers maintain a high enough concentration of nicotine to deactivate the receptors and slow down their recovery. This is why smokers develop a tolerance to nicotine and experience reduced pleasure from it.

In the absence of nicotine, after a period of smoking, all the nicotine receptors become functional again, and cholinergic neurotransmission in the brain is increased to an abnormally high level that affects all the cholinergic pathways in the brain. Smokers then experience the agitation and discomfort that leads them to smoke another cigarette.

Another substance in tobacco smoke inhibits monoamine oxydase B, an enzyme that breaks down dopamine after its reuptake. The result is a higher concentration of dopamine in the reward circuit, which also contributes to the smoker's dependence [7].

Pharmacokinetics

The substances in cigarette smoke can be divided into cigarette constituents (organic matter, nicotine alkaloids, additives) and pyrolysis products (CO_2, CO, tar). Carcinogens are found primarily in particulate smoke.

The smoke itself consists of *mainstream smoke*, which smokers inhale directly from cigarettes, and *sidestream smoke*, which enters the atmosphere from the lit ends of cigarettes. Smokers inhale both mainstream and sidestream smoke, and others, including nonsmokers, in the vicinity inhale sidestream smoke. Sidestream smoke also includes the smoke smokers exhale.

Of environmental tobacco smoke, 80% is sidestream smoke. It contains greater concentrations of various toxic and carcinogenic compounds than does mainstream smoke because it is unfiltered. Aldehydes, phenol, ammonia, and sulfur dioxide are surface irritants in cigarette smoke that cause some of its uncomfortable effects, such as eye and nasal mucosa irritation [8].

As smokers inhale, they pull air into cigarettes through the porous paper, diluting and cooling mainstream smoke. Filters trap some of the particulate matter. The amount of nicotine absorbed into the lungs depends on how much is inhaled, how deeply it is inhaled and for how long, and the pH of the smoke.

The average cigarette contains about 10 mg of nicotine. A variable amount, probably between 1 and 2 mg, is actually delivered to the lungs when the cigarette is smoked. A puff of smoke results in a measurable nicotine level in the brain in seconds.

With regular use, nicotine accumulates in the body during the day and persists overnight at a falling concentration. Thus, smokers are exposed to the effects of nicotine 24 h a day [9].

Nicotine is metabolized primarily in the liver. The major metabolites are cotinine and nicotine-1-N-oxide. These are rapidly eliminated by the kidneys. The half-life of nicotine after inhalation is 30–60 min. Cotinine, the major metabolite, has a half-life between 19 and 40 h [8, 10].

Through its direct effects on the medulla, nicotine causes a decrease in the strength of stomach contractions and nausea and vomiting. In the respiratory system, it causes local irritation and a decrease in ciliary motion.

Nicotine causes decreased strength of stomach contractions, decreased muscle tone, and weight loss. Acute cardiovascular effects include increased blood pressure, cutaneous vasoconstriction, increased heart rate, increased strength of heart contractions, and increased platelet adherence.

In the endocrine system, it causes release of epinephrine and norepinephrine from the adrenal glands and adrenergic axons. It also causes reductions in growth hormone (resulting in slightly decreased growth rate), cortisol, and antidiuretic hormone.

Nicotine has a direct effect on the brain, causing a generalized stimulating EEG pattern with low-voltage fast waves predominating.

In addition to its physical effects, nicotine exerts a strong behavioral influence. It may enhance an individual's level of alertness and speech [11].

Interactions with Other Drugs

Nicotine can alter the activity of many drugs, usually by induction of liver microsomal enzymes. Enzyme activity may remain elevated up to 6 months after patients stop smoking. Smokers may have reduced blood levels of theophylline, pentazocine, propranolol, phenothiazines, benzodiazepines, insulin, and some antidepressants. The rate of metabolism of warfarin may be increased. Smokers, especially heavy smokers, may need to have the dosages of their medications increased. In addition, smoking increases the potential for serious adverse effects of women taking birth control pills [9].

Factors That Influence Who Will Smoke Cigarettes

A number of factors contribute to whom will smoke cigarettes [12]. These include:

Genetics. The likelihood that an individual will start smoking and keep smoking may be partly inherited.

Home and peer influence. Children who grow up with parents who smoke are more likely to become smokers.

Mental illness. People who have depression, schizophrenia, posttraumatic stress disorder, or other forms of mental illness are more likely to be smokers and to have higher levels of smoking.

Substance use. People who abuse alcohol and illegal drugs are more likely to be smokers.

Age. Most people begin smoking during childhood or the teen years.

Health Risks

Health risks of smoking can be divided into those from active smoking and those from passive smoking (Table 8.4 [13]).

Smoking causes about 90% of all lung cancer deaths in men and women. About 80% of all deaths from chronic obstructive pulmonary disease (COPD) are caused by smoking. Smoking is estimated to increase the risk for coronary heart disease by two to four times, for stroke by two times or greater, and for developing lung cancer by 25 times [14].

Few women smoked prior to World War II. After the War, women began to feel liberated, which included driving and smoking. In 1970, the incidence of lung cancer deaths in women began to increase in a steady manner. Meanwhile, breast cancer deaths remained relatively stable. In 1987, the number of lung cancer deaths surpassed the number of lung cancer deaths in women (Fig. 8.2) [15].

Secondhand smoke exposure is higher among people with low incomes. Some groups have higher levels of secondhand smoke exposure, including blue-collar workers, service workers, and construction workers.

Most exposure to secondhand smoke occurs in homes and workplaces. People also are exposed to secondhand smoke in public places—such as in restaurants, bars, and casinos—as well as in cars and other vehicles. Since 1964, approximately 2,500,000 nonsmokers have died from health problems caused by exposure to secondhand smoke [16].

Benefits of Quitting Smoking

Within 20 min of giving up cigarettes, blood pressure and pulse rate drop to normal, and the temperature of the hands and feet returns to normal. Within 8 h, the carbon monoxide and oxygen levels in blood return to normal.

Table 8.4 Health risks from active and passive smoking (Based on [13])

Active smoking	
Cancer	Maternal smoking effects
Esophagus	Birth defects
Kidney and bladder	Hyperactivity in childhood
Lung	Increased infant mortality rate
Mouth and throat	Reduced birth weight
Pancreas	Risk of cancer later in life
Pulmonary	SIDS
Acute and chronic bronchitis	Spontaneous abortion
Aggravation of exercise induced asthma	Miscellaneous
Chronic cough	Adverse cardiovascular events in women taking oral contraceptives
Emphysema	Altered metabolism of some medications
Lung cancer	Decreased fertility
Vocal cord irritation and hoarseness	Decreased growth rate
Cardiovascular	Decreased sense of taste and smell
Aortic aneurysm	Decreased sperm count
Buerger's disease	Peptic ulcers
Cardiac arrhythmias	Smoker's skin
Coronary artery disease	
Myocardial infarction	

Passive smoking	
Adults	Children
Acute decline in lung function in persons with asthma	Bronchitis, pneumonia, and other pulmonary infections
Acute respiratory symptoms, including cough, wheezing, chest tightness, and difficulty breathing	Childhood cancers (leukemias, brain cancer, and lymphomas)
Atherosclerosis	Development of asthma
Breast cancer	Higher rates and worsening of asthma
COPD	Lower birth weight
Chronic respiratory symptoms	Lower level of lung function and lung complications during and after surgery
Development of asthma	Middle ear disease (otitis media, middle ear effusion)
Heart disease	Preterm delivery
Irritation of the eyes and nose	Respiratory symptoms including cough, phlegm, wheezing, and breathlessness
Lung cancer	Sudden infant death syndrome
Nasal sinus cancer	Worsening of cystic fibrosis
Small loss of lung function	
Stroke	
Worsening of asthma control	

Within 24 h, the chance of heart attack decreases. Within 48 h, nerve endings start to regrow, and the ability to smell and taste is enhanced. Within 2–3 months, circulation improves, walking becomes easier, and lung function increases by 30%.

Within 1–9 months, coughing, sinus congestion, fatigue, and shortness of breath decrease; cilia regrow in lungs, increasing the ability to handle mucus, clean the lungs, and reduce infection; and the body's overall energy increases.

One year after quitting smoking, the risk for a heart attack drops sharply. By 5 years, the lung cancer death rate for an average smoker (one pack a day) decreases by almost half. The risk of cancer of the mouth, throat, and esophagus decreases to half that of a smoker. By 10 years, lung cancer death rate is similar to that of nonsmokers. By 15 years, the risk of coronary heart disease is equal to that of a nonsmoker [17].

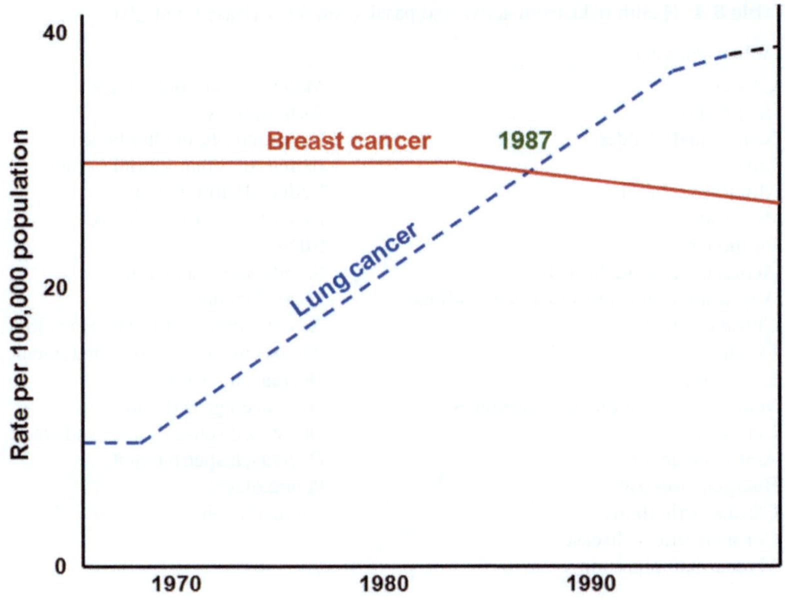

Fig. 8.2 Prevalence of breast and lung cancer deaths in women from 1960 to 2000 (Based on [15])

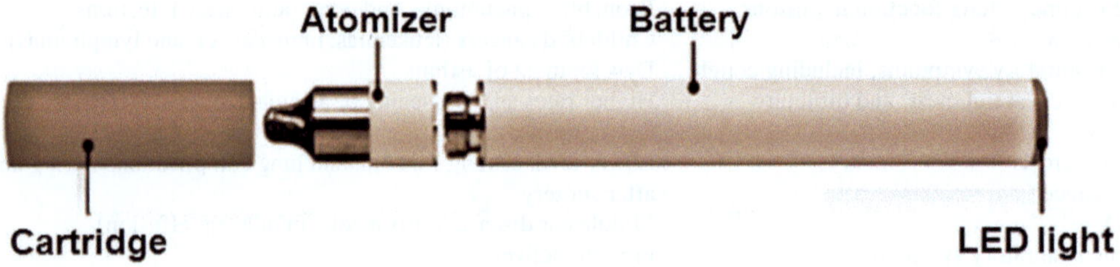

Fig. 8.3 Components of an e-cigarette

Electronic Cigarettes

Components

Electronic cigarettes (e-cigarettes) are devices used to simulate the experience of smoking. They have three components: a battery, a nicotine cartridge, and an atomizer (Fig. 8.3).

The battery is typically lithium-ion rechargeable. The battery contains circuitry for lighting the tip that simulates the glowing of a real cigarette.

The nicotine cartridge includes a mouthpiece and a reservoir for the nicotine solution. The cartridges can be purchased in various flavors (cherry, menthol, tobacco, vanilla, etc.) and levels of nicotine (zero, low, medium, high). The nicotine solution in the cartridge mainly consists of water and propylene glycol.

The atomizer is activated when the user takes a drag on the device. The atomizer consists of a "wicking" mechanism that is made of metal. This wick comes into contact with the liquid nicotine solution in the nicotine cartridge, and a small amount of nicotine solution flows down to heating element (filament). The filament is a small coil of high-resistance wire that becomes hot and vaporizes the nicotine solution [18].

A study has shown that e-cigarettes could lead to a 21% drop in deaths from smoking-related diseases when cigarette smokers are switched to them [19].

Poisoning from Liquid Nicotine

Fifty-one percent of poison calls involving e-cigarettes involve children aged five and younger, while 42% involve people aged 20 and older. The poisoning from liquid nicotine in e-cigarettes can occur in one of three ways: (1) by swallowing it, (2) by inhaling it, or (3) by absorbing it through the skin or membranes in the mouth and lips or eyes.

Nicotine poisoning can cause nausea, vomiting, and seizures. If liquid nicotine is spilled on the skin, the person should wash his or her skin in lukewarm water for about 20 min [20].

Illegal Use of Electronic Cigarette Cartridges

Any type of water-soluble drug can be inhaled through e-cigarette devices that heat up very quickly and vaporize whatever liquid is placed in the cartridge. Users can dissolve in water drugs like methamphetamine, powdered cocaine, and synthetic drugs like bath salts and use them in e-cigarettes. The vapor has little to no odor, making it hard for officials to detect [21].

Cigars and Pipes

One cigar may contain as much tobacco as an entire pack of cigarettes. Pipe and cigar smoking damages lung function in a manner similar to cigarettes and is associated with COPD. Cigar smoke is more concentrated and toxic than cigarette smoke. Smoking as little as one cigar a day increases the risk for cancer. Cigar and pipe smokers are at risk for early tooth loss. Cigar smoking has been linked to erectile dysfunction in men [22].

Smokeless Tobacco

Three percent of American adults are smokeless tobacco users (chewing tobacco, snuff).

Young adults between the ages of 18 and 25 are the most common smokeless tobacco users.

Table 8.5 Prevalence of use of smokeless tobacco by age range in 2015 (%) (From [3])

	Ages 12–17	Ages 18–25	Ages 26 or older
Lifetime	5.70	19.40	18.10
Past year	3.80	8.80	3.70
Past month	2.00	5.60	3.00

They run the same risks of gum disease, heart disease, and addiction as cigarette users but an even greater risk of oral cancer. Each year about 30,000 Americans are diagnosed with oral and pharyngeal cancers, and more than 8000 people die of these diseases [23, 24]. The prevalence of smokeless tobacco use for 2014 is given in Table 8.5.

Chewing Tobacco

Chewing tobacco is usually sold as leaf tobacco (packaged in a pouch) or plug tobacco (packaged in brick form). Each is placed between the cheek and gum. Users keep chewing tobacco in their mouths for several hours to get a continuous high from the nicotine in the tobacco [24].

Snuff

Snuff is a powdered tobacco (usually sold in cans) that is put between the lower lip and the gum. It is also referred to as "dipping tobacco." Just a pinch is all that is needed to release the nicotine, which is then swiftly absorbed into the bloodstream, resulting in a quick high.

Snuff also can be sniffed. *Snus* is finely ground tobacco snuff pasteurized to diminish nitrosamines.

In 1986, the US Surgeon General declared that the use of smokeless tobacco is not a safe substitute for smoking cigarettes [25].

Tolerance

Smokers develop tolerance to many of the effects of nicotine. However, they do not develop tolerance uniformly to all aspects of nicotine's actions. Most prominently, they develop tolerance for nausea, dizziness, and vomiting. People do not wake up 1 day smoking two packs of cigarettes per day. They build up to such a point over a period of time, usually years [26].

Dependence

Nicotine is a psychoactive substance whose continued use usually leads to dependence. The pharmacological and behavioral processes that determine nicotine dependence are similar to those that determine dependence to other drugs, such as heroin and cocaine [26]. Nicotine abstinence syndrome is defined by the American Psychiatric Association's DSM-5 criteria for dependence that was discussed in Chap. 1.

Abstinence Syndrome

Nicotine abstinence syndrome consists of irritability, frustration, anger, anxiety, difficulty concentrating, increased appetite, restlessness, depressed mood, and insomnia. These symptoms occur within hours of smoking cessation, peak in a few days, and disappear within a month. The physical symptoms of nicotine withdrawal also include weight gain due to increased appetite, decreased heart rate, slowing of the EEG, sleep problems characterized by altered REM pattern, and constipation. Nicotine craving can be very strong.

Most symptoms, which are most pronounced during the first week, decline over a 3–4 week period [27].

Quitting Smoking

Reasons for Quitting

Reasons for quitting smoking are varied. Patients may become aware of their general health and the effect smoking has on it, leading to decisions to lead healthier lives. Patients may have specific health reasons for wanting to quit, such as a strong family history of lung cancer related to smoking. Other smokers may decide to quit after they develop symptoms of a smoking-related disease. Parents may want to provide positive role models for their children, or they become aware of the health risks to their children from passive smoking. Pregnant women may want to stop smoking because of health risks to their fetus. For some people, smoking may simply become too expensive, and many simply want to gain better control of their lives. Others become aware that smoking no longer fills the function it once did.

Patients may have smoked initially because smokers were advertised as being sexy, accomplished, or independent. They may no longer need smoking for social acceptance or feel pressure to conform. Finally, some choose to quit smoking because it is now more socially acceptable to be a nonsmoker in some circles than to be a smoker [28]).

Five Stages of Quitting Smoking

Five stages of quitting smoking have been identified [28]. It is important for primary care physicians to be familiar with these.

1. *Precontemplation*. In this stage, patients are unlikely to be responsive to direct intervention. They have little concern about the negative aspects of smoking, and heavy-handed messages to this group may increase their resistance to quitting. If pushed hard they will simply find another physician. A calm, factual presentation of the risks in a low-key and matter-of-fact manner is the best approach.
2. *Contemplation*. In this stage, patients are much more open to receive information about smoking and its dangers. In fact, they may even ask for help.
3. *Action*. Smokers stop smoking.
4. *Maintenance*. This is the most difficult stage of all. It involves remaining abstinent from cigarette smoking.
5. *Relapse*. Relapse occurs so frequently in patients attempting to give up cigarettes that it has to be considered part of the quitting process. The average smoker attempts to quit six times before being successful.

Techniques to Help Patients Quit

Behavioral Techniques

Behavioral techniques primary care physicians can use to help their patients quit smoking include self-control strategies, stimulus control strategies, coping skills, and contingency management.

Self-Control Strategies

Self-control strategies consist of having smokers consistently remind themselves of why they want to stop smoking and having them smoke in the least pleasurable way possible. For instance, they can be told never smoke after meals, always smoke alone, or use their least favorite brand of cigarettes [25].

Stimulus Control Strategies

Stimulus control strategies involve limiting the number of cues for smoking and reducing the ability of cues to evoke the desire for a cigarette, a technique called "cue extinction." A cue may be a specific time, place, emotion, or social setting. One approach to cue extinction is for smokers, about 7–10 days before quitting, to select three cues they have identified as being the most difficult to endure without a cigarette. During this time they continue to smoke but do not smoke while experiencing a cue. This usually involves waiting at least 10 min after a cue has passed before lighting a cigarette [28].

Coping Skills

Coping skill*s* include learning to reduce stress and learning relaxation techniques, setting up rewards for success, and seeking out nonsmoking environments and social support. Useful techniques involve such things as thinking of the negative aspects of smoking and the positive aspects of not smoking, self-encouragement, avoiding situations where the temptation to smoke will be the greatest, and substituting other activities, such as having something low in calories to eat or drink as a substitute for a cigarette [29].

Contingency Management

Contingency management involves arranging for some reward or punishment that is contingent on not smoking during a specified time period after quitting smoking. This is best done by making a written contract with friends, family, or physician. Reward is usually more effective than punishment. The reward does not have to be large, but it should be frequent; for example, having the kids agree to clean the table each night a mother or father does not smoke [28].

Steps to Take Prior to the Quit Date

There are a number of steps a patient can take to help them prepare to quit smoking. These include:

- Buy cigarettes by single pack only.
- Cut down to a pack per day if more than that is smoked.
- Make a list of the times, places, and situations in which the urge to smoke is the greatest and then avoid these as much as possible.
- Don't smoke in the car.
- Smoke the least liked brand.
- Think about quitting 1 day at a time, not for the rest of one's life.
- Wait for 10 min to smoke after an urge to do so.

The Five-Step Smoking Intervention

The physician can follow these five steps to conduct a brief smoking intervention [30]:

Step 1. Discuss Smoking

Make asking about tobacco use a standard procedure. Always ask new patients, "Do you currently smoke or use other forms of tobacco?" Providing health risk information on continued smoking is an integral part of this step. Medical findings should be personalized whenever possible. The health effects of passive smoking on the patient's spouse and children should be included in the discussion.

Step 2. Assess Interest in Quitting
Assess the patient's interest in quitting and the patient's level of motivation and confidence in succeeding. If a patient is not ready to make an attempt, supply recommendations and material that may orient him toward quitting at a later date. If the patient is in the contemplation stage, determine why he is interested in quitting. They can then move on to the next step.

Step 3. Discuss Medications for Smoking Cessations, and Set a Quit Date
The physician may wish to discuss the nicotine replacement medications or bupropion (Zyban) or varenicline (Chantix). A quit date should be agreed upon by the patient and physician.

Step 4. Suggest Smoking Cessation Strategies
Furnish the patient self-help material, arrange to work with the patient using material available too, refer to a smoking cessation group or clinic if one is available, and prescribe smoking cessation medication if appropriate. The risk of becoming addicted to one of the nicotine replacement strategies is real. Simply prescribing one as if it were a magic bullet is ineffective. Other strategies should accompany the medication. Refer the patient of one of the free telephone help lines, such as 1-800-QUIT-NOW (1-800-784-8669).

Describe preparatory techniques to be used by the patient, such as listing reasons for quitting, becoming aware of smoking-related situations, seeking social support, and reducing the number of cigarettes before the quit date. Other things the patient can do are replacing cigarettes with low-calorie food or gum, planning to deal with weight gain, and planning to eliminate environmental cues for smoking.

The physician should discuss withdrawal symptoms with the patient, review strategies for dealing with high-risk situations, and schedule follow-up.

Step 5. Follow Up
Follow up regularly with patients who are trying to quit. Discuss possible slips and relapses. Taper the smoking cessation medication if indicated. If a slip or relapse occurs, encourage the patient to resume abstinence. And schedule follow-up appointments [31].

Triggers for Tobacco Use

To overcome dependence on tobacco, patients need to become aware of their triggers, so they can develop plans to deal with them. Behaviors and cues that may be associated with smoking include certain times of the day, such as first thing in the morning, morning coffee or breaks at work, after a meal, drinking alcohol, certain places or friends, talking on the phone, driving the car, sight or smell of a burning cigarette, stressful situations, and when they are feeling depressed.

Having smoked the last cigarette the evening prior to the quit date, they should throw away all cigarettes, cigarette lighters, and ashtrays and apply the first patch or start using the first nicotine gum or another nicotine replacement method. Some medications allow the smoker to start taking them 1–2 weeks prior to the quit date [32].

Steps to Take After the Quit Date

Steps patients can take after quitting include:

- Avoiding caffeine, which can make the patient feel jittery. They should try drinking water instead.
- Avoiding the times, places, and situations in which the urge to smoke is greatest, or making plans about how to deal with them if they cannot be avoided.
- Playing a relaxation tape from time to time if one tended to smoke when anxious.
- Playing with a pen to occupy the hand that usually has a cigarette in it.
- Rubbing the patch gently and saying "This is all the nicotine I need" when the urge to smoke occurs.
- Sucking air through a cut-off soda straw (cut to the length of a cigarette) when the urge to smoke is particularly strong.
- Taking five deep breaths and exhaling slowly when the urge to smoke occurs.
- Calling your local smoking hotline when you feel the need for support.

Nicotine Dependence Medications

Nicotine dependence medications include nicotine replacement therapy, bupropion (Zyban), and varenicline (Chantix).

Nicotine Replacement Therapy

Nicotine replacement therapy (NRT) works by partially replacing the nicotine previously obtained from tobacco. There are at least three mechanisms by which NRT works: (1) Reducing general withdrawal symptoms, thus allowing people to learn to get by without cigarettes; (2) reducing the reinforcing effects of tobacco-delivered nicotine; and (3) exerting some psychological effects on mood and attention states.

There are six types of nicotine replacement products currently on the market: (1) Transdermal nicotine patches, (2) nicotine nasal spray, (3) nicotine gum, (4) nicotine lozenges, (5) sublingual nicotine tablets, and (6) nicotine inhalers.

Transdermal nicotine patches are for continuous use (weeks to months). The other five are for intermittent use over the same period of time.

Transdermal Nicotine Patches

Nicotine patches (NicoDerm CQ, Habitrol) deliver nicotine through the skin at a relatively steady rate. For breakthrough cravings, intermittent therapies may be added. Nicotine patches come in 21 mg/24 h, 14 mg/24 h, and 7 mg/24 h. For the first 4 weeks, the user wears a nicotine patch that delivers 21 mg/24 h. For weeks 5 and 6, the user switches to the 14 mg/24 h patch. After that, the user moves to the 7 mg/24 h patch. Patients may wear the patch for 16–24 h a day.

If the patient smokes less than ten cigarettes per day, he should skip the 21 mg/24 h patch and go directly to the 14 mg/24 h patch. Physicians should encourage continued use of the nicotine patch during relapses. Nicotine patches are available without a prescription. Patients should follow the instructions on the boxes. Common side effects include skin irritation, insomnia, and vivid dreams [33–35].

Nicotine Nasal Spray

Nicotine nasal spray (Nicorette, Nicotrol NS) delivers nicotine to the brain more rapidly than other NRTs to provide relief of acute cravings. Each dose consists of two squirts to each nostril. Most patients start with one or two doses per hour, which may be increased up to the maximum of 40 doses per day.

Nasal and throat irritation, runny nose, sneezing, and coughing are common side effects. Nicotine nasal spray is a prescription medication [33–35].

Nicotine Gum

Nicotine gum (Nicorette) is also available without a prescription. It is available in 2 and 4 mg doses, which deliver approximately 1 and 2 mg of nicotine, respectively. It is chewed periodically to release the nicotine and then placed between the cheek and gum for a period of time until the next nicotine dose is needed.

Mouth irritation is a common side effect. Other side effects are often a result of overly vigorous chewing that releases nicotine too quickly. These include heartburn, nausea, and hiccups [33–35].

Nicotine Lozenges

Nicotine lozenges (Nicorette, NiQuitin) are available in 2 and 4 mg formulations. Nicotine from the lozenge is absorbed slowly through the buccal mucosa. The lozenge should not be chewed. The amount of nicotine absorbed per lozenge is somewhat higher than that absorbed from nicotine gum. The patient should avoid drinking anything right before, while using, or right after the lozenge.

Side effects include mouth irritation, as well as nicotine-related effects—heartburn, nausea, and hiccups [33–35].

Sublingual Nicotine Tablets

A small nicotine tablet (Nicorette, Nicofi) is held under the tongue where it is absorbed. The levels of nicotine obtained by using the 2 mg tablet are comparable to those obtained by using the 2 mg nicotine gum. One or two tablets each hour is recommended if the smoker smokes 20 or fewer cigarettes a day. Two tablets are recommended if the smoker smokes more than 20 cigarettes per day. The maximum number of tablets is 40 each day. It is recommended that smokers use the sublingual tablet regularly for at least 12 weeks, after which period the number of tablets used can be gradually tapered [36].

Nicotine Inhaler

The nicotine inhaler (Nicorette, Nicotrol) consists of a mouthpiece and a plastic cartridge containing nicotine. Each inhaler cartridge contains 10 mg of nicotine, of which 4 mg can be delivered; of the 4 mg delivered, 2 mg is absorbed. The nicotine is deposited and absorbed in the mouth as with nicotine gum. Most people use between 6 and 16 cartridges a day. Common side effects are mouth and throat irritation and occasional coughing [33–35].

Long-Term NRT

For some smokers, complete withdrawal from smoking may be difficult. In those individuals, it may be beneficial to continue NRT for longer periods, even indefinitely, to prevent relapse to smoking. Although nicotine is not entirely without risk, nicotine maintenance is clearly safer than cigarette smoking [32].

Non-nicotine Medications

Non-nicotine medications for smoking cessation include bupropion, varenicline, nortriptyline, and clonidine.

Bupropion

Bupropion (Zyban) acts by alleviating some of the symptoms of nicotine withdrawal. The recommended and maximum dosage of bupropion is 300 mg/day, given as 150 mg twice daily. Dry mouth and insomnia are the most common adverse events associated with its use. A very small risk of seizure exists. Those who have a seizure disorder should not use this medication [37].

Varenicline

Varenicline (Chantix) is a partial agonist that is selective for nicotinic acetylcholine receptors.

Its action is thought to result from binding to the receptors to prevent nicotine binding. Its agonistic activity is significantly lower than that of nicotine. The main adverse effect of varenicline is nausea, which usually subsides over time. The usual adult dose for smoking cessation is:

- Days 1–3—0.5 mg orally once a day
- Days 4–7—0.5 mg orally twice a day
- Days 8 to end of treatment—1 mg orally twice a day

The patient should set a date to stop smoking; dosing should start 1–2 weeks before this date. Rarely, varenicline has been associated with serious psychiatric symptoms, such as depressed mood and suicidal thoughts [37].

Long-Term Monitoring

Highly nicotine-dependent smokers may require initial therapy for 6 months or longer. Some individuals may require low-dose maintenance therapy for years. Long-term follow-up is recommended because individuals who successfully quit smoking are at high risk for relapse.

Relapse during the first year after achieving smoking cessation occurs in approximately 50% of patients, irrespective of therapeutic regimen. Immediately restarting medication might be helpful if a relapse occurs [37].

Second-Line Therapies

Clonidine

Clonidine (Catapres), an alpha$_2$-noradrenergic agonist, has been shown to diminish symptoms of opioid, alcohol, and nicotine withdrawal symptoms. The dose is 0.3 mg/day. The most common side effects of clonidine are constipation, dizziness, drowsiness, dryness of the mouth, and tiredness or weakness. The mechanism of action may involve decreased firing of alpha-2-noradrenergic cells in the locus coeruleus [38, 39].

Nortriptyline

The dosage of nortriptyline (Pamelor, Aventyl) is initially 25 mg/day, beginning 10–28 days before the quit date. The dose should be increased gradually to 75–100 mg/day. Then it should be continued at that dosage for at least of 12 weeks. The dose should be tapered at the end of this time to avoid withdrawal symptoms that may occur if it is stopped abruptly. Common side effects may include dry mouth, drowsiness, dizziness, and constipation [40].

Combination Pharmacotherapy

To improve smoking cessation, medications can be combined. For example, continuous nicotine delivery (transdermal patch) may be used in conjunction with another NRT medication that permits acute dosing (gum, nasal spray, tablet, or inhaler). Any of the NRT medications may be combined with Zyban, clonidine, or nortriptyline, but not Chantix [37].

Weight Gain

There are several steps that patients can take to maintain a healthy body weight. When people gain weight, it is usually because they start to eat more once they quit smoking.

Eating plenty of fruits and vegetables, fat-free or low-fat snacks like pretzels, sugar-free hard candy, and foods low in sodium, trans fat, and added sugar can be helpful. Patients should be instructed to read food labels and choose healthy options. They should drink lots of water and cut back on alcohol, sugar-sweetened beverages, and drinks with caffeine.

Walking and other exercises release stress and help control appetite. It improves mood and burns calories [41, 42].

Relapse

Because it occurs so often in those attempting to quit smoking, relapse must be considered part of a program to stop smoking. Circumstances leading to relapse generally vary with time from the moment of quitting. The most common reason given for relapse in the first week is withdrawal symptoms. After the first week, coping with crisis situations and exposure to smoking triggers, such as other smokers or drinking alcohol or coffee, are prominent reasons.

The majority of crises occur at work or involve family situations, most commonly arguments with the spouse or other family members. It may occur in response to a serious illness of a family member. Inactivity and boredom are also dangerous.

Relapse during the first week is more apt to occur at home and in the evening. After the second week, relapse is more apt to occur outside the home. In one study, over half of relapses occurred in the home, about a fourth occurred in the workplace, and another fourth occurred in other places, such as bars, restaurants, or friends' home [43].

Patients should not view relapse as a failure but should learn from the reason for the relapse. They should set another quit date and include the reason for relapse in their revised maintenance program. They should receive continued support and encouragement. The predictor of relapse may be the quality of support from family, friends, and coworkers [29, 43, 44].

Overdose

Nicotine is a potentially lethal poison at high exposure levels. Overdose occurs primarily as a result of accidental ingestion or skin exposure to nicotine-containing pesticides or in children after ingesting tobacco or tobacco juice.

Mild nicotine intoxication occurs in first-time smokers, in nonsmoking workers who harvest tobacco, and in people who chew excessive amounts of gum that contain nicotine. Mild overdose causes nausea, salivation, abdominal pain, diarrhea, vomiting, headache, dizziness, decreased heart rate, and weakness. In higher doses, these symptoms are followed by feelings of faintness, precipitous drops in blood pressure, decrease in respiration, convulsions, and death. Table 8.6 gives the symptoms of nicotine overdose [45].

Table 8.6 Symptoms of nicotine overdose (Based on Heller [45])

Abdominal cramps	Dizziness
Agitation, restlessness, or excitement	Drooling
Apnea	Syncope
Burning sensation in the mouth	Headache
Coma	Muscle twitching
Confusion	Nausea
Convulsions	Salivation
Death	Tachycardia followed by bradycardia
Depression	Rapid breathing
Diarrhea	Vomiting
Difficulty breathing	Weakness

Treatment

The initial treatment of nicotine poisoning may include the administration of activated charcoal to try to reduce gastrointestinal absorption if taken orally in the past hour. Treatment is mainly supportive, and further care can include control of seizures with the administration of a benzodiazepine, intravenous fluids for hypotension, and administration of atropine for bradycardia. Respiratory failure may necessitate respiratory support with rapid sequence induction and mechanical ventilation [45].

Summary

In the United States, 75% of adults make at least one visit to a physician each year, with the mean yearly number being about five. Thus, for the majority of physicians, the opportunity for helping people stop smoking will come in the office. The majority of smokers say they want to quit.

A history of smoking should be part of every medical history. It should include questions such as (1) does the patient smoke, if so, how much does he smoke; (2) how long has he been smoking; (3) how early each day does he begin smoking; (4) what type of cigarette does he smoke; (5) has he ever tried to quit; (6) reasons for success or failure; (7) whether he smokes in public or restricted places; (8) whether he smokes when ill; and (9) why does he smoke. These questions are aimed at determining the degree of nicotine addiction as well as past successes and failures.

During the physical examination, abnormalities related to smoking should be emphasized as they are found. These might include cigarette-stained fingers, smoker's lines and crow's feet on the face, pulmonary rales or rhonchi, and increased resonance on percussion. Patients who are ready to quit may sign a contract to do so. Patients who are not ready to sign a contract are not ready to quit.

A major obstacle to getting people to quit smoke, especially women, is that they fear they will gain weight. This must be addressed ahead of quitting. Exercise and good nutrition to prevent weight gain may be essential to success.

Some of the immediate consequences of quitting smoking include improved breathing, less coughing, better taste and smell, saved money, fresh breath, no burn holes, no ashtrays to empty, no more tobacco stains on teeth and fingers, better insurance risk and lower premiums, decreased risk of passive smoking on family and coworkers, and improved tolerance to exercise. Physicians can take advantage of these facts and use them as early positive reinforcement.

Physicians can prescribe a medication (nicotine replacement therapy, bupropion, varenicline) to improve their patient's chance of success.

Physicians should encourage patients to call them if they relapse to identify a reason for the relapse and to use it in revising their maintenance programs after they set a new quit date.

If a primary care physician chooses not to counsel patients about quitting smoking, their minimum intervention should be to explain the health risks to patients and to advise them to quit smoking. Between 5% and 10% of smoking, patients will quit simply on the advice of their physician.

References

1. Smoking and health. Report of the advisory committee to the surgeon general of the public health service. Rockville: U.S. Department of Health, Education, and Welfare; 1964.
2. History of tobacco. Health Literacy. http://healthliteracy.worlded.org/docs/tobacco/Unit1/2history_of.html
3. National survey on drug use and health: trends in prevalence of various drugs for ages 12 or older, ages

12 to 17, ages 18 to 25, and ages 26 or older. National Institute on Drug Abuse (NIDA). 2015. https://www.drugabuse.gov/national-survey-drug-use-health
4. Trends in current cigarette smoking among high school students and adults, United States, 1965–2014. Centers for Disease Control and Prevention (CDC). https://www.cdc.gov/tobacco/data_statistics/tables/trends/cig_smoking. March 30, 2016.
5. Current cigarette smoking among adults in the United States. Centers for Disease Control and Prevention (CDC). https://www.cdc.gov/tobacco/data_statistics/fact_sheets/adult_data/cig_smoking. December 1, 2016.
6. Greene HL, Goldberg RJ, Ockene JK. Cigarette smoking: the physician's role in cessation and maintenance. J Gen Intern Med. 1988;3:75–87.
7. Dubuc B. The brain from top to bottom: how drugs affect neurotransmitters. McGill University. 2012. http://thebrain.mcgill.ca/flash/i/i_03/i_03_m/i_03_m_par/i_03_m_par_amphetamine.html
8. American Medical Association (AMA). AMA drug evaluations. Philadelphia: W.B. Saunders; 1986. p. 157–60.
9. Chesebro MJ. Passive smoking. Am Fam Physician. 1988;37:212–8.
10. Henningfield JE, Nemeth-Coslett R. Nicotine dependence: Interface between tobacco and tobacco-related disease. Chest (Suppl). 1988;93:37–55.
11. Schuckit MA. Drug and alcohol abuse. New York: Plenum Press; 1984. p. 189–97.
12. Nicotine dependence. Mayo Clinic. http://www.mayoclinic.org/diseases-conditions/nicotine-dependence/home/ovc-20202596. May 3, 2016.
13. Diseases related to secondhand smoke. Quit.org. 2016. http://www.quit.org.au/about/frequently-asked-questions/faqs-passive-smoking/diseases-secondhand-smoke.html
14. Health effects of cigarette smoking. Centers for Disease Control and Prevention (CDC). https://www.cdc.gov/tobacco/data_statistics/fact_sheets/health_effects/effects_cig_smoking. December 1, 2016.
15. Prevalence of breast and lung cancer deaths in women from 1960 to 2000. Based on Cancer Facts & Figures 2015. American Cancer Society. 2015. https://old.cancer.org/acs/groups/content/@editorial/documents/document/acspc-044552.pdf
16. Secondhand smoke (SHS) facts. Centers for Disease Control and Prevention (CDC). https://www.cdc.gov/tobacco/data_statistics/fact_sheets/secondhand_smoke/general_facts. December 1, 2016.
17. Benefits of quitting. Centers for Disease Control and Prevention (CDC). https://www.cdc.gov/tobacco/quit_smoking/how_to_quit/benefit. December 5, 2014.
18. How do electronic cigarettes work? Electronic Cigarette Review. http://www.electroniccigarettereview.com/how-do-electronic-cigarettes-work
19. Clarke TE. Cigarettes could cut smoking deaths 21 percent. *Reuters,* July 14, 2016.
20. Reinberg S. Liquid nicotine in e-cigarettes rising cause of poisonings. WebMD. http://www.webmd.com/smoking-cessation/news/20140403/nicotine-in-e-cigarettes-a-growing-public-health-threat-cdc-says. April 3, 2014.
21. Baier E. As e-cigarette popularity leaps, worries of illegal drug use follow. *MPR News*. April 28, 2014.
22. Martin T. 6 surprising facts about cigar smoking. VeryWell. https://www.verywell.com/facts-about-cigar-smoking-2824739. April 21, 2016.
23. Smokeless tobacco. American Academy of Otolaryngology/Head and Neck Surgery (AAO-HNS). http://www.entnet.org/content/smokeless-tobacco
24. Chewing Tobacco (Smokeless Tobacco, Snuff). MedicineNet.com. http://www.medicinenet.com/smokeless_tobacco/article.htm. August 22, 2016.
25. Schuckit MA. Drug and alcohol abuse. New York: Plenum Press; 1984. p. 189–97.
26. The health consequences of smoking: nicotine addiction. Report of the surgeon general. Rockville: U.S. Department of Health and Human Services; 1988.
27. Hughes JR, Hatsukami DK, Skoog KP. Physical dependence on nicotine in gum. J Am Med Assoc. 1986;255:3277–9.
28. Fisher EB, Bishop DB, Goldmunz J, Jacobs A. Implications for the practicing physician of the psychosocial dimensions of smoking. Chest (Suppl). 1988;93:69–78.
29. Gritz ER. Cigarette smoking: the need for action by health professionals. CA Cancer J Clin. 1988;38:194–212.
30. Fiore MC. Treating tobacco use and dependence. U.S. Department of Health and Human Services/Public Health Service. https://bphc.hrsa.gov/buckets/treatingtobacco.pdf. May 2008.
31. Okuyemi N, Nollern NL, Ahluwalia JS. Interventions to facilitate smoking cessation. Am Fam Physician. 2006;74(2):262–71.
32. Milhorn HT. Nicotine dependence. Am Fam Physician. 1989;39:214–24.
33. FDA 101: smoking cessation products. U.S. Food and Drug Administration (FDA). https://www.fda.gov/ForConsumers/ConsumerUpdates/ucm198176.htm. March 9, 2015.
34. Nicotine replacement therapy for quitting tobacco. WebMD. http://www.webmd.com/smoking-cessation/nicotine-replacement-therapy-for-quitting-tobacco. August 21, 2015.
35. Nicotine replacement therapy. MedlinePlus. https://medlineplus.gov/ency/article/007438.htm
36. Nicotine replacement therapy products. Patient. http://patient.info/medicine/nicotine-replacement-therapy-products
37. Lande RG. Nicotine addiction treatment & management. In: Xiong GL, editor. Medscape. http://emedicine.medscape.com/article/287555-treatment. July 15, 2016.
38. Wei H, Young D. Effect of clonidine on cigarette cessation and in the alleviation of withdrawal symptoms. Br J Addict. 1988;83:1221–6.
39. Glassman AH, Jackson WK, Walsh BT, Roose SP, Rosenfeld B. Cigarette craving, smoking withdrawal and clonidine. Science. 1984;226:864–6.

40. Barclay L. Nortriptyline helpful in smoking cessation. Medscape. http://www.medscape.com/viewarticle/440502. August 23, 2002.
41. Fagerstrom KO. Reducing weight gain after stopping smoking. Addict Behav. 1987;12:91–3.
42. How can I avoid weight gain when I stop smoking? American Heart Association. http://www.heart.org/HEARTORG/HealthyLiving/QuitSmoking/Urges/How-Can-I-Avoid-Weight-Gain-When-I-Stop-Smoking_UCM_307852_Article.jsp#.WKdFCLGZM8Y. March 27, 2015.
43. Cummings KM, Jaen CR, Giovino G. Circumstances surrounding relapse in a group of recent smokers. Prev Med. 1985;14:195–202.
44. Shiffman S, Read L, Jarvik ME. Smoking relapse situations; a preliminary topology. Int J Addict. 1985;20:311–8.
45. Heller JL. Nicotine poisoning. MedlinePlus. https://medlineplus.gov/ency/article/002510.htm. May 10, 2016.

Cannabis Dependence

9

Key Chapter Points

- *Cannabis* is a genus of flowering plant that includes three species—C. sativa, C. indica, and C. ruderalis.
- To produce a mood-altering effect, cannabis is used in three main forms: (1) marijuana, (2) hashish, and (3) hash oil.
- Long-term health risks of marijuana use include immune system effects, cardiovascular effects, respiratory effects, reproductive effects, behavioral effects, and cancer.
- Three medicinal products are derived from marijuana: dronabinol, nabilone, and nabiximols.
- Depending on the state, patients may qualify for treatment with medical marijuana if they meet certain requirements.
- *Cannabis indica*, or "ganja," is smoked as a form of marijuana.
- The synthetic cannabinoids, known as Spice or K2, are lab-synthesized liquid chemicals that mimic the effect of *THC*.
- Hashish, or hash, is an extracted product from the cannabis plant that is composed of compressed or purified preparations of glandular resin hairs called trichomes.
- Hash oil is a resinous matrix produced by a solvent extraction of cannabis.
- Repeated use over days to weeks induces considerable tolerance to the behavioral and psychological effects of cannabis.
- Thirty percent of those who use marijuana may develop some degree of marijuana use disorder.
- Acute marijuana toxicity (bad trip) results in anxiety, agitation, difficulty with coordination, decreased muscle strength, postural hypotension, headache, sweating, and lethargy.

Cannabis is a genus of flowering plant that includes three species—C. sativa, C. indica, and C. ruderalis. *Cannabis sativa* and *Cannabis indica* products are used recreationally and as a source of fiber. *Cannabis ruderalis* is a species of *Cannabis* originating in Central Russia. It is less common than the other species of *Cannabis*. It has a lower tetrahydrocannabinol (THC) content than the other two, so it is rarely grown for recreational use. Its much shorter stature (about 2 ft) limits its application for hemp production. It is used traditionally in Russian and Mongolian folk medicine, especially for the treatment of depression [1].

Cannabinoids are organic substances present in the cannabis plant. More than 60 have been identified. The cannabis plant grows wild in many of the tropical and temperate areas of the world. It can be grown in almost any climate and is increasingly cultivated indoors. It consists of a male plant and a female plant. The male plant produces pollen, which pollinates the flowers of the female plant (Fig. 9.1). Once pollinated, the

H.T. Milhorn, *Substance Use Disorders*, DOI 10.1007/978-3-319-63040-3_9

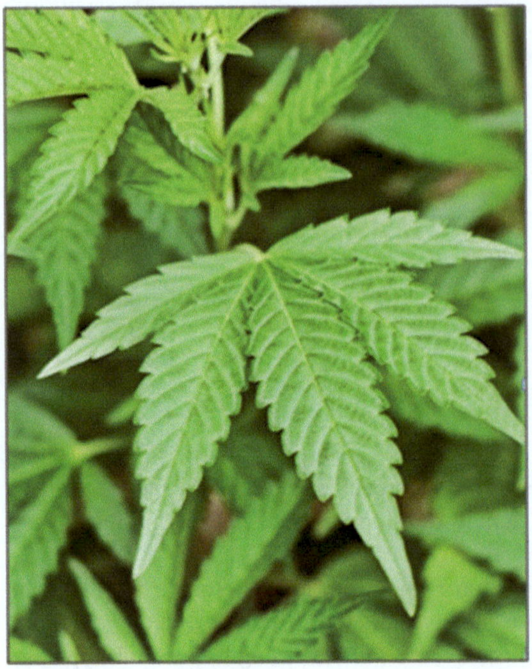

Fig. 9.1 Female *Cannabis sativa* plant

female plant produces seeds. If the female plant is not pollinated, the buds and flowers continue to develop and produce tetrahydrocannabinol (THC), which is the major psychoactive substance in the cannabis plant [2].

There were at least 2000 medicinal cannabis products produced by over 280 manufacturers at the turn of the century. Cannabis products were on the shelf of every pharmacy and were widely prescribed until medical use was prohibited in 1937 by the Marijuana Tax Act [2].

The Controlled Substances Act of 1970 classified marijuana, along with heroin and LSD, as a Schedule I drug.

Medical marijuana was legalized in California in 1996, and several other states have followed suit. In addition, several states, including California, have made recreational marijuana legal. Such laws are in direct disagreement with federal law prohibiting the possession of marijuana [3].

In states where marijuana has become legalized, more and more marijuana "edibles" are seen in retail establishments. Marijuana products include baked goods and candy that closely resemble well-known foods. Some of the names of these products are Rastateers, KeefKat, Munchy Way, and Rasta Reese's [4].

Table 9.1 Prevalence of marijuana plus hashish use in 2015 for various age ranges (%) (From [5])

	Ages 12–17	Ages 18–25	Age 26 and older
Lifetime	15.70	52.70	46.00
Past year	12.60	32.20	10.40
Past month	7.00	19.80	6.50

Prevalence of Use

Table 9.1 gives the prevalence of marijuana plus hashish for various age ranges [5]. To produce a mood-altering effect, cannabis is used in three main forms: (1) marijuana, (2) hashish, and (3) hash oil.

Marijuana

Marijuana is the most commonly used illicit drug in the United States. It is made from the dried flowers and leaves of the unpollinated female *Cannabis sativa* plant. It is the least potent of the three cannabis mood-altering products.

Marijuana is usually smoked in hand-rolled cigarettes (joints) or in special water pipes (bongs). Marijuana can also be mixed into food or brewed as tea and ingested. It also has been used as cigars called "blunts." It also may come in a "wax" form that resembles lip balm. It can be eaten or smoked [6].

Prevalence of Use

Marijuana use by 8th, 10th, and 12th graders have held steady in the past few years following several years of increase in the previous decade. In 2015, 11.8% of 8th graders reported marijuana use in the past year, and 6.5% were current users. Among 10th graders, 25.4% had used marijuana in the past year and 14.8% were current users. Among 12th graders, 34.9% had used marijuana during the prior year and 21.3% were current users. Six percent said they used marijuana daily or nearly daily. However, teens' perceptions of the risks of marijuana use have steadily declined over the past decade, possibly related to increasing public debate about legalizing or loosening restrictions on marijuana for medicinal and recreational use [7].

Street Names

Because marijuana is such a popular drug, it has a large number of street names. Some of the more popular ones are:

Bud	Sinsemilla	Joint	Reefer
Blunt	Grass	Loud	Skunk
Chronic	Green	Mary Jane	Smoke
Dope	Hash	MJ	Trees
Ganja	Herb	Pot	Weed

Marijuana is commonly laced with other psychoactive substances. Some of these street names are:

With tobacco	Kiff
With PCP	Chips, donk, illies, illing, lovelies, love leaf, killer supergrass, wack, woolies, zoom, fry, frios, yerba mala
With formaldehyde (embalming fluid)	Boat, loveboat, amp, drank, clickem, ill, illy, wet, water-water
With cocaine HCl	Chronic, banano, caviar, champagne, cocoa puff, gremmies, lace
With crack cocaine	Chronic, bazooka, cocktail, crack back, daddy, dirty, geek, gimmie, juice joint, liprimo, oolies, p-dogs, torpedo, turbo, woolies
With heroin	A-bomb

Pharmacology

Pharmacodynamics Cannabinoids exert their effect by interaction with specific endogenous neuronal cannabinoid receptors that are termed CB_1 receptors. These receptors have been found in the brain and peripheral nerves. A second cannabinoid receptor, the CB_2 receptor, is present in macrophages in the spleen and in other immune cells. The distribution of CB_1 receptors includes the cerebral cortex, limbic areas (including hippocampus and amygdala), basal ganglia, cerebellum, thalamus, and brain stem. The endogenous substance, named anandamide after the Sanskrit word for bliss (ananda), has a high affinity for CB_1 receptors and has most of the same actions of THC.

THC has been shown to increase the release of dopamine from the nucleus accumbens and prefrontal cortex. This effect may be the basis of cannabis's reinforcing properties and the cause of its recreational use.

It appears that there may be a whole system of multiple cannabinoid receptors and anandamide-related substances.

The sensations of slight euphoria, relaxation, and amplified auditory and visual perceptions produced by marijuana are due almost entirely to its effect on the cannabinoid receptors in the brain [8].

Pharmacokinetics In the United States, the content of marijuana was originally 1–2%. Selective breeding now yields marijuana with much higher THC concentrations. The average THC concentration in 2008 was 10.1%. The most potent marijuana is known as sinsemilla, with a THC concentration that may be 14% or higher.

To obtain maximal effect from marijuana, users must master a smoking technique that is different from that used to smoke regular cigarettes. Users inhale smoke as deeply into their lungs as possible and then hold their breath for 20–30 s to extract as much of the THC from the smoke as possible.

Various methods of smoking marijuana include rolling it into "joints" (marijuana cigarettes) or "blunts" (marijuana rolled into the leaf wrap of a hollowed-out cigar). Smoking it through a pipe, through a water pipe ("bong"), or a vaporizer are also common methods. While marijuana is most often smoked, it can also be ingested.

The effects of smoking are typically felt within a few minutes and can peak in 10–30 min. Short-term effects from smoking generally wear off within 2–3 h. About 50% of the THC in a joint of herbal cannabis is inhaled; nearly all of this is absorbed through the lungs, rapidly enters the bloodstream, and reaches the brain within seconds. Effects are perceptible within seconds and fully apparent in a few minutes.

When marijuana is ingested, its onset of action is within 30–60 min, and peak effects may not occur until the second or third hour. After oral ingestion, blood concentrations reached are 25–30% of those obtained by smoking the drug, partly because of first-pass metabolism in the liver.

THC is rapidly converted into its active metabolite 11-hydroxy-delta-9-tetrahydrocannabinol, which produces effects identical to the parent compound. The active metabolite is then converted to inactive metabolites and excreted in the feces (65%) and urine (25%). Very little unmetabolized THC is found in the urine.

Once absorbed, THC and other cannabinoids are rapidly distributed to all other tissues at rates dependent on the blood flow. Because they are extremely lipid soluble, cannabinoids accumulate in fatty tissues, reaching peak concentrations in 4–5 days. They are then slowly released back into other body compartments, including the brain. Because of the sequestration in fat, the tissue elimination half-life of THC is about 7 days, and complete elimination of a single dose may take up to 30 days. With repeated dosage, high levels of cannabinoids can accumulate in the body [9, 10].

Cannabis short-term effects include a burning sensation in the mouth, a dry throat, and bloodshot eyes. It produces euphoria and altered senses, such as seeing brighter colors. It produces muscle relaxation, slowed reflexes, an altered sense of time, and altered cognitive function. It decreases muscle coordination, causes a loss of short-term and working memory, increases heart rate, and increases appetite causing the "munchies." It negatively affects perception and judgment; increases chances of risky behavior, such as unprotected sex and trying more dangerous drugs; and creates difficulty problem solving.

Short-term pharmacological effects of marijuana are given in Table 9.2 [11]. Cardiovascular effects of marijuana include increased heart rate, increased systolic pressure, decreased blood pressure while erect, and a marked reddening of the conjunctiva due to blood vessel dilation. Sodium retention and expanded plasma volume occur.

Table 9.2 Short-term pharmacological effects of marijuana (From Milhorn [11]. Approved with permission, Springer)

Central nervous system
Altered perception of time (time seems to pass more slowly)
Antiemetic effect
Anxiety
Balance difficulty
Coordination problems
Decreased reaction time
Depersonalization
Difficulty carrying out tasks requiring multiple mental steps to reach a goal
Euphoria
Feelings of relaxation and sleepiness
Impaired perception, attention, and information processing
Impaired psychomotor sensation
Increased hunger
Increased risk of contracting sexually transmitted diseases
Increased sense of well-being
Keener sense of hearing
Paranoia
Psychosis
Sense of detachment
Senses of touch, taste, and smell seem to be enhanced
Short-term memory impairment
Subtle visual and auditory stimuli may take on novel characteristics
Vivid visual imagery
Peripheral effects
Increased heart rate
Increased systolic pressure in the supine position
Decreased blood pressure in the erect position
Marked reddening of conjunctiva
Plasma volume expansion
Increased body temperature due to impaired sweating
Decreased intraocular pressure
Dry mouth and throat
Muscle weakness
Tremors
Unsteadiness
Increased deep tendon reflexes

Muscle weakness, tremors, unsteadiness, and increased deep tendon reflexes occur. Intraocular pressure is decreased and an antiemetic effect occurs.

Marijuana is known to produce flashbacks in previous users of lysergic acid diethylamide (LSD).

Drugs that sometimes are mixed with marijuana to increase its effects include phencyclidine (PCP), opium, formaldehyde, and Raid insect spray [12].

Interactions with Other Drugs

Marijuana may increase the risk of bleeding when taken with drugs such as aspirin, warfarin (Coumadin), and heparin, antiplatelet drugs such as clopidogrel (Plavix), and nonsteroidal anti-inflammatory drugs such as ibuprofen (Motrin, Advil) or naproxen (Naprosyn, Aleve).

Marijuana may increase blood sugar levels by interacting with medications that are used for blood sugar control. Medication adjustments may be necessary.

Marijuana may cause low blood pressure, so caution is advised in people taking medications that lower blood pressure.

Marijuana may interfere with the way the body processes certain drugs using the liver's cytochrome P450 enzyme system. As a result, the levels of these drugs may increase in the blood and may cause increased effects or potentially serious adverse reactions.

Marijuana may increase the amount of drowsiness caused by benzodiazepines such as lorazepam (Ativan) or diazepam (Valium), barbiturates such as phenobarbital, narcotics such as hydrocodone, some antidepressants, and alcohol. In addition, marijuana may adversely affect the immune system.

Marijuana may interfere with agents that treat lung disorders, heart disorders, nausea or vomiting, nervous system disorders, psychiatric disorders, HIV, skin disorders, stomach disorders, cancer, and seizures.

Moderate interaction occurs with disulfiram (Antabuse), causing agitation, trouble sleeping, and irritability. Fluoxetine (Prozac) also interacts with marijuana. Taking marijuana with fluoxetine may cause a hypomanic state, consisting of irritability, nervousness, jitteriness, and excitability.

Marijuana may increase the risk of bleeding when taken with herbs and supplements that are believed to increase the risk of bleeding (*Ginkgo biloba*, garlic, saw palmetto) [13, 14].

Health Risks

Long-term health risks of marijuana use include immune system effects, cardiovascular effects, respiratory effects, reproductive effects, behavioral effects, and cancer. Marijuana use also puts users at risk for various types of accidents.

Coinciding with the increasing rates of cannabis use due to medical marijuana has been the recognition of a new clinical condition known as *cannabinoid hyperemesis syndrome*. This syndrome is characterized by cyclic episodes of nausea and vomiting and abdominal pain. Despite the well-established antiemetic properties of marijuana, there is increasing evidence of its paradoxical effects on the gastrointestinal tract and central nervous system.

The clinical course of cannabinoid hyperemesis syndrome consists of three phases: (1) prodromal, (2) hyperemetic, and (3) recovery phase. The hyperemetic phase usually ceases within 48 h after cessation of use, and treatment involves supportive therapy with fluid resuscitation and antiemetic medications. Patients often demonstrate the learned behavior of frequent hot bathing, which produces temporary cessation of nausea, vomiting, and abdominal pain [15, 16].

Marijuana affects the immune, cardiovascular, respiratory, and reproductive systems. It also has psychiatric/behavioral effects and can cause cancer. Motor vehicle accidents occur under the influence of marijuana [17].

Immune System

Long-term cannabis use can impair the immune system's ability to fight off microbial and viral infections. Both animal and human studies have shown that marijuana impairs the ability of T-cells in the lungs' immune defense system to fight off some infections [18].

Cardiovascular System

Users with preexisting coronary artery disease or cerebrovascular disease may experience myocardial infarctions, congestive heart failure, or stroke. Peripheral vasodilatation causes postural hypotension, which may lead to dizziness or syncope. Cannabis arteritis is a very rare peripheral vascular disease similar to Buerger's disease [18].

Respiratory System

The amount of tar in a marijuana cigarette is three times the amount in a tobacco cigarette, with one-third greater deposition in the respiratory tract. Chronic cannabis use is associated with bronchoconstriction, pharyngitis, sinusitis, bronchitis, squamous metaplasia of the tracheobronchial epithelium, and emphysema.

Several case reports suggest a link between cannabis smoking and cancer of the oropharynx and tongue, nasal and sinus epithelium, and larynx.

Some illegally obtained marijuana is contaminated with *Aspergillus* species, which can cause invasive pulmonary aspergillosis in immunocompromised users.

Smoking marijuana may increase the risk of opportunistic infections among those who are HIV positive, although it does not seem to effect the development of AIDS or lower white cell counts [18, 19].

Reproductive System

High doses of THC cause a drop in testosterone level, decreased sperm production, and compromised sperm motility and viability.

THC alters the normal ovulatory cycle by decreasing follicle-stimulating hormone, luteinizing hormone, and prolactin secretion. It crosses the placenta and impairs placental development, fetal nourishment, and placental gas exchange. For this reason, it is implicated in low birth weight, growth restriction, preeclampsia, spontaneous miscarriage, and stillbirth. It also accumulates in breast milk.

Children of chronic users (greater than five joints per week) were found to have lower verbal and memory scores at age 2 years [18].

A possible increased risk of nonlymphoblastic leukemia, rhabdomyosarcoma, and astrocytoma exists in children whose mothers use cannabis during their pregnancies.

Psychiatric/Behavioral

Long-term use of marijuana also can lead to a series of attitude and personality changes known as "amotivational syndrome." This syndrome is characterized by a diminished ability to carry out long-term plans, a sense of apathy, decreased attention to appearance and behavior, and decreased ability to concentrate for long periods of time. These changes can also include poor performance in school. Long-term marijuana use has been shown to cause a decline in IQ of up to eight points.

Marijuana use can cause relationship problems and antisocial behavior, such as lying and stealing money. It leads to lower life satisfaction, financial difficulties, and a greater chance of being unemployed.

Marijuana use has been shown to increase the risk of schizophrenia two fold in vulnerable individuals [18].

Cancer

Marijuana smoke contains some of the same cancer-causing compounds as tobacco, usually in higher concentrations. Someone who smokes five joints per day may be taking in as many cancer-causing chemicals as someone who smokes a full pack of cigarettes every day.

Cancer of the respiratory tract and lungs may be promoted by marijuana smoke, since it contains irritants and carcinogens. Tobacco smoke and marijuana smoke may work together to change the tissues that line the respiratory tract.

Marijuana smoking could contribute to early development of head and neck cancer in some people. Smoking marijuana has been linked to testicular cancer [20].

Accidents

Marijuana is the most common illegal drug reported in motor vehicle accidents. Fatal crashes involving marijuana use tripled during the previous decade. Marijuana also has been involved in other types of accidents [18, 21].

Medical Use

Dronabinol, Nabilone, and Nabiximols

Three medicinal products are derived from marijuana: dronabinol, nabilone, and nabiximols.

The synthetic THC product *dronabinol* (Marinol) is for the control of nausea and vomiting caused by chemotherapeutic agents and for stimulating the appetite of AIDS patients. A DEA Schedule II drug, dronabinol, is supplied as a 2.5, 5, and 10 mg capsule.

Nabilone (Cesamet) is used to treat severe nausea and vomiting caused by chemotherapy. Nabilone is a man-made drug similar to the natural substances found in marijuana. It works by decreasing the signals in the brain that lead to nausea and vomiting.

Nabiximols (Sativex) is used to treat spasticity caused by multiple sclerosis. It is composed of two compounds found in marijuana—THC and cannabidiol (CBD)—which isn't psychoactive. The drug, delivered through a vaporizer, is approved in 25 countries but isn't available in the United States [22].

Medical Marijuana

Although several states have decriminalized marijuana, it remains an illegal substance under federal law. Depending on the state, patients may qualify for treatment with medical marijuana if they meet certain requirements and have one of the following conditions [23]:

- Amyotrophic lateral sclerosis (ALS)
- Anorexia due to HIV/AIDS
- Chronic pain
- Crohn's disease
- Epilepsy or seizures
- Glaucoma, although the American Academy of Ophthalmology doesn't recommend medical marijuana
- Multiple sclerosis or severe muscle spasms
- Nausea, vomiting, or severe wasting associated with cancer treatment
- Terminal illness
- Tourette syndrome

Cannabis indica

Originally cultivated in the United States, *Cannabis indica*, or "ganja," is smoked as a form of marijuana. C. indica plants are short, dense plants, with broader, darker green leaves than the *Cannabis sativa* plant.

The plant is commonly referred to as "skunk" (for the pungent odor it produces while growing), northern lights, early girl, and many other names.

Cannabis indica and *Cannabis sativa* produce two greatly different effects. C. sativa produces a "high" effect, while C. indica produces a more relaxed, "stoned" effect.

Cannabis indica contains a higher amount of THC than *Cannabis sativa*, causing the psychological effects to be heightened [24].

Synthetic Cannabinoids

Spice

The synthetic cannabinoids, known as Spice or K2, are lab-synthesized liquid chemicals that mimic the effect of THC. The chemical ingredients of Spice are sprayed onto dried plant material, which consists of chopped up herbs in a mixture of colors including beige, cream red, and brown. The final product looks like colored marijuana or tobacco.

In 2015, 3.10% of 8th graders, 4.30% of 10th graders, and 5.20% of 12th graders reported past-year use of synthetic marijuana.

Spice was first sold as a recreational drug in 2004 in the United Kingdom. By 2006, it had gained a considerable hold on the market, and the brand name Spice (along with another brand K2) had become a generic term for all synthetic cannabis. Some synthetic cannabinoids are 100 times more potent than THC. This has resulted in a number of significant side effects, including hypertension, blurred vision, myocardial infarction, vomiting, severe anxiety, paranoia, seizures, and hallucinations.

In drug tests, the chemicals in synthetic marijuana are harder to detect than marijuana.

Spice is sold under a number of names, including Mojo, Scooby Snax, Black Mamba, and Annihilation. Vaping the liquid of synthetic marijuana using e-cigarette is a fast-rising trend.

Most Spice manufacturers do not follow high manufacturing standards, many of the chemicals being produced in cheap basement laboratories. Chemical impurities carry additional, and possibly much greater, risks. Deaths have been associated with use of the drug.

Spice is often sold as potpourri, room deodorizer, or incense, purporting to be an innocent product for scenting rooms and usually has the warning "Not for human consumption" on the packet.

It is estimated that there are well over 200 synthetic cannabinoids sold on the street, with about 50 of them currently listed as DEA Schedule I drugs.

Street names for synthetic cannabis include Spice, black mamba, K2, fake marijuana, and sexy monkey [25–27].

Hashish

Hashish, or hash, is an extracted product from the cannabis plant that is composed of compressed or purified preparations of glandular resin hairs called trichomes. It is made from the resin, which is a secreted gum. Hashish may be solid or resinous depending on the preparation; pressed hashish is solid, whereas water-purified hashish is often a paste-like substance with varying hardness and pliability. Its color, most commonly light to dark brown, can vary from transparent to yellow, tan, black, or red depending on the process and amount of solvent left over.

Hashish is usually smoked, but it also can be added to food and eaten. It may have 20–65% THC concentration.

The name hashish comes from an Arabic word meaning "grass." Massive hashish production for international trade originated in Morocco during the 1960s, where the cannabis plant was widely available. Northern India has a long social tradition in the production of hashish, known locally as *charas*. It is believed to be the same plant resin that was burned in the religious ceremonies of ancient Persia.

A 250–1000 mg ingestion of hashish can result in obtundation within 30 min. Street names for hashish include chocolate, hash, and shit [28, 29].

Hash Oil

Hash oil is a resinous matrix produced by a solvent extraction of cannabis. A wide variety of solvents can be used for the extraction, such as chloroform, dichloromethane, ether, naphtha, benzene, butane, methanol, ethanol, isopropanol, and olive oil.

One pound of marijuana yields from one-tenth to one-fifth of a pound of hash oil. It is a concentrated product with a high THC content, which generally varies between 20% and 60%, but can contain up to 80% THC.

Hash oil is traditionally a dark, golden hue. Related "honey oil" is a specific type of hash oil made from the more potent parts of the cannabis plant.

Hash oil is usually consumed by smoking, ingestion, or vaporization. Smoking or vaporizing hash oil is known as "dabbing" from the English verb to daub, which means "to smear with something adhesive." Dabbing devices include special kinds of water pipes ("oil rigs") and vaporizers similar in design to e-cigarettes.

Anxiety or panic is the most common bad reaction, occurring during or shortly after smoking hash oil, or they can appear more gradually 1–2 h after an oral dose. These reactions usually resolve without medical intervention. Hash oil can cause tightness in chest, nausea, hypotension, tachycardia, dry mouth, and lethargy. Deaths have occurred.

Flashbacks occasionally occur in which the original drug experience (usually dysphoria) is relieved weeks or months after use [30].

Wax is a new marijuana product that looks and feels like lip balm and is as strong as 15–20 joints of marijuana. The marijuana concentrate is also referred to as butane hash oil, honey oil, budder, dabs, and 710 (spelled upside down is oil). It is easy to conceal in lip balm jars. It can be eaten or smoked using a bong or an e-cigarette. It is made from the oils of marijuana plants. Highly flammable butane gas is used to extract the THC from the marijuana leaf and has resulted in home explosions, injuries, and deaths [31].

Tolerance

Repeated use over days to weeks induces considerable tolerance to the behavioral and psychological effects of cannabis. Regular marijuana smokers may require more potent cannabis or larger amounts of the drug to achieve the desired effects [32].

Dependence

Thirty percent of those who use marijuana may develop some degree of marijuana use disorder. People who begin using marijuana before the age of 18 are four to seven times more likely to develop a marijuana use disorder than those who begin smoking it in adulthood. Nine percent of people who use marijuana will become dependent on it, rising to about 17% in those who start using in their teens [33]. Diagnosis of cannabis dependence is based on the DSM-5 criteria discussed in Chap. 1.

Abstinence Syndrome

On cessation of cannabis use, withdrawal symptoms may develop. Users most commonly experience cravings, irritability, mild tremor, anxiety, and sleep disturbances. Other symptoms may include restlessness, anorexia and weight loss, nausea, sweating, salivation, mild hyperthermia, and tremor [34].

Overdose

Symptoms

Acute marijuana toxicity (bad trip) results in anxiety, agitation, difficulty with coordination, decreased muscle strength, postural hypotension, headache, sweating, and lethargy. It also results in slurred speech, confusion, amnesia, delusions, and hallucinations.

Treatment

In 2012, there were over 450,000 emergency department visits in the United States related to use of marijuana. Treatment depends on the clinical presentation, the age of the patient, and the presence of other legal or illicit substances. Immediate management should be supportive, including cardiovascular and neurological monitoring and placement in a quiet room. Most episodes of marijuana toxicity remit fairly quickly.

Gastric decontamination may be considered in children with an acute ingestion less than 2 h prior to presentation. Patients who are agitated or present with psychosis can be treated with a benzodiazepine [18].

Summary

Cannabis is a genus of flowering plant that includes three species—C. sativa, C. indica, and C. ruderalis. The male plant produces pollen, which pollinates the flowers of the female plant. Once pollinated, the female plant produces seeds. If the female plant is not pollinated, the buds and flowers continue to develop and produce THC, which is the major psychoactive substance in the cannabis plant. To produce a mood-altering effect, cannabis is used in three main forms: (1) marijuana, (2) hashish, and (3) hash oil.

Long-term health risks of marijuana use include immune system effects, cardiovascular effects, respiratory effects, reproductive effects, behavioral effects, and cancer.

Medical marijuana was legalized in California in 1996, and several other states have followed suit. Three medicinal products are derived from marijuana: dronabinol, nabilone, and nabiximols. Depending on the state, patients may qualify for treatment with medical marijuana if they meet certain requirements.

Cannabis indica, or "ganja," is smoked as a form of marijuana. The synthetic cannabinoids, known as Spice or K2, are lab-synthesized liquid chemicals that mimic the effect of *THC*.

Hashish, or hash, is an extracted product from the cannabis plant that is composed of compressed or purified preparations of glandular resin hairs called trichomes. Hash oil is a resinous matrix produced by a solvent extraction of cannabis.

Repeated use over days to weeks induces considerable tolerance to the behavioral and psychological effects of cannabis. Thirty percent of those who use marijuana may develop some degree of marijuana use disorder. People who begin using marijuana before the age of 18 are four to seven times more likely to develop a marijuana use disorder than adults.

Acute marijuana toxicity (bad trip) results in anxiety, agitation, difficulty with coordination, decreased muscle strength, postural hypotension, headache, sweating, and lethargy.

References

1. London D. What is Cannabis Ruderalis? Marijuana.com. http://www.marijuana.com/blog/news/2016/05/what-is-cannabis-ruderalis. May 12, 2016.
2. O'Brien R, Cohen S. The encyclopedia of drug abuse. New York: Facts on File; 1984.
3. Marijuana Timeline, PBS Frontline. http://www.pbs.org/wgbh/pages/frontline/shows/dope/etc/cron.html
4. Edible marijuana creates new cautions for a safe Halloween. McCook Gazette. http://m.mccookgazette.com/story/2355710.html. October 31, 2016.
5. National survey on drug use and health: trends in prevalence of various drugs for ages 12 or older, ages 12 to 17, ages 18 to 25, and ages 26 or older. National Institute on Drug Abuse (NIDA). 2015. https://www.drugabuse.gov/national-survey-drug-use-health
6. Marijuana. Partnership for Drug-Free Kids. 2017. http://www.drugfree.org/drug-guide/marijuana
7. Marijuana: What is the scope of marijuana use in the United States? National Institute on Drug Abuse (NIDA). November, 2016.
8. Dubuc B. The brain from top to bottom. McGill University. http://thebrain.mcgill.ca/flash/i/i_03/i_03_m/i_03_m_par/i_03_m_par_heroine.html#drogues. May 2012.
9. Ashton CH. Pharmacology and effects of cannabis: a brief review. Br J Psychiatry. 2001;178(2):101–6.
10. Schwartz RH, Hawks RL. Laboratory detection of marijuana use. J Am Med Assoc. 1981;254:788–92.
11. Milhorn HT. Chemical dependence: diagnosis, treatment, and prevention. New York: Springer; 1990.
12. Schwartz RH. Marijuana: an overview. Pediatr Clin N Am. 1987;34:305–17.
13. Wilford BB, editor. Major drugs of abuse. In: Drug abuse: a guide for the primary care physician. Chicago: American Medical Association; 1981.p. 21–84.
14. Marijuana (Cannabis Sativa). Mayo Clinic. http://www.mayoclinic.org/drugs-supplements/marijuana/selected-references/hrb-20059701. November 1, 2013.
15. Council on Scientific Affairs. Marijuana: its health hazards and therapeutic potentials. JAMA. 1981; 246:1823–7.
16. Galli JA, Sawaya RA, Friedenberg FK. Cannabinoid hyperemesis syndrome. Curr Drug Abuse Rev. 2011;4(4):241–9.
17. Morris RR. Human pulmonary pathophysiology changes from marijuana smoking. J Forensic Sci. 1985;30:345–9.
18. Russo L. Cannabinoid poisoning. Medscape. http://emedicine.medscape.com/article/833828-overview. June 24, 2016.
19. Wu TC, Tashkin DP, Djahed B, Rose JE. Pulmonary hazards of smoking marijuana as compared with tobacco. N Engl J Med. 1988;318:347–51.
20. What are the long-term effects of marijuana? VeryWell. http://www.verywell.com/long-term-effects-of-marijuana-63551. July 17, 2016.
21. Thompson D. Fatal car crashes involving pot use have tripled in U.S., study finds. WebMD. http://www.webmd.com/mental-health/news/20140204/fatal-car-crashes-involving-pot-use-have-tripled-in-us-study-finds#1. February 4, 2014.
22. Macaluso M. 3 prescription drugs that come from marijuana. USA Today, March 17, 2014.
23. Medical marijuana. Mayo Clinic. http://www.mayoclinic.org/healthy-lifestyle/consumer-health/in-depth/medical-marijuana/art-20137855. October 14, 2016.
24. Marijuana. Center for Substance Abuse Research (CESAR)/University of Maryland. http://www.cesar.umd.edu/cesar/drugs/marijuana.asp
25. Anderson, L. Synthetic marijuana – spice or K2. Drugs.com. https://www.drugs.com/illicit/synthetic-marijuana.html
26. What are synthetic cannabinoids?. National Institute on Drug Abuse (NIDA). November 2015.
27. Rael A. What is synthetic marijuana and how does it compare to traditional marijuana? The Huffington Post, September 11, 2013.
28. Hashish. MedLibrary. http://medlibrary.org/medwiki/Hashish
29. What is Hashish? Weed Street Journal. http://www.theweedstreetjournal.com/hashish. March 7, 2011.
30. Hash oil. WeedWiki. http://cannabis.wikia.com/wiki/Hash_Oil. September 28, 2015.

31. Dangerous new marijuana product looks like lip balm, packs big kick. Fox News/Health, August 17, 2014.
32. Hunt A, Jones RT. Tolerance and disposition of tetrahydrocannabinol in man. J Pharmacol Exp Ther. 1980;215:35–44.
33. Is marijuana addictive? National Institute on Drug Abuse (NIDA). January 2017.
34. Medina J. Cannabis (marijuana) withdrawal. PsychCentral. https://psychcentral.com/disorders/cannabis-marijuana-withdrawal. February 9, 2017.

Dissociative Drug Dependence 10

Key Chapter Points

- Phencyclidine (PCP) is a central nervous system depressant introduced as an anesthetic in the early 1950s but later abandoned because of unpredictable side effects, such as agitation, disorientation, and hallucinations.
- Medical consequences of PCP intoxication can include acute tubular necrosis secondary to rhabdomyolysis, acute hepatic necrosis secondary to hyperpyrexia, aspiration pneumonia, high-output cardiac failure, pulmonary edema, hypertensive encephalopathy, intracranial hemorrhage, convulsions, coma, and death.
- PCP use can lead to psychological dependence, craving, and drug-seeking behavior.
- Upon abrupt discontinuation of PCP, physical distress, lack of energy, and depression have been reported. Long periods of use may lead to memory loss, difficulties with speech and thinking, depression, and weight loss.
- The signs and symptoms of PCP intoxication or overdose are related to its dose, route of administration, and the individual's response to the drug.
- Much of the ketamine sold on the streets comes from veterinary offices.
- Illicit use of DXM is referred to on the street as "robo-tripping" or "skittling." These terms are derived from the most commonly abused products, Robitussin and Coricidin.

Dissociative drugs cause a disconnection between thoughts, identity, consciousness, and memory. They distort the user's perception of sight and sound and produce feelings of detachment from the environment and one's self. The major dissociative drugs are phencyclidine, ketamine, and the over-the-counter compound dextromethorphan.

Phencyclidine

Phencyclidine (PCP) is a central nervous system depressant introduced as an anesthetic in the early 1950s but later abandoned because of unpredictable side effects such as agitation, disorientation, and hallucinations. The drug can be synthesized easily by anyone with a basic knowledge of chemistry. It is abused because of its euphoric effects, ability to decrease inhibitions, ability to instill feelings of power and eliminate pain, and dissociative state in which altered perceptions of time space and body image occur [1–4].

Phencyclidine is produced inexpensively in clandestine laboratories set up in kitchens, garages, and basements. In addition to being used for its own effects, it is sometimes misrepresented by dealers as some other drug, most often LSD, mescaline, psilocybin, or THC. Because of its low cost and ease of manufacture, it is also used to adulterate other drugs [4].

H.T. Milhorn, *Substance Use Disorders*, DOI 10.1007/978-3-319-63040-3_10

Table 10.1 Prevalence of use of PCP in 2015 for various age ranges (%) (From [6])

	Ages 12–17	Ages 18–25	Ages 26 or older
Lifetime	0.2	0.80	2.90
Past year	0.10	0.10	0.00
Past month	0.00	0.00	0.00

A large number of precursors, derivatives, and analogs of phencyclidine have been manufacture over the years. Nearly all cause pharmacological effects similar to phencyclidine [5].

Prevalence of Use

The prevalence of use of PCP for various age ranges is given in Table 10.1 [6]. Emergency room visits related to PCP use increased more than 400%, from 14,825 to 75,538, between 2005 and 2011, the most recent available data [7].

Street Names

Street names for PCP include:

PCP	Angel dust, amoeba, amp, belladonna, animal trank, zoom, hog, peace pills, boat, sherm, sticks, super grass, STP, killer joints, cadillac, monkey dust, rocket fuel, zombie dust
PCP plus marijuana	Wet dust, blunt, happy stick, fry sticks, love boat, Illy dippers, supergrass, sherms
PCP plus MDMA	Elephant flipping, pikachu
PCP plus crack cocaine	Beam me up
PCP plus cocaine hydrochloride	Lovelies

Pharmacology

Pharmacodynamics

PCP works primarily as an N-methyl-D-aspartate (NMDA) receptor antagonist. The NMDA receptor is a type of glutamate receptor that participates in excitatory neurotransmission. NMDA receptors allow electrical signals to pass between neurons in the brain and spinal column; for the signals to pass, the receptor must be open. PCP closes the NMDA receptors by blocking them. This disconnection of neurons leads to loss of feeling and difficulty of moving. It affects a number of other neurotransmitters, including dopamine, serotonin, and norepinephrine.

PCP also causes CNS excitation via glutamate release at the presynaptic metabotropic receptors. A metabotropic receptor is an indirect receptor that initiates an intracellular biochemical cascade after it is triggered by an agonistic ligand.

Depending on the dosage, PCP can either excite or depress different areas of the brain to produce psychiatric and physical manifestations [8, 9].

Pharmacokinetics

In its pure form, phencyclidine is a white crystalline powder that dissolves easily in water or alcohol. Typically, it is sprayed onto leafy material, such as cannabis, mint, oregano, tobacco, parsley, or ginger leaves, and then smoked. As a liquid, it is clear, yellow, or tan. PCP is also mixed with dyes to produce colored powder, tablets, or capsules. It is often sold in vanilla extract bottles. It can be snorted or injected.

PCP is often mixed with crack, cocaine hydrochloride, and marijuana. Other drugs that may be combined with PCP include MDMA, formaldehyde, mescaline, ketamine, LSD, marijuana, and methamphetamine [1, 10].

PCP can quickly enter the bloodstream through smoking when it is sprinkled on tobacco, parsley, or mint. Marijuana cigarettes sometimes are dipped in a solution of PCP. PCP hydrochloride is usually insufflated. Because of an unpredictable response, it is rarely injected.

The onset of action and the length of time the effects last depend on the route of administration. When the powder form is snorted or smoked, the effects are felt within 2–5 min and last 4–6 h. PCP can be pressed into pills or put in capsules and swallowed. When ingested orally, effects are felt in 30–60 min and last 6–24 h. When PCP is injected, its time course of effects is similar to that of smoking [10].

PCP is a basic substance. As a result, it is better absorbed in the small intestine than in the acidic medium of the stomach. Its rate of excretion is increased in acidic urine. It is metabolized by the liver, and a small amount is excreted in the urine unchanged.

PCP that is excreted into the stomach from the blood is rapidly ionized by the stomach acid and trapped there because of the impermeability of membranes to ions. It again passes into the small intestine, where it reabsorbed. Thus, it is recirculated in the body. Regardless of its route of administration, PCP's gastric concentration may be several times its serum concentration.

PCP is lipophilic and therefore is rapidly removed from the blood and concentrated in adipose tissue and the brain. It remains in these storage sites for days to weeks. Therefore, blood and urine levels may be low while the effects of the drug persist [2, 5, 11, 12].

The most prominent pharmacological actions of phencyclidine are depression of the central nervous system and sympathetic actions. Variable cholinergic and anticholinergic effects also may occur [1, 12].

Chronic users sometimes binge, using PCP repeatedly for 2 or 3 days at a time without eating or sleeping. This is followed by a period of sleep. Flashbacks similar to those experienced by LSD users may occur [2, 10, 13].

Health Risks

Medical consequences of PCP intoxication can include acute tubular necrosis secondary to rhabdomyolysis, acute hepatic necrosis secondary to hyperpyrexia, aspiration pneumonia, high-output cardiac failure, pulmonary edema, hypertensive encephalopathy, intracranial hemorrhage, convulsions, coma, and death.

Physical harm can come from drowning (sometimes in shallow water), falls, automobile accidents, failure to flee fires and other imminent dangers, or self-inflicted injures. Deaths have been reported from accidental drowning, acute renal failure, disseminated intravascular coagulation, homicide, hyperthermia, leaping from tall buildings, motor vehicle accidents, violent episodes of self-mutilation, and suicide [13–18].

Tolerance

PCP use can lead to psychological dependence, craving, and drug-seeking behavior.

Dependence

Physical dependence to PCP probably occurs in humans. Experimental animals will administer it to themselves. The diagnosis of PCP dependence is based on the American Psychiatric Association's DSM criteria discussed in Chap. 1 [19].

Abstinence Syndrome

Upon abrupt discontinuation, physical distress, lack of energy, and depression have been reported. Long periods of use may lead to memory loss, difficulties with speech and thinking, depression, and weight loss. These can last up to a year after cessation of use (post-acute withdrawal syndrome) [7]. Nervousness, anxiety, and depression may occur. No medications are approved by the FDA to treat the PCP abstinence syndrome [2, 20].

Intoxication and Overdose

The signs and symptoms of PCP intoxication or overdose are related to its dose, route of administration, and the individual's response to the drug. Because the signs and symptoms vary greatly, trying to classify intoxication/overdose according to dosage is confusing and difficult. Dosage is rarely known or is impossible to determine. In many cases, patients are not even aware that PCP is the drug they took. Even when PCP blood levels can be measured, results are rarely available quickly enough to be of diagnostic or therapeutic value. For this reason, it is more helpful to divide PCP intoxication/overdose into stages based on the patient's signs and symptoms. As a rule, if patients are conscious their level is Stage I. If they are stuporous or mildly comatose, with active response to deep pain, their level is Stage II. Comatose patients with no response to deep pain are classified as Stage III [14, 21, 22].

Stage I (Intoxication)

Stage I generally corresponds to about 2–5 mg of ingested or smoked PCP and a serum concentration of 25–90 ng/ml [10].

Behavioral Manifestations The major manifestations of Stage I are behavioral. Patients are awake, and their behavior may be unpredictable. They may appear drunken and euphoric or they may be disoriented with alternating periods of lethargy and fearful agitation. They may have disorganized thoughts, and they can be combative and display sudden rage.

They misperceive distance and time and may feel dissociated from parts of their bodies. They may be catatonic and/or have stereotyped behavior, such as sucking, picking, and repetitive motor movements. They may stare blankly at their surroundings, appear to be unable to speak, or talk to themselves.

They may demonstrate echolalia (involuntary repetition of a word or phrase just spoken by another person) or hyperacusis (increased sense of hearing). They are usually unconcerned about their grooming. They may be socially uninhibited, obscene, and exhibit nudity.

PCP users' perception of imminent danger is impaired, and they may not flee from fires or avoid obvious danger. They have decreased perception of pain, and they may harm themselves with apparent lack of concern.

They may have delusion of invulnerability, may seem to possess inordinate strength, and may be without fear. They are capable of violent or self-destructive behavior. They have been known to set fire to themselves and stab or assault others.

Media reports of PCP-induced violence appear to be exaggerated. Incidents of violence are not common, and when they occur they are often limited to individuals with reputations for aggression regardless of drug use.

Symptomology may be indistinguishable from functional psychosis, paranoid schizophrenia, catatonia, or mania. Although visual, auditory, and tactile delusions may occur, patients seldom have true hallucinations [1, 11, 22, 23].

Physical Manifestations Physical manifestations of Stage I PCP intoxication include dysarthria, agitation, blunted pinprick response, ataxia, muscle rigidity, repetitive and purposeless movements, grimacing, and bruxism.

They may exhibit horizontal and even vertical nystagmus; blank stare; normal to mildly elevated temperature; mildly increased blood pressure and pulse rate; mildly increased respiratory rate, tidal volume, and minute ventilation; and clonus on deep tendon reflexes.

Autonomic signs include nausea, vomiting, diaphoresis, flushing, lacrimation, and hypersalivation [1, 11, 22, 24].

Stage II (Overdose)

Stage II usually results from 5 mg to 25 mg of ingested or inhaled PCP and a serum concentration of 90–300 ng/ml [13].

Behavioral Manifestations Because the prominent features of Stage II PCP overdose are stupor or a mildly comatose state, behavioral manifestations are not present [6].

Physical Manifestations Physical manifestations of Stage II include tonic-clonic seizures on stimulation, intact deep pain response, generalized muscle rigidity and twitching, nystagmus in any direction, roving eyes or fixed stare, and disconjugate gaze.

Blood pressure and pulse rate may be increased up to 25% above normal, respiratory rate may be increased up to 25% above normal, and deep tendon reflexes are further increased. Autonomic signs are also present, and vomiting may be protracted [1, 11, 13, 22, 24].

Stage III (Severe Overdose)

Stage III results from greater than 25 mg PCP ingested or injected and a serum level greater than 300 ng/ml [13].

Behavioral Manifestations Because the prominent feature of Stage III PCP severe overdose is deep coma, behavioral manifestations are not present [13].

Physical Manifestations Physical manifestations of Stage III include tonic-clonic seizures or status epilepticus; possible stroke; absent deep pain response; generalized myoclonic activity, opisthotonus, decerebrate posturing and muscle rigidity; nystagmus in any direction; open or closed eyes; increased pupillary size; disconjugate gaze; ptosis; and hippus (rhythmic contraction and dilation of the pupil).

Other findings may include hyperpyrexia with a temperature ranging from 103 °F to 108 °F, possible malignant hyperthermia, blood pressure and pulse rate increase as much as 100% above normal, spikes in blood pressure, and high-output cardiac failure [18].

Periodic breathing, apnea, aspiration pneumonia, and pulmonary edema may occur. Deep tendon reflexes are absent as are laryngeal/pharyngeal reflexes. The autonomic signs continue to be present. Rhabdomyolysis and cerebral hemorrhage have occurred [11, 14, 18].

Management

Management of PCP intoxication/overdose includes the use of general principles of drug intoxication or overdose, that is, controlling agitation or psychotic reactions, eliminating PCP from the body, treating muscle rigidity, managing medical complications, and treating hypertension, seizures, and hyperpyrexia. There is no antidote for PCP poisoning.

Level of consciousness should be assessed continually, and vital signs should be monitored closely in all stages of PCP intoxication/overdose. Blood and urine specimens should be obtained. If the patient is in a coma with a respiratory rate less than 12 breaths/min, a concomitant opioid overdose should be suspected and the patient be given naloxone (Narcan) 0.4 mg intravenously. In addition, the physician should consider giving 50 ml of 50% dextrose in water (D50W) to rule out hypoglycemia [2, 8, 17].

Laboratory Data

Other than drug screens if they can be rapidly obtained, other laboratory data are usually not helpful. An elevated WBC may be a nonspecific finding. When rhabdomyolysis occurs, creatine kinase (CK), aspartate aminotransferase (AST), and uric acid are elevated, and a urine analysis may indicate myoglobinuria. Liver enzymes may be elevated in the presence of acute liver necrosis. A blood glucose level should be obtained to rule out hypoglycemia. An EEG may be of diagnostic significance if it shows diffuse theta activity with periodic slow wave complexes.

A CT scan of the head should be considered to rule out an intracranial cause of altered mental status, and a lumbar puncture should be considered in patients with altered mental status and fever in whom the diagnosis is unclear [4].

Stage I (Intoxication)

Treatment of Stage I consists primarily of managing behavioral manifestations. External stimuli should be reduced whenever possible. Patients should be placed in a quiet room with minimal visual, auditory, and tactile stimuli. They may have hyperacusis, so treatment personnel should speak softly.

If a "talking down" strategy is not effective, or if the patient becomes more agitated, sometimes just leaving him alone may quiet him. If not, diazepam (Valium) in incremental intravenous doses of 2.5 mg given slowly at 10 min intervals up to a total of 25 mg is usually helpful. Cooperative patients can take the diazepam orally. If intramuscular injection is necessary, lorazepam (Ativan) in a 2–4 mg dose can be used. That said, benzodiazepines should be used with caution because they can delay the metabolism of PCP.

Psychosis is best treated with an antipsychotic medication, such as haloperidol (Haldol)

5–10 mg intramuscularly, but keep in mind that this may lower the seizure threshold.

Activated charcoal is usually not needed in Stage I. Urinary catheters, nasogastric tubes, and orotracheal intubation should be avoided if possible. Attempts to suction airways may precipitate laryngospasm, and so it should be avoided. Diphenhydramine (Benadryl) 50 mg intravenously may be given for localized dystonic reactions.

If symptoms continue to diminish with no cognitive impairment after 12 h, the patient may be discharged from the emergency department [5, 11, 17, 22–25].

Stage II (Overdose)

Stage II often requires admission to an intensive care unit from a few days to weeks, depending on the complications.

The patient's clothes should be removed, and sponging, ice packs, or fans should be used as necessary to encourage heat dissipation to try to avoid possible hyperthermic crisis. Because of the possibility of laryngospasm, deep oropharyngeal suctioning should be avoided when possible, but secretions should be gently suctioned orally as needed. Nasogastric and orotracheal tubes should be inserted only if absolutely necessary. Wheezing due to bronchospasm can be treated with an intravenous aminophylline infusion (250 mg over 20 min) if it's not possible for the patient to use an inhaled bronchodilator.

Some evidence suggests that restraints may lead to rhabdomyolysis and therefore should be used only when absolutely necessary. If restraints can't be avoided, totally immobilizing patients by rolling them in a sheet is probably the best method.

A continuous infusion of 5% dextrose in a Lactated Ringer's Solution (D5LR) should be started. Hypertension and tachycardia can be controlled by intravenous titration of a beta-blocker, such as labetalol 0.5–2 mg/min. Alternatively, hypertension can be controlled by hydralazine 10 mg slow intravenous bolus (maximum dose 20 mg) every 4–6 h as needed.

Since acute urinary retention may occur, a urinary catheter should be placed. A urine sample should be sent to a laboratory for analysis for myoglobin. Blood for blood gases, electrolytes, creatine kinase (CK), aspartate aminotransferase (AST), alanine aminotransferase (ALT), BUN, creatinine, and uric acid should be obtained and sent for analysis.

Urinary excretion of PCP may be enhanced by acidification of the urine to a pH of 5.0–5.5. This can be done by intravenous infusion of ascorbic acid 0.5–1.5 gm every 4–6 h as required. Acidification of the urine is contraindicated in the presence of myoglobinuria. Furosemide (Lasix) 20–40 mg intravenously at 6 h intervals can increase urinary output and hasten PCP excretion.

Extreme muscle rigidity not responsive to diazepam, especially in the face of rhabdomyolysis, may require neuromuscular blockade and mechanical ventilation [5, 16–18, 22].

Stage III (Severe Overdose)

In Stage III, intravenous fluids should be initiated, a urinary catheter inserted, and urinary output monitored as in Stage II. Orotracheal intubation should be performed. In this stage, vigorous tracheobronchial suctioning is indicated. A large bore gastric tube should be placed and gastric contents suctioned and saved for analysis. If the PCP was ingested within the past hour, activated charcoal 50–150 gm may be instilled into the stomach.

A nasogastric tube can be placed and connected to continuous suction to remove PCP secreted into the stomach from the bloodstream. Because of the possibility of electrolyte abnormalities with continuous suction, some prefer an alternate approach—putting 30–40 gm of activated charcoal in the stomach every 6–8 h to bind the PCP.

In the absence of contraindications, urinary acidification should be instituted, and furosemide should be given as in Stage II. Strict attention should be paid to the patient's core temperature, and measures should be instituted to control it when necessary.

Hypertension and tachycardia can be controlled by intravenous titration of a beta-blocker such as labetalol 0.5–2 mg/min. Alternatively, hypertension can be controlled by hydralazine 10 mg slow intravenous bolus (maximum dose 20 mg) every 4–6 h as needed.

Status epilepticus, should it occur, usually can be effectively treated with diazepam 5–10 mg slow IV push up to a total of 30 mg. Similarly, extreme muscle rigidity not responsive to diazepam may also require neuromuscular blockade and mechanical ventilation. Dialysis has been shown to be ineffective in removing PCP from the body.

Not only may PCP overdose be life threatening, but PCP itself tends to be the longest acting of any psychoactive substance. The entire picture may take up to 6 weeks to clear [5, 11, 17, 22, 25].

Differential Diagnosis

PCP intoxication can easily be confused with stimulant (amphetamine, cocaine) or hallucinogen (LSD, mescaline) intoxication and with psychotic states such as paranoid schizophrenia and catatonia or bipolar disorder. A drug screen may be the only way distinctions can be made.

Stimulants often cause severe tachycardia, hypertension, tremulousness, and hyperthermia, but are not associated with the increased muscle tone that PCP produces. In addition, the presence of nystagmus rules out stimulants. Frank hallucinations are more characteristic of hallucinogenic drugs. Fear (panic reactions) can occur with stimulant, hallucinogenic, and marijuana use as well as with PCP use.

Coma can result from a variety of central nervous system insults, including trauma, metabolic disturbances, and drug overdoses. The characteristic muscle rigidity of PCP overdose, coupled with tachycardia and hypertension, may be helpful with the diagnosis. Depressant drugs tend to lower pulse rate and blood pressure, whereas PCP raises them [21].

Polydrug Use

Patients often use other drugs in addition to PCP, and this always poses a problem. Drugs used together do not always act in the same fashion as each drug does when taken alone. Some drugs may enhance one another's effects, while other drugs may partially cancel some effects. For example, when drugs that depress the central nervous system (alcohol, barbiturates, benzodiazepines, opioids) are combined with PCP, vital signs that may be increased by PCP alone may be somewhat lower than expected. In addition, some symptoms of PCP intoxication, such as increased vital signs, ataxia, vomiting, and seizures, may be misinterpreted as part of an alcohol or solid sedative/hypnotic abstinence syndrome [25].

Emergence Phenomena

Physicians should remember that when patients emerge from one level of overdose to the next lowest level, they will exhibit the signs and symptoms of that stage. For example, patients emerging from Stage II may become violent or self-destructive as they enter Stage I if appropriate measures are not taken [22, 26].

Ketamine

Ketamine (Ketalar) is used as an intravenous surgery anesthetic for humans and animals. Much of the ketamine sold on the streets comes from veterinary offices. A recent study showed that ketamine successfully treated symptoms in patients with severe depression who had not responded to antidepressant medications. It was classified as a DEA Schedule III controlled substance in 1999 [27, 28].

Prevalence of Use

Ketamine is primarily a drug used by young people, generally less than 25 years of age. In 2011, the reported annual prevalence of ketamine use in grades 8, 10, and 12 was 0.8%, 1.2%, and 1.7%, respectively. In 2015, lifetime use of ketamine by high school seniors was reported at 1.5% [29].

Street Names

Street names for ketamine include:

Special K K Kit kat	Cat Valium Super C	Purple Green	Vitamin K Super acid

Pharmacology

Pharmacodynamics

Ketamine is pharmacologically similar to PCP. Like PCP, ketamine has activity at N-methyl-D-aspartate (NMDA) receptors. Relative to PCP, ketamine is less potent as an anesthetic and has a faster onset and shorter duration of action. Upon emergence from anesthesia, it produces changes in mood, body image, and hallucination but to a much lesser extent than PCP [30].

Pharmacokinetics

As a human anesthetic, it is used most often in children who appear less susceptible than adults to emergent delirium. In medical settings, it is injected intravenously or intramuscularly depending on its clinical use.

As an illicit drug, ketamine is insufflated, smoked, injected, or taken orally. It comes as a liquid and a white powder. Most oral users of ketamine take an average dose of 100 mg.

Over the past few years, ketamine has become popular as a club drug, most commonly encountered at nightclubs and raves. It also has gained a reputation as a date rape drug. Illicit ketamine has the perception among users as being medically safe to use because it is made and packaged by pharmaceutical companies, although most often for veterinary use.

Ketamine is typically used with other drugs; however, sole use of ketamine does occur. The effects from injection generally take between 1 min and 5 min, the effects from snorted ketamine between 5 min and 15 min, and the effects from oral ingestion between 5 min and 30 min. The hallucinatory effects of ketamine last 1 h or less, but the user's senses, judgment, and coordination may be affected for up to 24 h. Euphoria and hallucinosis peak effects occur in roughly 2.5 h. Doses of ketamine as large as 900–1000 mg given intravenously or intramuscularly are lethal.

Although ketamine is often self-administered by insufflation, studies suggest an emerging problem of young people injecting it. These young people may be more likely to engage in multiple injections, share bottles of ketamine, and use syringes obtained from secondary sources—practices that increase risk for hepatitis C, HIV, and other infectious diseases [31].

Ketamine induces coma in a dose-dependent manner. The clinical effects of ketamine are similar to PCP.

Health Effects

Short Term

In the short term, ketamine causes problems with attention, learning, and memory. It also causes dreamlike states, hallucinations, sedation, confusion, speaking problems, loss of memory, and moving problems progressing to becoming immobile. Raised blood pressure, unconsciousness, and slowed breathing can occur. Overdose can cause death [32].

Long Term

Ketamine dependence can causes long-term damage to the bladder and urinary tract that can result in a condition known as ketamine bladder syndrome. The syndrome may cause ulcers in the bladder, blood in the urine, and incontinence. Ketamine can also cause kidney problems, stomach pain, and depression [32].

Tolerance, Dependence, and Abstinence Syndrome

Evidence supports the potential for tolerance and physical dependence. A common feature of ketamine dependence is that of repeated binges in which the user indulges in excessive amounts of the drug over a short period of time.

Large doses of ketamine may produce what users refer to as a *K-hole*. A K-hole is generally reached when the user is on the brink of being fully sedated and is likened to an out-of-body or near-death experience [33].

Ketamine abstinence syndrome is similar to that of PCP. There are no FDA-approved medications to treat addiction to ketamine dependence.

Intoxication and Overdose

Intoxication and overdose symptoms are similar to those of PCP, only much milder. Treatment uses many of the same principles.

Dextromethorphan

Dextromethorphan (DXM) is a synthetic analog of codeine. More than 120 DXM-containing products are available to consumers. When the recommended dose is taken, DXM has few adverse side effects. It has a long history of safety and effectiveness.

In 2010, the FDA approved the combination product dextromethorphan and quinidine for the treatment of pseudobulbar affect, whose main symptom is emotional lability [34].

Street Names

Street names for DXM include:

Dex Robo	Skittles Triple C	Tussin

Illicit use of DXM is referred to on the street as "*Robo-tripping*" or "*skittling*." These terms are derived from the most commonly abused products, Robitussin and Coricidin.

Pharmacology

Legal users consuming DXM-containing cough syrups (such as Robitussin) for medical reasons typically ingest 10–20 mg every 4–6 h or 30 mg every 6–8 h. On the other hand, a single dose for recreational users can range from 240 to 1500 mg. Heavier users have been known to ingest up to three or four bottles a day.

In addition to the legal forms, there is evidence that DXM is being sold over the Internet in powder, capsule, and pill forms. These are snorted or ingested orally. Powders and pills have an effect similar to syrups without the need to consume large quantities of the substance in a short time period. DXM can be associated with psychosis at doses of 300–600 mg. Serotonin syndrome has also been reported [34].

Health Risks

High doses of dextromethorphan can cause impaired vision, sweating, rapid breathing, tachycardia, elevated blood pressure, dysrhythmias, nausea and vomiting, and diarrhea. They also can cause slurred speech, impaired judgment, memory loss, rapid eye movements, hallucinations, dissociative effects, and coma.

Users often abuse DXM in combination with other drugs. The interaction between DXM and other substances (alcohol, ecstasy, and other OTC cough medicines) produces a synergistic effect that can be dangerous. Ingredients of cough medicines other than DXM, like acetaminophen, are hazardous when consumed in high doses and can cause liver damage.

DXM can be found in the form of a bromide salt, which can lead to bromide poisoning if large quantities are taken. Bromide poisoning is manifested by behavior changes, headaches, apathy, irritation, slurred speech, psychosis, tremors, ataxia, hallucinations, weight loss, can-like rash, and coma.

Abuse can cause serious adverse events, such as heart attack, seizure, loss of consciousness, irregular heartbeat, stroke, and even death. Serotonin syndrome has been reported [35].

Tolerance, Dependence, and Abstinence Syndrome

When it is abused regularly, DXM can actually cause some of the symptoms (insomnia and dysphoria) that it is designed to treat. In addition, high-dose chronic use of DXM can lead to the development of toxic psychosis, as well as other physiological and behavioral problems.

It is not known what effect frequent use of low-dose DXM has on the user, although anecdotal reports include moderate physical dependence and tolerance. Withdrawal symptoms include anxiety, restlessness, insomnia, diarrhea, vomiting, severe weight loss, and upset stomach [34].

Overdose

Symptoms

Overdose symptoms include jerky muscle movements of the extremities, nausea, vomiting, dizziness, and unsteadiness. It can also cause changes in vision, tachycardia, hot flashes, seizures, difficulty breathing, hallucination, and coma. It can cause disassociation from the body. Additional ingredients (decongestants, antihistamines, acetaminophen, bromides) can cause other problems [36].

Treatment

Activated charcoal can be given to patients who have overdosed on dextromethorphan in the past hour. Intravenous fluids should be given as indicated. For patients who are sedated or comatose, naloxone in the usual doses for opioid overdose can be given intravenously. An intravenous benzodiazepine can be given for seizures, and external cooling measures can be used for hypothermia that may result from serotonin syndrome [36].

Summary

Dissociative drugs cause a disconnection between thoughts, identity, consciousness, and memory. They distort the user's perception of sight and sound and produce feelings of detachment from the environment and one's self. Phencyclidine (PCP) is a central nervous system depressant introduced as an anesthetic in the early 1950s but later abandoned because of unpredictable side effects such as agitation, disorientation, and hallucinations.

Medical consequences of PCP intoxication can include acute tubular necrosis secondary to rhabdomyolysis, acute hepatic necrosis secondary to hyperpyrexia, aspiration pneumonia, high-output cardiac failure, pulmonary edema, hypertensive encephalopathy, intracranial hemorrhage, convulsions, coma, and death. Physical dependence to PCP probably occurs in humans. Experimental animals will administer it to themselves. Upon abrupt discontinuation of PCP, physical distress, lack of energy, and depression have been reported. Long periods of use may lead to memory loss, difficulties with speech and thinking, depression, and weight loss.

The signs and symptoms of PCP intoxication or overdose are related to its dose, route of administration, and the individual's response to the drug.

Much of the ketamine sold on the streets comes from veterinary offices. Large doses of ketamine may produce what users refer to as a "*K-hole*." A K-hole is generally reached when the user is on the brink of being fully sedated and is likened to an out-of-body or near-death experience.

Illicit use of DXM is referred to on the street as "robo-tripping" or "skittling." These terms are derived from the most commonly abused products, Robitussin and Coricidin. In addition to the legal forms, there is evidence that DXM is being sold over the Internet in powder, capsule, and pill forms.

References

1. Aniline O, Pitts FN Jr. Phencyclidine (PCP): a review and perspectives. CRC Crit Rev Toxicol. 1982;10:145–77.
2. Miller NS, Gold MS, Millman R. PCP: a dangerous drug. Am Fam Physician. 1988;38(3):215–8.
3. Robinson B, Yates A. Angel dust: medical and psychiatric aspects of phencyclidine intoxication. Ariz Med. 1984;41:808–11.
4. Young T, Lawson GW, Gacono CB. Clinical aspects of phencyclidine (PCP). Int J Addict. 1987;22:1–15.
5. Woolf DS, Vourakis C, Bennett G. Guidelines for management of acute phencyclidine intoxication. Crit Care Update. 1980;7:16–24.

6. National survey on drug use and health: trends in prevalence of various drugs for ages 12 or older, ages 12 to 17, ages 18 to 25, and ages 26 or older. National Institute on Drug Abuse (NIDA). 2015. https://www.drugabuse.gov/national-survey-drug-use-health
7. Alexander B. Return of angel dust? ERs see spike in PCP, synthetic drugs. NBC News. http://www.nbcnews.com/health/health-news/return-angel-dust-ers-see-spike-pcp-synthetic-drugs-f2D11674428. December 3, 2013.
8. Johnson KM. Neurochemistry and neurophysiology of phencyclidine. In: Meltzer HY, editor. Psychopharmacology. 3rd ed. New York: Raven Press; 1987. p. 573–1579.
9. Koek W. N-methyl D-aspartate antagonists and drug discrimination. Pharmacol Biochem Behav. 1999;64(2):275–81.
10. Phencyclidine (PCP). Center for Substance Abuse Research (CESAR)/University of Maryland. http://www.cesar.umd.edu/cesar/drugs/pcp.asp
11. Aronow JN, Miceli JN, Done AK. A therapeutic approach to the acutely overdosed PCP patient. J Psychedelic Drugs. 1980;12:259–67.
12. Davis BL. The PCP epidemic: a critical review. Int J Addict. 1982;17:1137–55.
13. Milhorn HT. Diagnosis and management of phencyclidine intoxication. Am Fam Physician. 1991;43(4):1293–30.
14. Armen R, Kanel G, Reynolds T. Phencyclidine-induced malignant hyperthermia causing submassive liver necrosis. Am J Med. 1984;77:167–72.
15. Bessen HA. Intercranial hemorrhage associated with phencyclidine abuse. J Am Med Assoc. 1982;248:585–6.
16. Giannini AJ, Eighan MS, Loiselle RH, Giannini MC. Comparison of haloperidol and chlorpromazine in the treatment of phencyclidine psychosis. J Clin Pharmacol. 1984;24:202–4.
17. McCarron MM, Schulze BW, Thompson GA, Condor MC, Goetz WA. Acute phencyclidine intoxication: clinical patterns, complications, and treatment. Ann Emerg Med. 1981;10:290–7.
18. Patel R, Connor G, Drew CR. A review of thirty cases of rhabdomyolysis associated renal failure among phencyclidine users. Clin Toxicol. 1986;23:547–56.
19. Phencyclidine (PCP). Drugs and human performance fact sheets. National Highway Traffic Safety Administration. https://one.nhtsa.gov/people/injury/research/job185drugs/phencyclidine.htm
20. Balster RL. In: Meltzer HY, editor. The behavioral pharmacology of phencyclidine. Psychopharmacology: the third generation of progress. New York: Raven Press; 1987. p. 581–1587.
21. Gibson MS. Phencyclidine intoxication. Ear Nose Throat J. 1983;62:75–80.
22. Rappolt RT, Gay GR, Farris RD. Phencyclidine (PCP) intoxication: diagnosis in stages and algorithms of treatment. Clin Toxicol. 1980;16:509–29.
23. Done AK, Aronow R, Miceli JN. Pharmacokinetic bases for the diagnosis and treatment of acute PCP intoxication. J Psychedelic Drugs. 1980;12:253–8.
24. Pearlson GD. Psychiatric and medical syndromes associated with phencyclidine (PCP) abuse. Johns Hopkins Med J. 1981;148:25–33.
25. Shuckit MA. Drug and alcohol abuse: a clinical guide to diagnosis and treatment. New York: Plenum Press; 1984. p. 152–60.
26. Milhorn HT. Phencyclidine overdose: a case report. J Miss State Med Assoc. 1990;31:37–40.
27. Castillo M. Ketamine may be quick, effective treatment for untreatable depression. CBS News. http://www.cbsnews.com/news/ketamine-may-be-quick-effective-treatment-for-untreatable-depression. May 20, 2013.
28. Date rape drugs fact sheet. WomensHealth. https://www.womenshealth.gov/publications/our-publications/fact-sheet/date-rape-drugs.html#a. July 16, 2012.
29. Witmer D. What parents should know about teen use of the drug special K, VeryWell. https://www.verywell.com/ketamine-drug-use-statistics-and-facts-among-teens-3963099. September 03, 2016.
30. Ketamine. Ketamine has activity at N-methyl-d-aspartate (NMDA) receptors. Drug Enforcement Administration (DEA). https://www.deadiversion.usdoj.gov/drug_chem_info/ketamine.pdf
31. Mathias R. Study suggests ketamine injection poses new disease risk for street youths. National Institute on Drug Abuse (NIDA). https://archives.drugabuse.gov/NIDA_Notes/NNVol18N4/Study.html. November 2003; 18(4).
32. Anderson L. Ketamine. Drugs.com. https://www.drugs.com/illicit/ketamine.html. May 18, 2014.
33. Ketamine. Center for Substance Abuse Research (CESAR)/University of Maryland. http://www.cesar.umd.edu/cesar/drugs/ketamine.asp
34. Dextromethorphan (DXM). Center for Substance Abuse Research (CESAR)/University of Maryland. http://www.cesar.umd.edu/cesar/drugs/dxm.asp
35. Dextromethorphan. Office of Alcoholism and Substance Abuse Services (OASAS). http://www.oasas.ny.gov/AdMed/FYI/dmx.cfm
36. Dextromethorphan overdose. MedlinePlus. https://medlineplus.gov/ency/article/002628.htm. October 15, 2015.

11 Inhalant Dependence

Key Chapter Points

- The inhalant drugs are volatile solvents and aerosols, gases, and nitrites.
- Adolescent males most commonly use solvents and aerosols recreationally because they have easy access to many common household products.
- Solvents and aerosols are highly lipid soluble; they easily cross the alveolar membrane of the lungs and of the blood-brain barrier to reach high concentrations in the brain.
- Sudden sniffing death syndrome is an event in which the heart beats quickly and irregularly and then suddenly stops. Physicians should strongly suspect solvent and aerosol abuse in the setting of sudden collapse during adolescent group activities.
- Nitrous oxide is a gas that is usually used in combination with a potent halogenated inhalational anesthetic, along with oxygen, to produce general anesthesia for surgery.
- Nitrous oxide overdose symptoms include light-headedness; confusion; cough and/or wheezing; eye, nose, or throat irritation; dyspnea; chest tightness; cheat pain; diaphoresis; and blue in the lips, fingers, or toes. In severe cases, loss of consciousness, coma, and death may occur.
- The three alkyl nitrites of abuse importance in primary care medicine are amyl nitrite, butyl nitrite, and cyclohexyl nitrite.
- Taking Viagra with nitrites can cause a serious decrease in blood pressure, leading to fainting, stroke, or myocardial infarction.

Many products readily found in the home or workplace, such as spray paints, glues, and cleaning fluids, contain volatile substances that have psychoactive properties when inhaled. Inhalants also include gases, such as ether and nitrous oxide, and alkyl nitrites, such as amyl and butyl nitrite. These substances are used at room temperature by volatilization or from a pressurized container and do not include drugs that are sniffed after burning or heating, such as crack cocaine [1].

Prevalence of Use

Prevalence of use of inhalants in 2015 by age range is given in Table 11.1 [2].

The Inhalant Drugs

Inhalants fall into one of the four categories [3]:

1. *Volatile solvents.* Volatile solvents are liquids that become gases at room temperature. They are found in numerous household cleaning products and industrial items.
2. *Aerosols.* Aerosols are sprays that contain propellants and solvents. They include spray

H.T. Milhorn, *Substance Use Disorders*, DOI 10.1007/978-3-319-63040-3_11

   paint, hair spray, and various other types of sprays.
3. *Gases*. Gases may be in household or commercial products or used in the medical field as anesthetics. These include butane lighter fluid, ether, and nitrous oxide.
4. *Nitrites*. Nitrites primarily act to dilate blood vessels and relax the muscles. These are used mainly to enhance sexual experiences. The two most commonly abused nitrites are amyl nitrite and butyl nitrite.

There are more than 3000 products containing volatile chemicals that are legal and readily obtained, easy to purchase, easy to conceal, and are found in every household or garage [4]. Some inhalants are given in Table 11.2.

Solvents and Aerosols

Adolescent males most commonly use solvents and aerosols recreationally because they have easy access to many common household products and do not have access to more conventional drugs. Some of these are shown in Fig. 11.1 [5].

Table 11.1 Prevalence of use of inhalants in 2015 by age range (%) (From [2])

	Ages 12–17	Ages 18–25	Ages 26 or older
Lifetime	9.10	13.10	9.60
Past year	2.70	4.10	0.30
Past month	0.70	0.90	0.10

Most users inhale either directly from a bottle or can that contains a solvent, from a solvent-soaked rag, or from a mist produced by an aerosol spray. Another method, known as "bagging," involves placing a piece of cotton or a rag soaked with solvent in the bottom of a paper bag. The bag is then placed over the mouth and nose and inhaled from. Solvent and aerosol inhalation is *known as huffing*. *Dusting* is inhaling vapors directly from electronic equipment cleaning aerosols. *Sniffing* or *snorting* involves inhaling spray fumes directly from an aerosol container [4, 6].

Although inhalants are not regulated under the Controlled Substances Act, most states have placed restrictions on the sale and distribution to minors of certain products that are commonly abused as inhalants.

Pharmacology

Solvents and aerosols are highly lipid soluble; they easily cross the alveolar membrane of the lungs and of the blood-brain barrier to reach high concentrations in the brain. Inhalation avoids first-pass hepatic metabolism, so the onset is fast.

The inhaled concentration depends on the mode of administration. With sniffing, onset occurs in a few seconds, with a peak plasma concentration 15–30 min after inhalation. The effects last a few minutes to an hour, depending on the substance and the dosage. Sniffing gives the lowest blood concentration, followed by huffing. Bagging gives the highest blood concentration.

Table 11.2 Some inhalants (Based on [5])

Volatile solvents	Aerosols	Gases	Nitrites
Correction fluid (White Out) Electronic contact cleaner Felt-tip marker fluid Paint thinner Nail polish remover Degreaser Dry cleaning fluid Gasoline Contact cement Rubber cement	Deodorant spray Fabric protector spray Hair spray Spray paint	Nitrous oxide Ether Butane lighters Propane tanks Refrigerant gases	Amyl nitrite Butyl nitrite Cyclohexyl nitrite

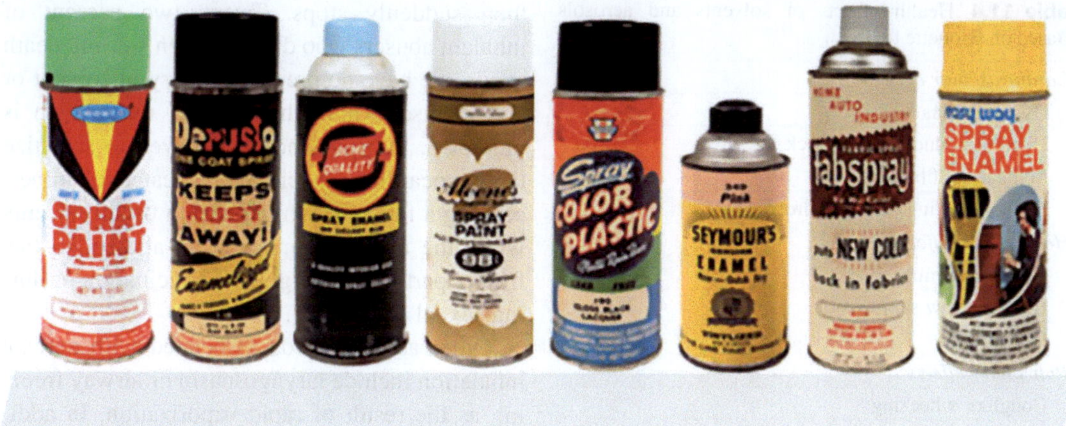

Fig. 11.1 Some common solvents and aerosols

Table 11.3 Hazardous chemicals in commonly abused solvents and aerosols (From [7]; Approved with permission, Williams & Wilkins)

Chemical	Inhalant
Toluene	Paint thinner, spray paint, airplane glue, rubber cement, nail polish remover, shoe polish
Butane	Lighter fluid, fuel, spray paint, hair spray, room freshener, deodorants
Fluorocarbons	Asthma sprays, analgesic sprays, spray paint, hair spray, deodorants, room fresheners
Chlorinated hydrocarbons	Dry-cleaning agents, spot removers, degreasers, correction fluid
Acetone	Nail polish remover, rubber cement, permanent markers

Elimination from the body occurs primarily through the lungs, with many inhaled compounds eliminated unchanged by exhalation. Most solvents and aerosols leave the body quickly, but others remain for a long time because they are absorbed by fatty tissues, including the brain and spinal cord.

Solvents and aerosols usually are not detected with urine or blood drug screening tests for two reasons: (1) inhalants are not included in the usual drug screen and (2) many of them have been eliminated from the body by the time a specific test is done.

Because the high lasts only a few minutes, users often try to make the feeling last longer by inhaling repeatedly over several hours. Inhalants often contain more than one chemical [4, 6].

Hazardous chemical substances in commonly abused solvents and aerosols are given in Table 11.3.

Symptoms of Solvent and Aerosol Intoxication

Symptoms of solvent and aerosol intoxication are similar to those of alcohol, and consist of confusion, disorientation, euphoria, sedation, lowered inhibitions, and incoordination. They also include psychomotor retardation, slurred speech, and unsteady gait [6].

Health Risks

Health effects of abusing solvents and aerosols are given in Table 11.4 [7]. Some damage may not be reversible.

Long-term use of solvents and aerosols also can cause bone marrow damage, hearing loss, and nerve problems, such as numbness, tingling of the hands and feet, and tremors [5].

Sudden sniffing death syndrome is an event in which the heart beats quickly and irregularly and

Table 11.4 Health effects of solvents and aerosols (Based on Brouette [8])

Cardiovascular effects
Dysrhythmias
Hypoxia-induced heart block
Myocardial fibrosis
Sudden sniffing death syndrome
Hematologic effects
Aplastic anemia
Bone marrow suppression
Leukemia
Pulmonary effects
Cough or wheezing
Dyspnea
Emphysema
Goodpasture's syndrome
Pneumonitis
Dermatologic effects
Burns
Contact dermatitis
Perioral eczema
Neurological effects
Ataxia
Cerebellar degeneration
Change in speech
Nystagmus
Peripheral neuropathy
Sensorimotor polyneuropathy
Tremor
White matter degeneration
Gastrointestinal effects
Hepatotoxicity
Nausea or vomiting
Neuropsychiatric effects
Apathy
Dementia
Depression
Insomnia
Memory loss
Poor attention
Psychosis
Renal effects
Acid-base disturbance
Acute renal failure
Fanconi's syndrome
Renal tubular acidosis

then suddenly stops. Twenty-two percent of inhalant abusers who die of sudden sniffing death syndrome have no previous history of solvent or aerosol use. Although the exact mechanism is unknown, the substance is believed to sensitize the myocardium to circulating catecholamines, causing a fatal arrhythmia. Death usually occurs while the user is running in an attempt to flee from a particularly frightful hallucination or during sexual activity [8].

Other acute hazards associated with aerosol inhalation include laryngospasm or airway freezing as the result of rapid vaporization. In addition, Freon can block oxygen diffusion at the pulmonary membrane.

Asphyxiation can result from the displacement of oxygen in the lungs by prolonged or repeated inhalations. Suffocation can occur if a plastic bag is placed over the head to enhance inhaling fumes and the user becomes unconscious. Suffocation also has occurred when the user loses consciousness and falls face down on a cloth containing the solvent. Death can occur because of complications of the intoxication, such as choking on aspirated gastric contents.

Fire-related injuries from inhalant combustion or fatal injuries suffered as a result of high-risk behaviors can occur [4, 6].

Deaths have even occurred from sniffing typewriter correction fluid (Liquid Paper) [8]. Some of the findings on presentation of solvent and aerosol users are given in Table 11.5.

Tolerance and Dependence

Physical dependence to solvents and aerosol with regular and prolonged inhalation can occur. Psychological dependence is common. Tolerance is known to occur [6].

Abstinence Syndrome

Solvent and aerosol withdrawal symptoms are similar to those of alcohol. They include anxiety, agitation, elevated blood pressure and body tem-

Table 11.5 Solvent and aerosol use clinical presentation (Based on Jauch [4])

Skin	
Paint or stains on the face, hands, or clothing Huffer rash—erythematous "frost bite" eruption on the face and oral mucosa caused by severe drying and cracking of the skin and resultant bacterial infection	Thermal or chemical burns on the face or hands Conjunctival injection Jaundice (with chronic hepatic injury) Cyanosis (with methemoglobinemia)
Respiratory	
Chemical odor in the breath Wheezing, rhonchi, or rales Oral or airway burns	Rhinitis Respiratory distress with aspiration of gastric contents
Neurologic/psychiatric	
Slurred speech Diplopia Blurred vision Nystagmus Euphoria Psychomotor retardation Disorientation Sense of invulnerability Distortion of space and time	Auditory or visual hallucinations with paranoid ideations Photophobia Weakness Impaired memory Peripheral neuropathy (typically stocking-glove distribution) Seizures Agitated coma
Cardiovascular	
Arrhythmias, including premature ventricular contractions (PVCs) or supraventricular tachycardia (SVT)	Tachycardia or bradycardia Hypotension
Gastrointestinal tract	
Nausea and vomiting Diarrhea Flank pain (suspect renal injury in chronic abusers)	Abdominal pain (suspect hepatic injury if the pain is in the right upper quadrant, especially in a chronic abuser)

perature, headache, tremor, and impaired concentration, memory, and judgment. They also include irritability, nausea and vomiting, restlessness, tachycardia, and visual disturbances. In severe cases, these may progress to psychosis and seizures [9].

Overdose

Symptoms

Physicians should strongly suspect solvent and aerosol abuse in the setting of sudden collapse during adolescent group activities. Family or friends may report empty chemical or spray containers found at the scene. Chemical-soaked rags or clothes may be found. Strange smells may have been present at the time of the collapse. Sometimes co-ingestion occurs, suggested by pill bottles found at the scene.

With acute intoxication, neurologic, cardiac, and pulmonary symptoms predominate. Acute neurologic symptoms resemble alcohol intoxication and include euphoria, slurred speech, ataxia, dizziness, diplopia, confusion, and CNS depression. Other effects may include headache, vertigo, auditory and visual hallucinations, seizures, stupor, and coma.

Acute cardiac effects include heart palpitations and tachycardia. Respiratory effects include dyspnea, wheezing, and coughing. Asphyxiation and direct lung damage due to pneumonitis may occur. Most symptoms resolve within 2 h [4, 10].

Laboratory Studies

The laboratory workup depends on the severity of the illness [8]. For moderate to severe intoxication, pulse oximetry should be done to assess for oxygenation impairment. Chest radiography helps identify the etiology of respiratory difficulties associated with inhalant abuse, such as pneumothorax, aspiration pneumonia, or chemical pneumonitis. Cardiopulmonary monitoring is recommended because of the risk of apnea and cardiac arrest after acute exposure.

Serum chemistry should include sodium, potassium, chloride, bicarbonate, BUN, creatinine, and CBC.

Inhalants that contain toluene, such as paint thinner, airplane glue, rubber cement, and nail polish, cause distal renal tubular acidosis, with a resultant elevated anion gap, hyperchloremia, hypokalemia, and hypophosphatemia. Hyaline casts, elevated white blood cell counts, elevated red blood cell counts, or abnormal glucose and protein levels in the urine may suggest renal injury.

Azotemia also is common with chronic exposure but resolves with abstinence. Hypoglycemia may occur. Pregnancy testing should be done in all solvent-abusing females.

Chronic users may exhibit bone marrow suppression, thrombocytopenia, and aplastic anemia.

Elevated urobilinogen suggests hepatic involvement. Creatine kinase is useful in patients with muscle tenderness or myoglobinuria to evaluate for the presence of rhabdomyolysis.

Chronic abusers might exhibit cardiomegaly and pulmonary edema. They may show signs of cerebral or cerebellar atrophy on CT scan. Significant acidosis, hypoxemia, or hypercarbia might indicate the need for intubation.

Many inhalants are proarrhythmic; therefore, acutely intoxicated patients should have continuous ECG monitoring. The ECG often shows tachycardia, bradycardia, arrhythmias, or cardiac ischemia.

Methylene chloride found in paint stripper can cause carboxyhemoglobin formation, so this should be checked for [4].

Chronic gasoline sniffing formerly was associated with lead poisoning, but the advent of the catalytic converted spelled the death of leaded gasoline [11, 12].

Specific toxicologic tests of inhalant agents are not readily available in all laboratories and may take several days to weeks to get results, so they are not helpful in the immediate diagnosis [4].

Treatment

For most patients, treatment is supportive. Beta blockers can be administered early to protect the catecholamine-sensitized heart. Acid-base and metabolic disturbances should be corrected. One-hundred percent oxygen is indicated in the presence of carboxyhemoglobin.

Many acute neurologic findings are reversible after cessation of inhalants, but some neurologic sequelae (dementia, cerebral or cerebellar dysfunction) may be permanent and difficult to manage.

Long-term solvent and aerosol users should be referred to an addictionist at a treatment center for evaluation and treatment [4].

Gases

Nitrous Oxide

Nitrous oxide is a gas that is usually used in combination with a potent halogenated inhalational anesthetic, along with oxygen, to produce general anesthesia for surgery. It has been used in the past for pain relief during childbirth and it is used by dentists. It is used as an oxidizer in rocketry and in motor racing to increase the power output of engines and used as the propellant in whip cream canisters. The propellants for whip cream canisters are called *whippets* (Fig. 11.2). Nitrous oxide is abused for its euphoric effect.

In the United States, possession of nitrous oxide is legal under federal law and is not subject to DEA purview. It is, however, regulated by the Food and Drug Administration. Anyone over the age of 18 can legally purchase the gas in large tanks or in the small canisters intended for food-related use. Prosecution is possible under the "misbranding" clause, prohibiting the sale or distribution of nitrous oxide for the purpose of human consumption [6].

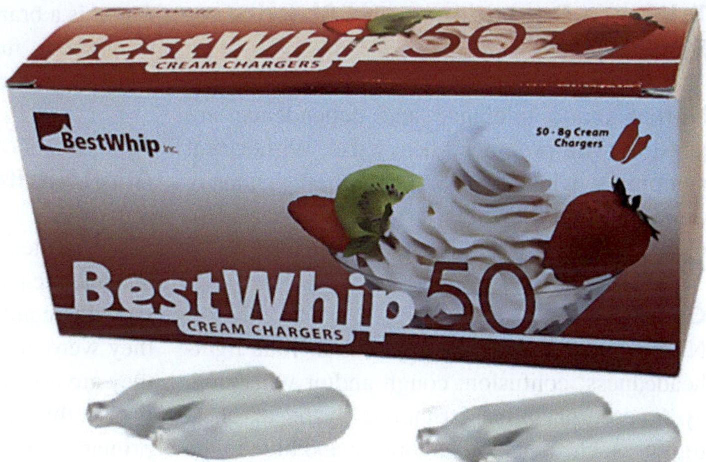

Fig. 11.2 Whippets

Street Names

Street names for nitrous oxide include laughing gas, whippets, buzz bomb, hippy crack, and NOX (nitrous oxide plus MDMA).

Pharmacology

At room temperature, nitrous oxide is a colorless, nonflammable gas with a slightly sweet odor and taste. When inhaled, it rapidly dissolves into the bloodstream and arrives at the brain in a matter of seconds. Its onset of action is in 2–3 min, and it has a duration of 3–5 min. A concentration of nitrous oxide in oxygen less than 50% produces sedation. In a concentration of 50–75%, it causes analgesia.

When used as an anesthetic, breathing 70% nitrous oxide will achieve 90% saturation of tissues within 15 min. It is excreted unchanged by the lungs. After completion of the surgery or dentistry procedure, the nitrous oxide is washed out of the body by inhalation of 100% oxygen over 5 min.

Nitrous oxide has little effect on the respiratory, gastrointestinal, muscular, and renal systems. It has mixed effects on the cardiovascular system. It causes mild cardiac depression and indirect sympathetic stimulation. Little change in blood pressure occurs because the mild cardiac depressant effect is offset by a mild increase in peripheral resistance [13–15].

Nitrous oxide intoxication causes euphoria, dizziness, dulling of the senses, decreased pain sensation, and distorted audiovisual processes.

Health Risks

Individuals who have inhaled large amounts of nitrous oxide daily for long periods of time may suffer peripheral nerve and brain damage secondary to vitamin B_{12} deficiency. Although treatment with vitamin B_{12} usually is effective, some damage may be irreversible. Less severe cases of vitamin B_{12} deficiency caused by nitrous oxide abuse, such as depression, forgetfulness, and fatigue, tend to go undiagnosed. Subacute combined degeneration has been reported.

Deaths from nitrous oxide have occurred. I know of one case of death from trying to inhale the gas directly from a nitrous oxide tank without the use of a pressure reduction valve. This resulted in high pressure damage to the lungs. Another method of death from nitrous oxide is asphyxiation. Nitrous oxide has to be administered along with oxygen. If the oxygen runs out leaving only the nitrous oxide inhalation, death soon occurs [15, 16].

Tolerance, Dependence, and Absence Syndrome

Nitrous oxide tolerance and dependence are possible with prolonged heavy use. Withdrawal symptoms, when they occur, consist primarily of excitement. Seizures have been reported in mice [17].

Overdose

Nitrous oxide overdose symptoms include lightheadedness; confusion; cough and/or wheezing; eye, nose, or throat irritation; dyspnea; chest tightness; cheat pain; diaphoresis; and blue in the lips, fingers, or toes. In severe cases, loss of consciousness, coma, and death may occur [18].

Treatment of nitrous oxide overdose is primarily supportive. Mechanical ventilation may be temporarily required. Breathing 100% oxygen for 5 min, if required, will wash the nitrous oxide out of the body [17].

Other Gases

Other abused gases include butane, propane, ether, and Freon. They are much less abused than nitrous oxide; however, deaths have occurred from all of them.

Butane is a colorless, flammable gas (C_4H_{10}) that is a saturated aliphatic existing in two isometric forms. It is used chiefly in the manufacture of rubber and as fuel. It is colorless [18].

Propane is a flammable gas (C_3H_8) of the alkane series occurring in petroleum and natural gases. It is used chiefly as a fuel and in organic synthesis. Its primary form of abuse is from butane cigarette lighters [18].

Ether is a colorless, highly volatile, flammable liquid ($C_4H_{10}O$) having an aromatic odor and a sweet, burning taste. It is derived from ethyl alcohol by the action of sulfuric acid. It is used as a solvent and, formerly, as an inhalant anesthetic [18].

Freon is a brand name for any of a class of liquid or gaseous fluorocarbon or chlorofluorocarbon product used chiefly as refrigerants [18].

Alkyl Nitrites

Alkyl nitrites were initially used as medications and chemical reagents, practices that began in the late nineteenth century. In their use as medicine, they were inhaled for relief of angina. However, they are now used as recreational drugs.

The three alkyl nitrites of abuse importance in primary care medicine are amyl nitrite, butyl nitrite, and cyclohexyl nitrite. Unlike most other inhalants, which act directly on the central nervous system (CNS), alkyl nitrites act primarily to dilate blood vessels and relax the muscles, including the anal sphincter. As a result they are a popular substance used by gay men and often considered a party or sex drug. Amyl nitrite is used medically as an antidote to cyanide poisoning [19–21].

Common brand names for over-the-counter nitrites include Liquid Gold, Buzz, Purple Haze, and Rush (Fig. 11.3).

Street Names

Street names for the alkyl nitrites include:

Amyl nitrite	Amies, amys, pearls poppers, snappers
Butyl nitrite	Banapple gas, locker popper, jock aroma, rush bolt, bullet, locker room, climax, thrust

Pharmacology

Organic nitrites are prepared from alcohols and sodium nitrite in a sulfuric acid solution. They decompose slowly on standing, the decomposition products being oxides of nitrogen, water, the alcohol, and polymerization products of the aldehyde.

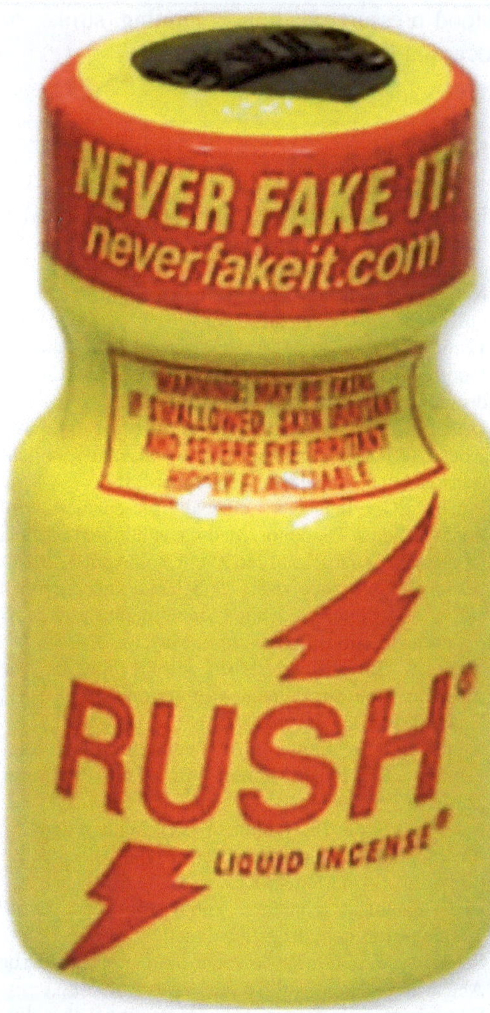

Fig. 11.3 Over-the-counter nitrite liquid incense sold by the brand name Rush

Alkyl nitrites decompose in gastric secretions, so they are ineffective when taken orally. When inhaled, their effects begin in 15–30 s and last a few minutes. They rapidly cross the pulmonary membrane to reach the bloodstream where they cause relaxation of vascular smooth muscle. The antianginal effect results from dilation of peripheral blood vessels and reduced venous return to the heart, resulting in decreased cardiac preload [22].

The effects of alkyl nitrite inhalation are instantaneous and brief but intense. They are caused by a sudden surge of blood to the heart and brain. Light-headedness, giddiness, heat flush or heightened sensual awareness may also result and is known as a "head rush." Some users may also experience the impression of time slowing down. The effects fade 2–5 min after use. Users are often left with a headache. It was widely reported that poppers can enhance and prolong orgasms [21].

Health Risks

Acute intake of alkyl nitrites may cause asphyxia, cardiac arrhythmias, cardiovascular depression, carbon monoxide poisoning, hepatorenal toxicity, skin irritation, and facial dermatitis. With chronic use, neurological damage may occur.

Accidental aspiration of alkyl nitrites may lead to the development of lipoid pneumonia. Swallowing alkyl nitrates can cause serious acute medical complications and may result in death.

Taking Viagra with nitrites can cause a serious decrease in blood pressure, leading to fainting, stroke, or myocardial infarction.

Alkyl nitrites can also increase intraocular pressure, resulting in glaucoma. Rarely methemoglobinemia and hemolysis may occur. Other risks include burns if spilled on skin, headache, and red or itching rashes around the mouth and nose.

Alkyl nitrites have been associated with unsafe sexual practices, which increase the risk of contracting and spreading infectious diseases like HIV/AIDS and hepatitis B [19, 23, 24].

Tolerance, Dependence, and Abstinence Syndrome

Tolerance and dependence almost certainly occur. It is uncertain whether or not an abstinence syndrome exists.

Overdose

Overdose symptoms include nausea, vomiting, hypotension, hypoventilation, and shortness of breath. Syncope, especially when the person becomes erect, can occur.

Treatment of alkyl nitrite overdose is generally symptomatic. If methemoglobinemia is present, slow intravenous infusion of methylene blue in distilled water or isotonic saline should be given [22].

Summary

The inhalant drugs are volatile solvents and aerosols, gases, and nitrites. Adolescent males most commonly use solvents and aerosols recreationally because they have easy access to many common household products. Solvents and aerosols are highly lipid soluble; they easily cross the alveolar membrane of the lungs and of the blood-brain barrier to reach high concentrations in the brain. Solvent and aerosol inhalation is known as *huffing*. *Dusting* is inhaling vapors directly from electronic equipment cleaning aerosols. *Sniffing* or *snorting* involves inhaling spray fumes directly from an aerosol container. Sudden sniffing death syndrome is an event in which the heart beats quickly and irregularly and then suddenly stops. Physicians should strongly suspect solvent and aerosol abuse in the setting of sudden collapse during adolescent group activities.

Nitrous oxide is a gas that usually is used in combination with a potent halogenated inhalational anesthetic, along with oxygen, to produce general anesthesia for surgery. It is most commonly abused as the propellant in whip cream canisters called *whippets*. Nitrous oxide overdose symptoms include light-headedness; confusion; cough and/or wheezing; eye, nose, or throat irritation; dyspnea; chest tightness; cheat pain; diaphoresis; and blue in the lips, fingers, or toes. In severe cases, loss of consciousness, coma, and death may occur.

The three alkyl nitrites of abuse importance in primary care medicine are amyl nitrite, butyl nitrite, and cyclohexyl nitrite. Because they relax the anal sphincter, they are used by gay men and often considered a party or sex drug. Taking Viagra with nitrites can cause a serious decrease in blood pressure, leading to fainting, stroke, or myocardial infarction.

References

1. Inhalants. Center for Drug Abuse Research (CESAR)/University of Maryland. http://www.cesar.umd.edu/cesar/drugs/inhalants.asp
2. National survey on drug use and health: Trends in prevalence of various drugs for ages 12 or older, ages 12 to 17, ages 18 to 25, and ages 26 or older. National Institute on Drug Abuse (NIDA). 2015. https://www.drugabuse.gov/national-survey-drug-use-health
3. Drug Facts: inhalants. National Institute on Drug Abuse (NIDA). https://www.drugabuse.gov/publications/drugfacts/inhalants. September 2012.
4. Jauch EC. Inhalants clinical presentation. In: Ramachandran TS, editor. Medscape. http://emedicine.medscape.com/article/1174630-clinical. April 3, 2014.
5. Borke J. Substance use – inhalants. In: Zieve D, editor. MedlinePlus. https://medlineplus.gov/ency/patientinstructions/000794.htm. May 14, 2016.
6. Cohen S. Solvent and aerosol intoxication. In: The substance abuse problems: volume one. New York: Haworth Press; 1981. p. 40–5.
7. Anderson CE, Lumis GA. Recognition and prevention of inhalant abuse. Am Fam Physician. 2003;68(5):869–74.
8. King GS, Smile JE, Troutman WG. Sudden death in adolescents from the inhalation of typewriter correction fluid. J Am Med Assoc. 1985;253:1604–6.
9. Drug Factuals: inhalants. Youth on drugs. http://youthondrugs.com/drugs/inhalants
10. Schuckit MA. Glues, solvents, and aerosols. Drug Abuse and Alcoholism Newsletter. July 1989.
11. Edminister SC, Bayer MJ. Recreational gasoline sniffing: acute gasoline intoxication and latent organ lead poisoning. J Emerg Med. 1985;3:365–70.
12. Fortenberry DJ. Gasoline sniffing. Am J Med. 1985;8:36–51.
13. Marshall BE, Woolman H. General anesthetics. In: Gilman AG, Goodman LS, Rall TW, Murad F, editors. Goodman and Gilman's the pharmacological basis of therapeutics. New York: Macmillan; 1985. p. 276–301.
14. O'Brien R, Cohen S. The encyclopedia of drug abuse. New York: Facts on File; 1984.
15. Shlafer M, Marieb EN. General anesthetic agents. In: The nurse pharmacology, and drug therapy. Redwood City: Addison-Wesley; 1989. p. 314–31.
16. Gillman MA. Nitrous oxide, an opioid addictive agent. Am J Med. 1986;81:97–102.
17. Kamangar N. Nitrogen dioxide toxicity. Medscape.http://emedicine.medscape.com/article/302133-overview. January 10, 2017.

18. Dictionary.com. http://www.dictionary.com
19. Cheng D. Amyl nitrites: a review of history, epidemiology, and behavioral usage. J Stud Res. 2013;2(1):17–21.
20. Cohen S. Amyl nitrite rediscovered. In: The substance abuse problems: volume one. New York: Haworth Press; 1981. p. 51–5.
21. Cohen S. The volatile nitrites. J Am Med Assoc. 1979;241:2077–8.
22. Cohen S. Inhalants and solvents. In: Escher GM, Friedman AS, editors. Youth drug abuse. Lexington: Lexington Books; 1979.
23. Bogart L, Bonsignore J, Carvalho A. Massive hemolysis following inhalation of volatile nitrites. Am J Hematol. 1986;22:327–9.
24. Wood RW. The acute toxicity of nitrite inhalants. Natl Inst Drug Abuse Res Monogr Ser. 1988;83:23–38.

Hallucinogen Dependence

12

Key Chapter Points

- Hallucinogens can be divided into lysergamides, phenylethylamines, indolealkylamines, amphetamine-related hallucinogens, and other hallucinogens.
- LSD is the most potent of the hallucinogenic drugs. Despite its potency, it has a very large safety margin.
- Mescaline is the psychogenic substance found in the peyote cactus (*Lophophora williamsii* or *Lophophora diffusa*), which is a spineless cactus with small protrusions called "buttons" that are used for hallucinogenic purposes.
- *Salvia divinorum* is an herb in the mint family. Its active ingredient is salvinorin A.
- Psilocybin and psilocin are naturally occurring compounds produced by at least 75 species of mushrooms.
- Several species of toads produce venom that has psychoactive properties due to mappine and 5-MeO-DMT.
- MDMA, most commonly known as ecstasy, has a structure similar to methamphetamine. It is known as *Adam* on the street. MDEA is used recreationally in a similar manner as MDMA. It is known as *Eve* on the street.
- N-bomb is a powerful synthetic hallucinogen sold as an alternative to LSD or mescaline. Smiles results from the substitution of one iodine atom for a chlorine atom on N-bomb.
- Hallucinogen persisting perception disorder (HPPD) is an involuntary recurrence of some aspect of a hallucinatory experience occurring weeks or months after using the hallucinogen that produced the original effect and without subsequent ingestion of the substance.

Hallucinogens are a diverse group of drugs that have different chemical structures, different mechanisms of action, and different adverse effects. They cause an alteration in perception, thought, and mood. Most hallucinogens do not cause outright hallucinations [1–3].

The Hallucinogens

The hallucinogenic drugs can be divided into five groups [2]:

Lysergamides The lysergamides include lysergic acid diethylamide (LSD) and lysergic acid hydroxyethylamide (morning glory and Hawaiian baby woodrose seeds).

Phenylethylamines The phenylethylamines include mescaline (peyote cactus) and *Salvia divinorum*.

Indolealkylamines The indolealkylamines include psilocybin and psilocin, both from mushrooms, and bufotenine and 5-MeO-DMT from toad frogs.

Amphetamine-Related Hallucinogens The amphetamine-related hallucinogens include 3,4-methyl-

H.T. Milhorn, *Substance Use Disorders*, DOI 10.1007/978-3-319-63040-3_12

enedioxymethamphetamine (MDMA) and methylenedioxyethylamphetamine (MDEA).

Other Hallucinogens Other hallucinogens include muscimol and ibotenic acid from mushrooms, myristicin and elemicin from nutmeg, atropine and scopolamine from the nightshade plant, 25I–NBOMe (N-bomb), 2,5-dimethoxy-4-iodophenethylamine (Smiles), and ibogaine.

Prevalence of Use

The highest rate of hallucinogen use occurs in persons aged 18–25 years. Hallucinogens continue to be among the most frequently abused class of drugs in high school students, after alcohol and marijuana.

Hallucinogen use in 2015 by age range is given in Table 12.1. Hallucinogen use is most common in non-Hispanic whites and most frequently by males. There is also a high lifetime prevalence rate of hallucinogen use among American Indian and Alaska Natives. Hallucinogens are often referred to as psychedelic drugs.

Lysergamides

The lysergamides include LSD (D-lysergic acid diethylamide) and lysergic acid hydroxyethylamide, which is a naturally occurring psychedelic found in morning glory and Hawaiian baby woodrose seeds.

LSD

LSD was initially derived from the alkaloid lysergic acid, which is found in ergot, a parasite fungus contaminant of wheat, rye, and other grains. It is now produced as a semisynthetic organic compound, $C_{20}H_{25}N_3O$, that is soluble in water.

The most common form of LSD is a liquid that has been transferred onto a small paper square known as "blotter" or as a microdot tablet. It also is found as a powder or crystal that is dried on gelatin sheets, in capsules, on sugar cubes, or laced on other drugs.

In its pure form, it is a white, odorless crystalline material, but street preparations usually are mixed with colored substances. It is soluble in water.

LSD is the most potent of the hallucinogenic drugs. Despite its potency, it has a very large safety margin; no deaths associated with isolated LSD ingestion have been reported despite ingestions of several thousand micrograms of the drug.

Gelatin squares impregnated with LSD are known as *windowpanes*. Tiny tablets containing LSD are known as *microdots*. Although usually ingested in blotter form, LSD also can be used via intranasal, sublingual, parenteral, inhalational, or even the conjunctival route as eye drops [4]. It is classified as a DEA Schedule I drug.

Prevalence of Use

LSD use by age range is given in Table 12.2.

Pharmacology

LSD acts on serotonin and dopamine receptors in the brain. The neurotransmitter serotonin modulates mood, pain, perception, personality, sexual activity, and other functions. LSD's net effect is that of a serotonin agonist.

Table 12.1 Prevalence of hallucinogen use in 2015 by age range (%) (From [2])

	Ages 12–17	Ages 18–25	Ages 26 or older
Lifetime	3.10	18.60	16.20
Past year	2.10	7.00	0.80
Past month	0.50	1.80	0.20

Table 12.2 Prevalence of LSD use in 2015 by age range (%) (From [2])

	Ages 12–17	Ages 18–25	Ages 26 or older
Lifetime	1.30	7.70	10.70
Past year	1.00	2.80	0.10
Past month	0.20	0.60	0.00

LDS is manufactured as pills, capsules, and liquid and almost always is used orally. Because small amounts produce the desired effects, it is usually put on sugar cubes, blotter paper, and small gelatin squares. Typical street doses are 25–150 mcg.

The onset of effects occurs 30–60 min after ingestion. Effects peak at approximately 5 h and lasts up to 12 h.

The effects of LSD depend on the quantity of the drug taken and the user's psychological and emotional state, as well as the setting in which the drug is used [2].

Lysergic Acid Hydroxyethylamide

Lysergic acid hydroxyethylamide occurs in various species in the Convolvulaceae family; that is, morning glory and Hawaiian baby woodrose seeds. The seeds contain a naturally occurring tryptamine.

The Aztecs were the first to discover the hallucinogenic properties of morning glory seeds, whose effects in doses of 200–300 seeds are somewhat like those of LSD. The seeds are consumed orally, either directly or pulverized and soaked in water; the liquid is then strained and drank.

Effects of lysergic acid hydroxyethylamide occur in 25–40 min after ingestion and last up to 6 h. The drug is about one tenth as potent as LSD.

Side effects include nausea, vomiting, intense headache, drowsiness, diarrhea, chills, impaired vision, decreased blood pressure, and the risk of shock.

The sale of morning glory seeds and Hawaiian baby woodrose seeds are not regulated by law [2, 5, 6].

Phenylethylamines

The phenylethylamines include mescaline (peyote cactus) and *Salvia divinorum*.

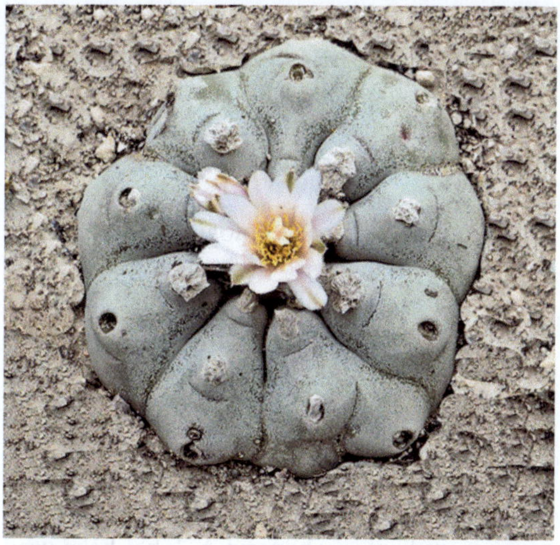

Fig. 12.1 Peyote cactus

Mescaline

Mescaline is the psychogenic substance found in the peyote cactus (*Lophophora williamsii or Lophophora diffusa*), which is a spineless cactus with small protrusions called "buttons" that are used for hallucinogenic purposes (Fig. 12.1). Mescaline can also be produced in a laboratory by chemical synthesis.

Native Americans have used peyote for more than 5000 years. Members of the Native American Church are still permitted to use the drug in religious ceremonies.

The peyote cactus is native to northern Mexico and Texas. Mescaline was isolated in 1897, and its chemical structure was identified in 1918. It is considerably less potent than LSD.

Mescaline is thought to induce hallucinations by an amphetamine-like action, although the precise mechanism is unknown. The drug is usually ingested but can be inhaled by smoking ground-up peyote buttons. Peyote buttons are the dried bitter fleshy tops of the cactus. More rarely mescaline is injected.

At low doses (ingestion of 6–12 peyote buttons), the user begins to feel effects in 30 min to 2 h.

At higher doses, the drug may cause fever, headache, vomiting, hypotension, ataxia, diaphoresis, and depressed cardiac and respiratory function. These effects may precede the hallucinogenic effects. The hallucinogenic effect may last 8–12 h.

Tolerance and psychological dependence develop with repeated doses, as does cross-tolerance to LSD. LSD and phencyclidine may be sold on the street as mescaline [2, 7, 8].

Salvia divinorum

Salvia divinorum is an herb in the mint family. Its active ingredient is salvinorin A. It has been used for centuries in religious ceremonies by the Mazatec Indians, a native people who live in Oaxaca, Mexico. The Mazatecs believe it is an incarnation of the Virgin Mary [9].

Pharmacology

Salvia divinorum is widely available through smoke shops and on the Internet in concentrated form. It is used in cigarettes and incense. As a recreational drug, *Salvia divinorum* produces hallucinations when inhaled, when the leaves are chewed, or when extracts are placed under the tongue. It rivals the potency of LSD.

Dried leaves of Saliva can be smoked like marijuana in a bong or pipe or as a joint, with effects lasting up to 15–25 min. It has been described as a 20 min acid trip.

Fresh leaves of Salvia also can be chewed and swallowed or chewed as a quid. When chewed as a quid, the leaves of Salvia produce extraction of salvinorin A. The extraction is absorbed through the oral mucosa and produces visual hallucinations that last 1–2 h; the longer the herb remains in the mouth, the stronger is the effect. A quid is something that is to be chewed but not swallowed.

When Salvia's leaves are crushed and salvinorin A extracted, it can be mixed with water and drank.

Since salvinorin A is partially deactivated by the gastrointestinal system before entering the bloodstream, oral use may produce a more moderate effect than other methods of use.

The extract also can be vaporized and inhaled. To do so, salvinorin A is heated on a piece of tinfoil, and the vapors are inhaled through a glass pipe [9].

Effects

Intense hallucinations such as sensations of traveling through time and space or floating or flying may occur. Sensations of twisting and spinning, heaviness or lightness of the body, and soreness also are common.

Other effects include awkward sentence patterns, bradycardia, chills, dizziness, lack of coordination, nausea, and slurred speech.

Neither *Salvia divinorum* nor its active ingredient salvinorin A is listed as controlled substances by the DEA. However, they are illegal in some states [9].

Indolealkylamines

The indolealkylamine group includes psilocybin and psilocin and mappine and 5-MeO-DMT. They all appear to cause their psychogenic effects through activity at the serotonin receptor.

Psilocybin and Psilocin

Psilocybin and psilocin are naturally occurring compounds produced by at least 75 species of mushrooms. The most potent mushrooms are members of the genus *Psilocybe* (Fig. 12.2).

Often growing on cow dung, the mushrooms are found in most areas of the United States, with the exception of arid regions.

Although psilocybin and psilocyn are Schedule I drugs under the Controlled Substances Act of 1970, the mushrooms themselves are not scheduled.

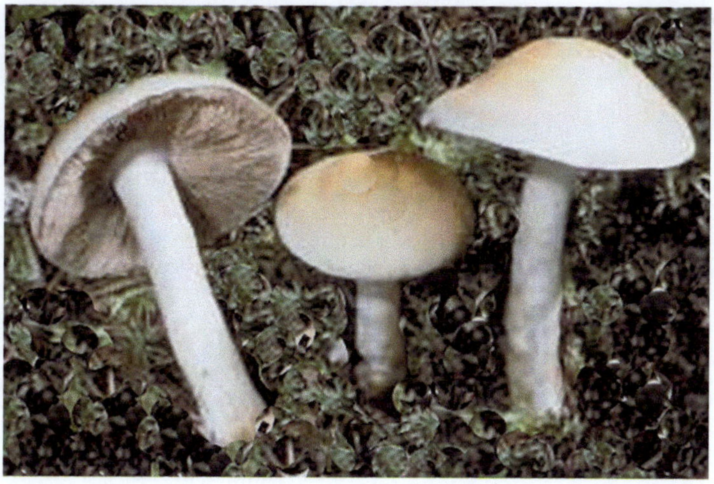

Fig. 12.2 Hallucinogenic mushrooms

Pharmacology

In its pure powder form, psilocybin can be prepared in capsules, tablets, or solution. Psilocybin can be consumed orally, sniffed, smoked, or injected. Fresh or dried psilocybin mushrooms can be sprinkled on top of food or brewed as a tea. The effects of psilocybin last approximately 4–6 h.

The mushrooms cause fewer adverse reactions than LSD, although cases of hyperthermia, seizures, and coma have been reported.

Misidentification of the mushrooms in the wild and on the street is common. Only one third of "magic mushrooms" bought on the street contain psilocybin. Many are simply store-bought mushrooms laced with PCP [2, 10, 11].

Mappine and 5-MeO-DMT

Several species of toads produce venom that has psychoactive properties due to mappine and 5-MeO-DMT (Fig. 12.3).

Mappine (bufotenine) is a hallucinogenic alkaloid, $C_{12}H_{16}N_2O$, found in the skin glands of toads of the genus *Bufo* and some mushrooms. 5-MeO-DMT is a psychedelic tryptamine found in a wide variety of plant species and a single psychoactive toad species, the Colorado River toad.

The toads are either licked or milked for their venom, which may then be ingested or smoked. Their dried skin also may be smoked. The drug has been injected.

Like their close relative, mappine, toad venom has been used for religious or spiritual purposes by South American shamans for thousands of years [2, 6]. 5-MeO-DMT and mappine are DEA Schedule I drugs.

Amphetamine-Related Hallucinogens

The hallucinogenic amphetamines are structural analogs of mescaline and amphetamine. Most were derived from their parent compounds in an effort to avoid US Drug Enforcement Agency prosecution. They all have similar psychogenic effects and toxicity. They include MDMA and MDEA.

MDMA

MDMA (3,4-methylenedioxymethamphetamine), most commonly known as ecstasy, has a structure similar to methamphetamine. MDMA affects serotonin neurotransmission at presynaptic and postsynaptic sites.

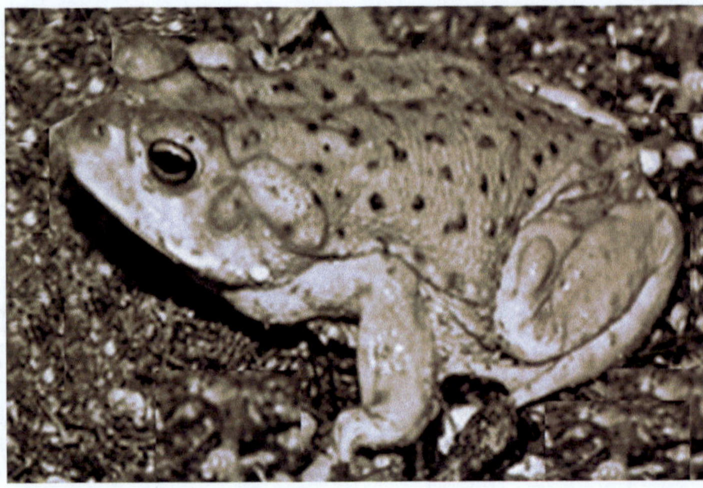

Fig. 12.3 Hallucinogenic toad frog

Table 12.3 Prevalence of MDMA use in 2015 by age range (%) (From [2])

	Ages 12–17	Ages 18–25	Ages 26 or older
Lifetime	1.40	13.10	6.50
Past year	0.80	4.10	0.50
Past month	0.10	0.90	0.10

Although MDMA usually does not cause hallucinations, it does cause changes in mood and increases interpersonal communication and fosters feelings of intimacy and empathy.

People who use MDMA usually take it as a capsule or tablet, although some swallow it in liquid form or snort the powder. It can be smoked.

In oral doses of 100 mg, it produces euphoria and enhanced self-awareness; in higher doses, it acts as a CNS stimulant. MDMA may cause permanent degradation of serotonergic neurons. This degradation is thought to be cumulative and dose-related.

In 1988, the DEA placed it in Schedule I; however, it is still available on the illicit market.

MDMA is presently the drug of choice at "raves," which are popular in the United States and the United Kingdom. Users often can be seen hugging or massaging one another, as physical sensitivity is extremely heightened. It is known on the street mainly as *Adam* [12, 13].

Prevalence of Use

Prevalence of MDMA use in 2015 by age range is given in Table 12.3.

Effects

Many of the toxicities of MDMA are identical to those of amphetamines. Sympathomimetic effects predominate, with hypertension and tachycardia being common. Hyperthermia is also common and occasionally is a serious complication.

The combination of sympathomimetic effects, strenuous physical activity, dehydration, and high ambient temperatures found at raves all contributes to hyperthermia. The hyperthermia may result in rhabdomyolysis, renal failure, and disseminated intravascular coagulation (DIC). The dehydration leads to increased water intake. Media coverage has resulted in the belief that water is the antidote to MDMA. The consumption of large amounts of water, combined with an intrinsic SIADH-like effect of MDMA, can lead to hyponatremia.

Users can often be seen with water and pacifiers, which are items used to counteract the side effects of MDMA, such as dry mouth, dehydration, and jaw or teeth clenching. Lollipops and chewing gum also may be used for the same reasons. Other complications of MDMA use are serotonin syndrome, seizures, hepatotoxicity, and tachydysrhythmias.

Molly is the name given to the most-refined, crystalline form of MDMA. Deaths also have occurred from molly use [14].

There have been reports of a combination of drugs that has been hitting the streets and club scenes. Ecstasy and Viagra are being used in a combination known as *sextasy* or *trail mix.* By combining the two drugs, users attempt to avoid the impotence side effect of ecstasy by increasing sexual functioning. These two drugs together can produce priapism, possibly resulting in permanent penile damage [2, 14]. Deaths have occurred from MDMA use [15].

MDEA

3,4-Methylenedioxyethamphetamine (MDEA) is used recreationally in a similar manner as MDMA. The effects are milder and shorter-lasting. MDEA recreational use began in 1985 as a legal substitute for the banned MDMA. It is most frequently consumed orally. Recreational doses of MDEA are in the range 100–200 mg. Deaths have occurred from its use [15]. MDEA was made a DEA Schedule I substance in 1987. It is known as *Eve* on the street.

Other Hallucinogens

Muscimol and Ibotenic Acid

Several mushrooms of the genus *Amanita* possess hallucinogenic effects. These include *Amanita muscaria*, *Amanita pantherina*, and *Amanita cothurnata.* These are not to be confused with the deadly *Amanita phalloides* group. *Amanita muscaria* has been used as a psychotropic by Siberians for centuries.

The active substances in the mushroom, muscimol and ibotenic acid, are thought to act on GABA receptor sites.

The drug is excreted unchanged in the urine, leading to the Siberian practice of drinking the urine of persons or reindeer that have eaten the mushroom. Effects begin approximately 20 min after ingestion and last for 6–12 h. Visual hallucinations and mania alternate with periods of deep sleep [2, 16].

Atropine and Scopolamine

The plant family Solanaceae (nightshade) contains atropine and scopolamine, which can cause hallucinations. These effects may be unpleasant and dissociative in nature. Scopolamine has the potential for abuse. Hallucinations are the most common neurological effect, with amnesia being the next most common.

Scopolamine has been used by criminals to sedate victims, mainly in Colombia, where the tree from which it derives proliferates. Slipped into drinks or sprinkled on food, it renders its victims so submissive that they have been known to empty their bank accounts and help thieves rob their homes.

Common side effects of scopolamine include dry mouth and skin, sleepiness, dizziness, restlessness, blurred vision, dilated pupils, dry or itchy eyes, constipation, and decreased sweating. In overdose, it can cause confusion, agitation, rambling speech, hallucinations, and paranoia [2].

Myristicin and Elemicin

Nutmeg is the dried seed of *Myristica fragrans*, an evergreen tree indigenous to East India. Mace, its seed root, has similar properties. Both are common cooking spices. The active ingredients, myristicin and elemicin, are related to mescaline.

Because of their unpleasant side effects, nutmeg and mace have limited popularity, being used primarily by adolescents as substitutes for illegal drugs.

The usual dose is less than 20 mg in tea, hot chocolate, or orange juice. This produces euphoria similar to mescaline. In doses greater than 20 mg, the drugs can produce visual hallucinations, fear, anxiety, and sometimes panic.

Physical effects begin about 45 min of ingestion and psychological effects after 1–2 h. The effects usually last 2–4 h and then begin to subside.

Side effects include vomiting, abdominal pain, chest pain, coldness of extremities, delirium, difficulty breathing, dizziness, increased body temperature, tachycardia, excessive thirst, bloodshot eyes, constipation, and difficulty urinating.

High doses of nutmeg can cause psychotic episodes, such as delusions and hallucinations. Anxiety, fear, and a feeling of impending doom are common during a nutmeg high, as are feelings of detachment from reality and visual hallucinations, which take the form of time, color, or space distortions. The sale of nutmeg and mace is not regulated by law [5, 16, 17].

N-Bomb and Smiles

N-Bomb

25I–NBOMe (N-bomb) is a powerful synthetic hallucinogen sold as an alternative to LSD or mescaline. There are several variations of this drug, but 25I–NBOMe is its most abused and the more potent form.

N-bomb is sold in liquid and powder form or on soaked blotter paper. Effects of a tiny amount of the drug can last 12 h or longer. The negative effects and aftereffects of the drug appear to be worse than those of LSD. The drug also mimics the effects of methamphetamine. It has a strong bitter metallic taste, and some dealers add mint or fruit flavoring to the liquid and blotter varieties.

As N-bomb creates no effect if swallowed, users place it under their tongue where it is absorbed. Some users inject it, smoke the powdered form, vaporize and inhale it, or insert it rectally. N-bomb is so toxic that it requires a filter mask, gloves, and glasses while handling it [18, 19].

Smiles

Similar to N-bomb, 2,5-dimethoxy-4-iodophenethylamine (Smiles), also known as 2C-1, results from the substitution of one iodine atom for a chlorine atom on N-bomb. Smiles is one of the 2C group of drugs; others include 2C-B, 2C-E, and 2C-T-7.

It is available in pill, liquid, and powder form. It can be taken orally or snorted in a powder form. Orally, Smiles takes 45–75 min to take effect. The primary effects of Smiles last 5–8 h when taken orally. The effects are said to be similar to a mix of ecstasy and LSD, but with a longer high.

Smiles causes hallucinations and can cause seizures and panic attacks. A number of deaths have occurred from Smiles use. The federal government has declared the entire 2C class of drugs as DEA Schedule I substances [20].

Ibogaine

Ibogaine is a naturally occurring psychoactive alkaloid, $C_{20}H_{26}N_2O$, found in plants in the Apocynaceae family, such as *Tabernanthe iboga.* Indian tribes in South America use ibogaine in a rite of passage into adulthood and call the drug the "ordeal bean." The people of West Africa and the Congo region have used iboga extracts or chewed the root of the plant in order to remain calm but alert while stalking game.

Howard Lotsof, a 19-year-old heroin addict, is responsible for introducing ibogaine to the Western world. In 1962, he procured the drug from a chemist friend and ingested it looking for a recreational high. It was isolated in 1901 and synthesized in 1966.

Ibogaine hydrochloride is a crystalline salt, soluble in alcohol and in water. It is an indole hallucinogen that blocks the action of serotonin. It was proposed for medical use as an antidepressant, but it was rejected in favor of more practical and less toxic drugs.

Ibogaine prolongs the QT interval, increasing the risk for ventricular tachycardia. Its use has been associated with serious side effects and death.

One of the first noticeable effects of a large dose of ibogaine ingestion is ataxia. Xerostomia, nausea, and vomiting may follow. These symptoms may last from 4 to 24 h. Ibogaine is sometimes administered per rectum to avoid nausea and vomiting.

In Africa, iboga root bark is sometimes chewed, releasing small amounts of ibogaine to produce a stimulant effect. Ibogaine currently is used as an alternative medicine treatment for

Table 12.4 Street names for hallucinogens (From Milhorn [22]. Approved with permission, Springer)

LSD	Acid, Beavis and Butthead. Big D, blotter, blotter acid, blue acid, blue heaven, cubes, dots, microdots, paper acid, sugar cubes, wedges, windowpanes
Morning glory seeds	Bindweed, blue star, flying saucers, pearly gates, wedding bells
Mescaline	Bad seed, beans, big chief, half moon, mesc, mescal, moon, nubs, topi buttons, cactus, cactus buttons
Salvia divinorum	Sage of the seers, magic mint, diviner's mint, seer's sage, Maria Pastora, diviner's sage, magic mint, Sally-D, the female, leaves of the shepherdess, herb of the shepherdess, leaves of Mary
Psilocybin and psilocin	Magic mushrooms, sacred mushrooms, shrooms, silly putty
MDMA	X, E, XTC, Adam, beans, candy, dancing shoes, disco biscuits, doves, E-bomb, egg rolls, happy pill hug, drug, love drug, Malcolm X, Molly, Scooby snacks, Smartees, sweets
MDEA	Eve
N-bomb	25I, 25C, 25B, N-bomb, BOM-CI, dime, cimbi-5, solaris
Mappine	Yopo, cohoba

drug addiction in some countries [6, 21]. It a DEA Schedule I drug.

Street Names

Street names for hallucinogens are given in Table 12.4 [22].

Hallucinogen Persisting Perception Disorder

Hallucinogen persisting perception disorder (HPPD) is an involuntary recurrence of some aspect of a hallucinatory experience occurring weeks or months after using the hallucinogen that produced the original effect and without subsequent ingestion of the substance.

The terms flashback and HPPD are usually used interchangeably; however, some people do make a distinction. Flashback is viewed as a short-term, non-distressing, spontaneous, recurrent, reversible, and benign condition accompanied by a pleasant affect. In contrast, HPPD is viewed as a generally long-term, distressing, spontaneous, recurrent, pervasive, either slowly reversible or irreversible, and non-benign condition accompanied by an unpleasant dysphoric affect.

The flashback or HPPD may consist of geometric hallucinations, false perceptions of movement in the peripheral visual fields, flashes of color, intensified colors, trails of images of moving objects, positive afterimages, halos around objects, and macropsia and micropsia. With macropsia everything is perceived by the eye appears to be larger than it really is, and with micropsia everything perceived by the eye appears to be smaller than it really is.

These symptoms can disappear as quickly as they appeared or last for several minutes or hours and may continue to occur repeatedly for an indefinite period of time [23, 24].

Tolerance, Dependence, and Abstinence Syndrome

Tolerance, dependence, and abstinence syndrome are not known to occur with hallucinogens.

Overdose

Symptoms

Most users who seek medical attention related to hallucinogens do so because of a massive overdose, an acute panic reaction, or an accidental ingestion. Users may have a blank stare, be agitated or violent, and show no regard for pain. A history of recent hallucbinogen use can often be obtained from the patient or the patient's friends and family. Organic causes for altered mental state, acute psychosis, and agitation should be ruled out.

Hallucinogen use may manifest with tachycardia, hypertension, and hyperthermia. Hypotension, hypoxia, and marked tachycardia or bradycardia are strong clues that imply serious overdose. Findings also may include mydriasis, sweating, ataxia, and vomiting. Sympathomimetic effects are common and often precede the hallucinogenic effects.

Affect, speech, appearance, presence of auditory or visual hallucinations, delusional thinking, and suicidal or homicidal ideation should be carefully assessed. Most persons experiencing the effects of a hallucinogen are awake, alert, and oriented. Obtunded patients or those with a focal neurologic examination should prompt an aggressive search for an organic etiology.

Persons who present following LSD ingestions most often do so because of a bad trip, characterized by disturbing visual hallucinations, anxiety, and paranoid delusions.

Patients who ingest peyote often have pronounced gastrointestinal effects (nausea and vomiting), diaphoresis, and ataxia before the onset of hallucinations. Users of hallucinogenic amphetamines, such as ecstasy, often give a history of rave attendance. Bruxism is also a common finding; many users carry something to put in their mouths. An 18-year-old with a pacifier in his mouth should be a clue.

A history of mushroom ingestion should prompt a thorough attempt to identify the ingested mushroom and to differentiate it from more toxic varieties.

Toad licking may cause profound drooling, seizures, and cyanosis. Severe hyperthermia may be observed with MDMA use. MDMA also may cause hyponatremia, rhabdomyolysis, and subsequent myoglobinuric renal failure. Trauma resulting from drug-induced behavior is common [2].

Laboratory Studies

In general, laboratory studies do not play a large role in the diagnosis and treatment of hallucinogen poisoning. Hallucinogenic drugs generally don't show up on standard drug screens. The exception is MDMA, which gives a positive test for amphetamine [22].

Imaging Studies

A CT scan of the head is indicated in all patients with an unexplained alteration in mental status.

Treatment

For any person presenting with hallucinations or psychosis, dextrose, thiamine, and naloxone should be given. Patients presenting with an acute panic reaction should be placed in a quiet non-threatening environment with minimal stimuli. Patients should be reassured that their anxiety is caused by the drug and that the effect will wear off in several hours.

Restraints should be avoided if at all possible. Prolonged or excessive physical restraint can contribute to hyperthermia, rhabdomyolysis, and acidosis and can exacerbate the patient's paranoia. Aggressive cooling measures should be undertaken if significant hyperthermia is noted.

Benzodiazepines can be used for anxious or agitated patients. Diazepam (Valium) 5–10 mg by mouth or intravenously or lorazepam (Ativan) 1–2 mg by mouth, intravenously, or intramuscularly can be given as needed. The hypertension and tachycardia associated with hallucinogens rarely require treatment beyond a benzodiazepine.

For severe agitation or psychosis, haloperidol (Haldol) may be used, but keep in mind that it may decrease the seizure threshold.

Rhabdomyolysis, if diagnosed, should be treated with intravenous fluids and alkalinization of the urine.

Patients that should be admitted to the hospital after several hours of observation include those who remain anxious or agitated, have continued hallucinations, remain a danger to themselves or others, or who are not be able to care for themselves [2].

Summary

Hallucinogens can be divided into lysergamides, phenylethylamines, indolealkylamines, amphetamine-related hallucinogens, and other hallucinogens. LSD is the most potent of the hallucinogenic drugs. Despite its potency, it has a very large safety margin. Mescaline is the psychogenic substance found in the peyote cactus (*Lophophora williamsii* or *Lophophora diffusa*), which is a spineless cactus with small protrusions called "buttons" that are used for hallucinogenic purposes. *Salvia divinorum* is an herb in the mint family. Its active ingredient is salvinorin A.

Psilocybin and psilocin are naturally occurring compounds produced by at least 75 species of mushrooms. Several species of toads produce venom that has psychoactive properties due to mappine and 5-MeO-DMT. MDMA, most commonly known as ecstasy, has a structure similar to methamphetamine. It is known as *Adam* on the street. MDEA is used recreationally in a similar manner as MDMA. It is known as *Eve* on the street.

N-bomb is a powerful synthetic hallucinogen sold as an alternative to LSD or mescaline. Smiles results from the substitution of one iodine atom for a chlorine atom on N-bomb.

Hallucinogen persisting perception disorder (HPPD) is an involuntary recurrence of some aspect of a hallucinatory experience occurring weeks or months after using the hallucinogen that produced the original effect and without subsequent ingestion of the substance.

References

1. Brown RT, Braden NJ. Hallucinogens. Pediatr Clin N Am. 1987;34:341–7.
2. Parish BS. Hallucinogen use. Medscape. http://emedicine.medscape.com/article/293752-overview. November 23, 2015.
3. National survey on drug use and health: trends in prevalence of various drugs for ages 12 or older, ages 12 to 17, ages 18 to 25, and ages 26 or older. National Institute on Drug Abuse (NIDA) 2015. https://www.drugabuse.gov/national-survey-drug-use-health
4. LSD. Center for Substance Abuse Research (CESAR)/University of Maryland. http://www.cesar.umd.edu/cesar/drugs/lsd.asp. October 29, 2013.
5. O'Brien R, Cohen S. The encyclopedia of drug abuse. New York: Facts on File; 1984.
6. Wilford BB, editor. Major drugs of abuse. Drug abuse: a guide for the primary care physician. Chicago: American Medical Association; 1981. p. 21–84.
7. Peyote/Mescaline. Center for Substance Abuse Research (CESAR)/University of Maryland. http://www.cesar.umd.edu/cesar/drugs/peyote.asp. October 29, 2013.
8. Schwartz RH. Mescaline: a survey. Am Fam Physician. 1988;37:122–4.
9. Salvia divinorum. Center for Substance Abuse Research (CESAR)/University of Maryland. http://www.cesar.umd.edu/cesar/drugs/salvia.asp. October 29, 2013.
10. Beck JE, Gordon DV. Psilocybin mushrooms. Pharm Chem Newsletter. 1982;4:1–4.
11. Schwartz RH, Smith DE. Hallucinogenic mushrooms. Clin Pediatr. 1988;27:70–3.
12. Clinko RP, Roehrich H, Sweeney DR, Al-Razi J. Ecstasy: a review of MDMA and MDA. Intl J Psychiatry Med. 1987;6:359–72.
13. Schonberg SK, editor. Specific drugs. Substance abuse: a guide for professionals. Elk Grove: American Academy of Pediatrics; 1988. p. 115–82.
14. MDMA (Ecstasy/Molly). National Institute on Drug Abuse (NIDA). https://www.drugabuse.gov/publications/drugfacts/mdma-ecstasymolly. October 2016.
15. Dowling DG, McDonough ET, Bost RO. Eve and ecstasy: a report of five deaths associated with MDEA and MDMA. J Am Med Assoc. 1987;257:1615–7.
16. Nutmeg abuse. Maryland Poison Center/ToxTidbits. http://www.mdpoison.com/media/SOP/mdpoisoncom/ToxTidbits/2011/March%202011%20ToxTidbits.pdf. March 2011.
17. Rolston-Cregler L, Weiner SW. Hallucinogenic mushroom toxicity. In: Tarabar A, editor. Medscape. http://emedicine.medscape.com/article/817848-overview#a4. April 8, 2015.
18. Hastings D. New drug N-bomb hits the street, terrifying parents, troubling cops. NY Daily News. May 6, 2013.
19. What is N-bomb? Foundation for a drug-free world. www.drugfreeworld.org/drugfacts/synthetic/what-is-n-bomb.html
20. Wilkerson M. Meet "Smiles": the next scary designer drug. The Fix. https://www.thefix.com/content/designer-drug-smiles90667. September 24, 2012.
21. Ibogaine. Chem Europe. http://www.chemeurope.com/en/encyclopedia/Ibogaine.html
22. Milhorn HT. Chemical dependence: diagnosis, treatment, and prevention. New York: Springer; 1990.
23. American Psychiatric Association. Hallucinogen persisting perception disorder (DSM-5). Arlington: American Psychiatric Publishing; 2013.
24. Litjens RP, Brunt TM, Alderliefste GJ, Westerink RH. Hallucinogen persisting perception disorder and the serotonergic system: a comprehensive review including new MDMA-related clinical cases. Eur Neuropsychopharmacol. 2014;24(8):1309–23.

13 Anabolic Steroid Dependence

Key Chapter Points

- Anabolic steroids are more accurately called anabolic-androgenic steroids because they produce an anabolic effect, which is protein synthesis for building muscle, and an androgenic effect, which is masculinization.
- Common patterns of illegal steroid use include cycling, stacking, and pyramiding.
- Anabolic steroids are synthetic derivatives of testosterone with enhanced anabolic activity and reduced androgenic activity.
- Users of anabolic steroids can become both physically and psychologically dependent on the drugs as evidenced by drug-seeking behavior, continued use even with adverse effects, and physical withdrawal symptoms.
- Denial plays a major role in illegal steroid dependence. They do not believe that the drugs are causing harm to anyone—a "victimless crime."
- The anabolic-steroid abstinence syndrome consists primarily of depression, which may be severe.
- The 10–25 pounds they lose on cessation of anabolic steroid use takes on an exaggerated importance, a phenomenon that has been termed *megarexia*.
- A number of drugs are used as alternatives to anabolic steroids.

Anabolic steroids are more accurately called anabolic-androgenic steroids because they produce an *anabolic effect*, which is protein synthesis for building muscle, and an *androgenic effect*, which is masculinization. The drugs are used illicitly in an attempt to increase muscle mass and athletic performance.

Most healthy males normally produce between 2 and 10 mg of testosterone a day, and females produce considerably less. The hormone's anabolic effect promotes retention of nitrogen and this helps muscle growth. It helps the male reproductive system grow and develop during puberty, assists with the growth of body hair, and causes deepening of the voice. During puberty, the testes increase testosterone production 20- or 40-fold compared to early childhood levels.

The most common illegal source of anabolic steroids is from smuggling steroids into the United States from other countries, such as Mexico and European countries. Smuggling from these areas is easier because a prescription is not required for the purchase of steroids. Less often, steroids found in the illicit market are from legitimate sources obtained by theft and inappropriate prescribing. Another source of steroids is clandestine laboratories [1, 2].

Prevalence of Use

Between one million and three million people are thought to have misused anabolic steroids in the United States at some time in their lives. It has been estimated that more than 80% of athletes

H.T. Milhorn, *Substance Use Disorders*, DOI 10.1007/978-3-319-63040-3_13

Table 13.1 Prevalence of anabolic steroid use in 2015 for 8th, 10th, and 12th graders (%) (From [3])

	8th graders	10th graders	12th graders
Life time	0.90	1.30	1.60
Past year	0.50	0.70	1.00
Past month	0.30	0.30	0.07

involved in bodybuilding, national and international weightlifting, powerlifting, and field events, such as shot put and discus throw, have used steroids. One-half of professional football linemen and linebackers were thought at one time to use the drugs. A number of female athletes, especially those involved in body building and powerlifting, are thought to be steroid users. Estimates of steroid use among college athletes have ranged from 5% to 20% [2].

Table 13.1 [3] gives the prevalence of steroid use in 2015 for 8th, 10th, and 12th graders in 2015.

Most anabolic steroid users are nonathletic, middle-class men with a median age of about 25 years who use the drugs to increase their muscle size and strength and reduce body fat, which they believe improves their personal appearance.

People who abuse anabolic steroids usually take them orally or inject them intramuscularly.

The doses may be 10–100 times higher than the doses prescribed for medical conditions [4].

The Anabolic Steroids

Anabolic steroids come in tablet and injectable forms. Some of the more common ones are given in Table 13.2. Boldenone undecylenate is a veterinary medicine.

Injectable steroids are absorbed directly into the bloodstream, thereby avoiding the first-pass effect by the liver. The first-pass effect refers to the fact that ingested drugs must pass from the intestines through the liver in order to reach the bloodstream. The liver metabolizes a major part of the oral dose in this process. In addition, by avoiding the first-pass effect, injectable steroids are less toxic to the liver than the oral ones [2].

Table 13.2 Anabolic steroids (Based on [1])

Oral steroids	Injectable steroids
Oxymetholone (Anadrol)	Nandrolone decanoate (Deca Durabolin)
Oxandrolone (Oxandrin)	Nandrolone phenylpropionate (Durabolin)
Methandrostenolone (Dianabol)	Testosterone cypionate (Depo-Testosterone)
Stanozolol (Winstrol)	Boldenone undecylenate (Equipoise)

Legal forms of testosterone come in transdermal patches, injectable liquid, tablets, creams, and jells.

Legal Uses

Anabolic steroids are available legally as prescribed medications for treating a number of conditions [5].

Bone Marrow Problems

For decades, anabolic steroids were used to treat hypoplastic anemia. They largely have been replaced for this use by synthetic hormones, such as epoetin alfa, that selectively stimulate growth of blood cell precursors.

Gender Dysphoria

Anabolic steroids are used to produce secondary male characteristics in women transitioning to male sex.

Growth Stimulation

Anabolic steroids have been used to treat children with growth failure. However, the availability of synthetic growth hormone, which has fewer side effects, makes this now a secondary treatment.

Induction of Male Puberty

Androgens are given to young males for delayed puberty. Testosterone now is the only androgen used for this purpose.

Stimulation of Appetite and Muscle Mass

Anabolic steroids have been used for chronic wasting conditions, such as cancer and AIDS.

Treatment of Testosterone Deficiency

In adult men, treatment for low testosterone is aimed at maintaining secondary sex characteristics; improving energy, strength, mood, and feelings of well-being; and preventing bone degeneration.

Patterns of Illegal Use

Common patterns of illegal steroid use include cycling, stacking, and pyramiding [6, 7].

Cycling

Cycling involves alternating periods of anabolic steroid use with periods of no use or the use of lower doses of the drug. Cycling periods usually last from 6 to 16 weeks. Reasons given for cycling include insuring peak performance at the time of competition, preventing detection of steroid use, reducing adverse effects, and reducing tolerance.

Stacking

Stacking is the concurrent use of two or more steroids. Injectable steroids may be stacked with oral steroids. Short-acting steroids may be stacked with longer-acting steroids.

Pyramiding

With pyramiding, there is a progressive increase in the doses of steroids in the first half of the pyramid and a gradual reduction in the doses in the latter half of the pyramid. Pyramiding is believed to give the optimal, desired steroid effect while decreasing the likelihood of detection.

Example of Pyramiding and Stacking

To maximize the anabolic effect, while minimizing the health risks and likelihood of being detected by drug screens, a regimen called *pyramiding* is often used by athletes. For example, an individual might use the first 3 weeks of a 12-week regimen before a competition to inject himself weekly with 200 mg of testosterone cypionate and ingest 10 mg of one of the oral forms daily. During the next 3 weeks, the dose of the injected drug might be increased to 400 mg and the dose of the oral drug to 15 mg.

For weeks 7 and 8, the weekly dose of the testosterone cypionate might be raised to 600 mg, the oral drug to 20 mg, and a second oral drug added, a process known as *stacking*. During weeks 9 and 10, the dose of the injected drug is reduced to 200 mg/week. The oral doses remain the same. During week 11, the first oral drug is discontinued, as is the injectable one. During week 12, the second oral drug is discontinued. To avoid being caught by a urine drug screen, no drugs are used the final week before the competition. Athletes have been known to use 10–40 times the normal daily dose [6, 7].

Doses of Illegal Anabolic Steroids

Steroid abusers select doses depending upon their particular objectives. For athletes, the doses selected are to some extent determined by the sporting event. Endurance athletes use at or slightly below replacement levels of 5–10 mg/day; sprinters use 1.5–2 times replacement levels; weightlifters and body builders use 10–100 times normal doses; and women, regardless of the sport, tend to use lower doses than men [1].

Actions

Individuals who use anabolic steroids do so in the belief that these drugs cause the effects given in Table 13.3. Whether anabolic steroids actually do all of these things is debatable. Research has shown that they do not improve performance in aerobic athletic events, such as the sprint races. They do seem to increase strength in weightlifters who have undergone intensive training before beginning anabolic steroid use.

Table 13.3 Effects anabolic steroid users believe to occur because of the drug use (Based on Milhorn [2])

Increase body mass
Increase muscle mass
Increase strength
Increase aggressiveness
Improve times in running events
Reduce recovery time after a workout
Increase the length of workout periods
Increase intensity at which weight training can be done
Promote rapid healing of injuries
Allow them to keep up with their opponents
Give them the winning edge
Make them look more attractive to the opposite sex

Street Names

Street names for anabolic steroids include:

Abolic	Hammer	Sauce	Therobolin
Anadrol	Junk	Slop	Weight trainers
Arnolds	Equipoise	Pumpers	Winstrol V
Bolasterone	Gym candy	Proviron	Roids
Dihydrolone	Juice	Stackers	Pumpers

Pharmacology

Anabolic steroids are synthetic derivatives of testosterone with enhanced anabolic activity and reduced androgenic activity. No anabolic steroid is devoid of androgenic effects. Activation of androgen receptors in cells and tissues mediate the anabolic and androgenic effects.

Anabolic steroids diffuse through cell membranes of target organs and combine with receptor proteins in the cytoplasm. The receptor-hormones migrate into the cell nucleus and bind to nuclear chromatin, stimulating the production of a messenger RNA. The messenger RNA then regulates the enzyme synthesis responsible for the physiologic activity of the anabolic steroid. Anabolic steroids stimulate and maintain a positive nitrogen balance by reducing renal elimination of nitrogen, sodium, potassium, chloride, and calcium. Production of myosin, sarcoplasm, and myofibrillar protein is enhanced [8, 9].

Table 13.4 Adverse effects of anabolic steroids in males and females (Based on [1])

Males	Females
Atrophy of the testicles Breast and prostate enlargement Decreased hormone levels Decreased sperm count Decreased sperm production Loss of sexual drive Sterility	Diminished breast size Deepened voice Enlargement of the clitoris Increased facial hair Infertility Menstrual irregularities

Health Risks

A number of adverse health effects can result from anabolic steroid use. Many of them are irreversible. Table 13.4 gives the adverse effects of anabolic steroids on males and females.

Adverse effects from anabolic steroids that occur in both sexes are given in Table 13.5. Peliosis hepatis is venous lakes in the liver which are prone to rupture. Steroid use can cause accelerated atherosclerosis, which can lead to myocardial infarction or stroke.

In children, anabolic steroids cause premature sexual development and early closure of the epiphyseal growth plates resulting in decreased height.

The aggressive behavior produced by anabolic steroids can be a significant problem. The author was told of one young athlete who, in a "roid rage," walked along the street bashing parked cars with a crowbar. When confronted by the police, he attacked them with the crowbar. Despite being shot repeatedly, he kept coming after them before finally falling dead at their feet [7].

Tolerance

Steroid abuse can cause downregulation of androgen receptors, thereby reducing the effects of testosterone and other androgens [7].

Table 13.5 Adverse consequences of anabolic steroids in both sexes (Based on [1])

Physical	Behavioral
Acne Alterations in cholesterol and other lipids Altered glucose metabolism Cholestatic jaundice Enlarged heart Fluid retention Heart attack and stroke High blood pressure Kidney disease Liver disease (tumors, cysts, cancer, peliosis hepatis) Male pattern baldness Premature closure of epiphyseal growth plates Risk of viral (including HIV) or bacterial infections due to unsterile injections Severe acne Stunted growth in teens	Aggression Anger Changes in libido Delusions Decreased fatigue Depression Euphoria Extreme mood swings Impaired judgment Irritability Manic-like symptoms of nervousness Paranoia Rage

Dependence

Users of anabolic steroids can become both physically and psychologically dependent on the drugs as evidenced by drug-seeking behavior, continued use even with adverse effects, and physical withdrawal symptoms [10].

Dependence on steroids is different from other drugs. Users don't become high when using them. They keep using steroids despite the harmful effects on their bodies and lives. In addition, they typically spend a large amount of time and money obtaining the drugs [11, 12].

Long-term steroid use can alter brain neurotransmitter levels, such as serotonin, that are affected by other drugs. This may result in a significant effect on mood and behavior.

Some anabolic steroid users turn to other drugs, such as opioids, to reduce sleep problems and irritability caused by anabolic steroids. This can result in a significant effect on mood and behavior [13]. Anabolic steroid dependence is not addressed in DSM-5 [14].

Denial

Denial plays a major role in illegal steroid dependence. They do not believe that the drugs are causing harm to anyone—a "victimless crime." They feel that they must use the drugs if they want to compete seriously with others whom they believe are using the drugs. They deny that anabolic steroid use has significant adverse health consequences.

Users make statements like "Every drug, even aspirin, has side effects." They condemn those who criticize the use of anabolic steroids by saying "People who are against steroid use are not athletes. They just don't understand."

They appeal to higher loyalties, sort of a code of commitment to the sport. Those competing at the international level may view anabolic steroid use as a patriotic act [2].

Abstinence Syndrome

The anabolic-steroid abstinence syndrome consists primarily of depression, which may be severe. Suicides have been reported. Other symptoms are mood swings, fatigue, restlessness, loss of appetite, insomnia, reduced sex drive, and steroid cravings. Depressive symptoms can persist for up to 1 year after the user stops taking the steroid.

Another withdrawal symptom is viewed as being the opposite of anorexia nervosa. Those suffering from anorexia nervosa see themselves as overweight despite being merely skin and bones. Anabolic steroid abusers see themselves as being undermuscled despite the fact that they may appear to others as having a tremendous physique. The 10–25 pounds they lose on cessation of anabolic steroid use takes on an exaggerated importance, a phenomenon which has been termed *megarexia* [2, 4, 11].

Drugs Used to Mask Anabolic Steroid Use

Steroid users often use other drugs in an attempt to mask anabolic steroids on drug screens as given in Table 13.6.

Alternatives to Anabolic Steroids

A number of drugs are used as alternatives to anabolic steroids [1, 15].

Table 13.6 Drugs used in an attempt to mask anabolic steroids on drug screens (Based on [1])

Drug group	Drug or effect	How drug masks steroid use
Uricosuric agents	Probenecid	Decreases entry of steroids into the urine
Diuretics	Spironolactone, furosemide	Dilutes steroid concentration in the urine
Epitestosterone	Decreases testosterone to epitestosterone ratio	Reduces detection of testosterone usage

Clenbuterol

Clenbuterol is a synthetic beta-receptor agonist used in the treatment of asthma and other respiratory diseases and in veterinary obstetrics. It also promotes the growth of muscle and decreases fat content. It is used illegally by athletes to enhance performance.

Creatine

Creatine is a compound the body synthesizes and then utilizes to store energy. It is abused by athletes to increase muscle bulk. It may produce small gains in short-term bursts of power.

Erythropoietin

Erythropoietin (*EPO*) is a hormone secreted by the kidneys that increases the rate of production of red blood cells in response to falling levels of oxygen in the tissues. It is abused to increase the oxygen carrying capacity of the blood above the normal level.

Gamma Hydroxybutyrate

Gamma hydroxybutyrate (*GHB*) is a naturally occurring neurotransmitter and a psychoactive drug. Athletes abuse it to raise growth hormone levels.

Human Chorionic Gonadotropin

Human chorionic gonadotropin *(hCG)* is a hormone made by chorionic cells in the fetal part of the placenta. It is directed at the gonads and stimulates them.

Human Growth Hormone

Human growth hormone (*HGH*) is released by the human pituitary gland to promote growth. A synthetic form of this hormone produced by recombinant DNA technology is used to treat a deficiency of growth hormone and certain other medical conditions. It is often used illegally, especially to improve athletic performance.

Insulin

Insulin is a hormone produced in the pancreas by the islets of Langerhans that regulates the amount of glucose in the blood. It is abused for its anabolic properties.

Insulin-Like Growth Factor

Insulin-like growth factor is either of two peptides that are structurally similar to insulin and are involved in the regulation of cell growth; insulin-like growth factor is used to increase muscle mass.

Vitamins and Amino Acids

Athletes use vitamins and minerals to supply the building blocks of protein in attempts to increase muscle mass.

Summary

Anabolic steroids are more accurately called anabolic-androgenic steroids because they produce an anabolic effect, which is protein synthesis for building muscle, and an androgenic effect, which is masculinization. Between one million and three million people are thought to have misused anabolic steroids in the United States at some time in their lives.

Common patterns of illegal steroid use include cycling, stacking, and pyramiding.

Anabolic steroids are synthetic derivatives of testosterone with enhanced anabolic activity and reduced androgenic activity. Legal forms of testosterone come in transdermal patches, injectable liquid, tablets, creams, and jells. Users of anabolic steroids can become both physically and psychologically dependent on the drugs as evidenced by a drug-seeking behavior, continued use even with adverse effects, and physical withdrawal symptoms.

Denial plays a major role in illegal steroid dependence. They do not believe that the drugs are causing harm to anyone—a "victimless crime." The aggressive behavior produced by anabolic steroids can be a significant problem. The anabolic-steroid abstinence syndrome consists primarily of depression, which may be severe. The 10–25 pounds they lose on cessation of anabolic steroid use takes on an exaggerated importance, a phenomenon which has been termed *megarexia*. A number of drugs are used as alternatives to anabolic steroids.

References

1. A guide for understanding steroids and related substances. Drug Enforcement Administration (DEA) website. U.S. Department of Justice/Diversion Control Division website. https://www.deadiversion.usdoj.gov/pubs/brochures/steroids/professionals. March 2004.
2. Milhorn HT. Drug and alcohol abuse: the authoritative guide for parents, teachers, and counselors. New York: Da Capo Press; 2003.
3. Steroids (anabolic). National Institute on Drug Abuse (NIDA) website. https://www.drugabuse.gov/drugs-abuse/steroids-anabolic. December 2012.
4. Drug facts: anabolic steroids. National Institute on Drug Abuse (NIDA) website. https://www.drugabuse.gov/publications/drugfacts/anabolic-steroids. March 2016.
5. Kishner S. Anabolic steroid use and abuse. Medscape website. http://emedicine.medscape.com/article/128655-overview. May 27, 2015.
6. Anabolic steroids. Drug Enforcement Administration (DEA)/Office of Diversion Control/Drug and Chemical Evaluation Section website. https://www.deadiversion.usdoj.gov/drug_chem_info/anabolic.pdf. August 2013.
7. Milhorn HT. Anabolic steroids: another form of drug abuse. J Miss State Med Assoc. 1991;32:293–7.
8. Dowling PM. Anabolic steroids. In: Merck veterinary manual. Kenilworth: Merck & Co., Inc.; 2016.
9. Lukas SE. The pharmacology of anabolic androgenic steroids. In: Ries RK, Fiellin DA, Miller SC, Saitz R, editors. Principles of addiction medicine. 4th ed. Philadelphia: Lippincott Williams & Wilkins; 2009. p. 251–63.
10. Anderson L. Anabolic steroids—abuse, side effects and safety. Drugs.com website. https://www.drugs.com/article/anabolic-steroids.html. May 4, 2014.
11. Tsuang JW. Psychiatric complications and dependence potential of anabolic steroids. J Fam Pract Recert. 1993;15:67–73.
12. Volkow ND. Anabolic steroid abuse. National Institute on Drug Abuse (NIDA) website. https://www.drugabuse.gov/publications/research-reports/anabolic-steroid-abuse. August 2006.
13. Drug facts: anabolic steroids. National Institute on Drug Abuse for Teens website. https://teens.drugabuse.gov/drug-facts/anabolic-steroids. September 30, 2016.
14. Kanayama G, Brower KJ, Ruth D, Wood I, Hudson JI, Pope HG Jr. Issues for DSM-V: clarifying the diagnostic criteria for anabolic-androgenic steroid dependence. Am J Psychiatr. 2009;166(6):642–5.
15. Jenkinson DM, Harbert AJ. Supplements and sports. Am Fam Physician. 2008;78(9):1039–46.

Part III

Diagnosis, Treatment, Recovery, Relapse, and the Family

14 Diagnosis

Key Chapter Points

- Many physicians underdiagnose substance dependence. Common problems that interfere with a physician's making the diagnosis of substance dependence include undereducation, false beliefs, denial, and feelings of inadequacy.
- A number of diagnostic tools are available to help physicians diagnose addiction to alcohol or other drugs. These include screening questionnaires, a patient's personal and family history, a physical examination, and laboratory tests.
- Signs and symptoms can be very helpful in acquiring an idea of which substance a patient has been abusing.
- Drug screening can be done on the urine, blood, hair, saliva, sweat, and nails. Urine is most often used for drug screening because it is easy to collect, collecting it is noninvasive, it is easier to analyze than blood or other fluids, and it can be refrigerated and stored.
- Two screening tests are currently in use—thin-layer chromatography and immunoassays. Confirmatory techniques include gas chromatography/mass spectrometry (GC/MS) and high-pressure liquid chromatography.
- Few addicts use only one drug; however, virtually all can identify the drug they most prefer (drug of choice).
- Discussing the diagnosis of substance dependence with a patient is never easy. The major barrier is the patient's denial, which physicians should view as a symptom of the disease in the same way that thirst is a symptom of diabetes.

Substance use disorders are common among patients in primary care settings. However, many physicians underdiagnose substance dependence. They do so for a variety of reasons. They may feel that substance dependence is a weakness rather than a disease, or they may believe that addicts differ in appearance from other patients. Patients, family members, and personal physicians frequently deny the existence of a problem. Some physicians are reluctant to make the diagnosis of a disorder they don't know how to treat.

Diagnosis is aided by a patient's medical, psychological, and social history, as well as the patient's presentation, physical examination, and laboratory findings. Questionnaires are useful for routine screening of patients. The ultimate diagnosis of substance dependence depends on the criteria of DSM-5 that were discussed in Chap. 1.

As with any chronic progressive disease, the earlier in its course the diagnosis of substance dependence is made, the better is the outcome.

Problems in Diagnosis

Common problems that interfere with a physician's making the diagnosis of substance dependence include undereducation, false beliefs, denial, and feelings of inadequacy.

H.T. Milhorn, *Substance Use Disorders*, DOI 10.1007/978-3-319-63040-3_14

Undereducation

Physicians and patients are products of the same culture, one in which most people believe that substance dependence is a weakness rather than a disease. As a result, many physicians believe that when they recognize addiction in a patient, they are accusing the patient of bad behavior, rather than making a medical diagnosis. The belief largely results from inadequate education about substance dependence in medical schools. Only about 3% of the nation's medical schools offer a separate course in substance dependence, and physicians generally receive little training in the behavioral sciences, including family function and dysfunction. As a result of this inadequate education, medical students have been found to have little expertise in substance dependence.

Most physicians can recognize the late-stage symptoms of addiction (gastrointestinal bleeding, jaundice, ascites) but are unable to recognize the early symptoms, which are behavioral. Because substance dependence is a chronic, progressive disease that responds well to early detection and early treatment, the failure to recognize the early symptoms of addiction represents a major oversight on the part of medical professionals. In most cases, this failure to diagnose addiction early in its course ensures that the substance-dependent person's disease will progress to more advanced, less treatable stages even while under the care of a physician. Effective physician education has been found to increase the diagnosis of substance dependence [1–3].

False Beliefs

There is a common belief that substance-dependent people differ from other patients in appearance. The myth persists that most substance-dependent people appear as skid row bums. In actuality, these individuals may account for as few as 3% of substance-dependent people. The other 97%, for the most part, are employed and on the surface appear to be doing well. Having accepted popular views of addiction and the resulting social stigma, physicians may be less likely to make diagnoses that they perceive to be embarrassing or demeaning to patients.

The false perception that alcoholism and other drug dependencies are hopeless conditions may prevent many physicians from making a diagnosis of addiction and taking the steps to get a substance-dependent person the professional help he needs. Studies have shown that interns and residents are significantly more pessimistic about the outcome of treatment for alcoholics than first-year medical students. This general pessimism arises from unpleasant experiences on clinical wards with intoxicated individuals going through withdrawal and who are immediately discharged from the hospital once they are stable.

Interns and residents, for the most part, have little or no experience with substance-dependent people with years of recovery. A number of studies have shown that many patients completing treatment are still drug-free after several years. Physicians need to be aware of these encouraging statistics and need to become aware of treatment programs in their local areas. Treatment offers hope for substance-dependent people and their families [4, 5].

Denial

Diagnosis is further complicated by denial, a hallmark of substance dependence. Addicts may firmly believe that their problem is not drugs and continue to use them in spite of medical, psychological, or social problems. Denial is a subconscious defense mechanism; it is not pathological lying but a predictable symptom of addiction. It is not used only by substance-dependent people. Frequently, spouses and children cover up for addicts out of misguided love and a reluctance to face the embarrassment of admitting the truth. Physicians must be careful not to become part of this denial system.

When patients refuse to acknowledge their illness, physicians face a considerably more difficult task. They need to be aware of the scope and subtleties of addictive denial so that they are not misled by addict's manipulative behavior or caught off guard by addicts' persuasiveness, congeniality, or defensiveness. When physicians recognize that substance-dependent people are trapped within their own substance-altered perceptions, they more easily can maintain the emotional detachment that is necessary to make diagnoses and direct patients to the professional help they need [6].

Feelings of Inadequacy

Many physicians face an additional problem. They are uncomfortable diagnosing an illness they don't know how to treat. Consequently, they limit their responsibility to treating the late medical stages of addiction and only warn patients that the offending agents are damaging their bodies and that they should quit using them. Physicians frequently do not realize that the problem is not that simple. Addicted people cannot stop on their own. If they could, they would [5, 7].

Making the Diagnosis

A number of diagnostic tools are available to help physicians diagnose addiction to alcohol or other drugs. These include screening questionnaires, a patient's personal and family history, a physical examination, and laboratory tests. Also, a patient's behavior during an office or emergency department visit may be a clue to the possibility of substance dependence.

Screening Questionnaires

Alcoholism

Anyone who consumes alcoholic beverages is at risk for developing alcoholism. Therefore, anyone who answers "yes" to the question "Do you drink?" should be screened. Ideally, screening should be part of every new patient's medical history and part of what is added to that history with each periodic physical examination [8].

Three short, self-administered questionnaires are suitable for this—the Short Michigan Alcohol Screening Test (SMAST), the CAGE questionnaire, and the Alcohol Use Disorders Identification Test (AUDIT).

The SMAST (Table 14.1) is a shortened 13-question version of the original 24-question Michigan Alcohol Screening Test (MAST). Scoring is as follows: a "no" answer to questions 1, 4, and 5 and a "yes" response to the other questions each earns one point. Two points indicate a possible problem. Three points indicate a probable problem. The SMAST has been shown to be as effective as the MAST and to have greater than 90% sensitivity. It can be administered to a patient or the patient's spouse. As with all screening tests, some false-positive results do occur. The SMAST deals with the consequences of drinking rather than the quantity, frequency, or duration of drinking [9].

The CAGE questionnaire (Table 14.2 [10]) is even shorter and easier to administer than the SMAST; however, it is more likely to give false-positive results. A "yes" answer to each question

Table 14.1 The Short Michigan Alcohol Screening Test (SMAST) (From Selzer [9]. Approved with permission, Journal of Studies on Alcohol)

1.	Do you feel you are a normal drinker?
2.	Do your spouse or parents worry or complain about your drinking?
3.	Do you ever feel bad about your drinking?
4.	Do friends or relatives think you are a normal drinker?
5.	Are you always able to stop drinking when you want to?
6.	Have you ever attended a meeting of Alcoholics Anonymous?
7.	Has drinking ever created problems between you and your spouse?
8.	Have you ever gotten into trouble at work because of drinking?
9.	Have you ever neglected your obligations, your family, or your work for 2 or more days in a row because you were drinking?
10.	Have you ever gone to anyone for help about your drinking?
11.	Have you ever been in the hospital because of drinking?
12.	Have you ever been arrested even for a few hours because of drinking?
13.	Have you ever been arrested for drunk driving or driving after drinking?

Table 14.2 The CAGE questionnaire (From Ewing [10]. Approved with permission, JAMA)

1.	Have you ever felt you should *cut down* on your drinking?
2.	Have people *annoyed* you by criticizing your drinking?
3.	Have you ever felt bad or *guilty* about your drinking?
4.	Have you ever had a drink first thing in the morning to steady your nerves or to get rid of a hangover (*eye-opener*)?

gets one point. A score of two or more is considered significant. Like the SMAST, the CAGE has a high degree of sensitivity. Either test is acceptable as a screening tool.

The Alcohol Use Disorders Identification Test (AUDIT) is a ten-question test developed by a World Health Organization-sponsored collaborative project to determine if a person may be at risk for alcohol abuse problems (Table 14.3 [11]). Scoring is as follows: 0–7 is a lower risk, 8–15 is an increasing risk, 16–19 is a higher risk, and 20+ means possible dependence. Audit has been validated across genders and in a wide range of racial/ethnic groups.

Other Drug Dependencies

Two commonly used screening tests for other drug dependencies are the CAGE-AID and the Drug Abuse Screening Test (DAST-10). CAGE-AID is given in Table 14.4 [12]. It covers alcohol as well as other drugs. Each "yes" answer counts one point. One point indicates a possible problem. Two points indicate a probable problem.

Another drug screening test is the DAST-10 (Table 14.5 [13]). Unlike CAGE-AID, it does not include alcoholic beverages. Each "yes" response gets one point. If the score is zero, then no problem is present, a score of 1–2 represents a low level of probability, a score of 3–5 represents a moderate level of probability, and a score of 6–8 represents a substantial level probability that the person has drug dependence.

Because most screening questionnaires have been developed for people in middle age, they are less appropriate for use with adolescents and the elderly.

Personal and Family History

As part of a personal history related to substance dependence, physicians should cover alcohol history, other drug history (including prescription drugs), social functioning, psychological functioning, and sexual functioning. In addition, a standard medical history should be taken, with special attention paid to medical problems associated with alcoholism and other drug addictions. The review of systems also may identify problems directing attention to substance dependence. Family history may be helpful [14].

Questions about substance use should begin with the least threatening subjects. Thus, start with questions about substances that are culturally acceptable, such as the number of cups of coffee a patient drinks a day. This can progress to the number of cigarettes a patient smokes a day and then to the patient's daily intake of alcohol and other drugs. A change in a patient's style of response can be a clue to addiction. Patients will freely tell you how many cups of coffee they drink a day or how many cigarettes they smoke, but when asked about alcohol or other drugs, substance-dependent people often switch from precise answers to vague ones such as "I drink a few beers now and then," "I drink socially," or "I've tried cocaine once or twice." Anger, evasiveness, or glib conversation from patients giving their substance use history should be regarded as suspicious.

Information about substance use that may be helpful includes (1) when a patient last drank or used other drugs; (2) how much the person drank or used on that occasion; [3] if the person drinks or uses drugs every day and, if not, how often he does so; (4) how much the person averages drinking or using on these occasions; (5) how long the person has been drinking or using drugs in this manner; and (5) how old the person was when he took a first drink or tried another drug. How much a patient is willing to admit depends to a great extent on the examiner's attitude. It should be emphasized that answers to these kinds of questions are only of secondary importance. The most important questions relate to what substance abuse is doing to a patient's life [8, 15].

Table 14.3 The Alcohol Use Disorders Identification Test (AUDIT) (From Higgins-Biddle [11]. Approved with permission, World Health Organization)

Points	0	1	2	3	4
How often do you have a drink containing alcohol?	Never	Monthly or less	2–4 times per month	2–3 times per week	4+ times per week
How many units of alcohol do you drink on a typical day when you are drinking?	1–2	3–4	5–6	7–9	10+
How often have you had six or more units if female, or eight or more if male, on a single occasion in the last year?	Never	Less than monthly	Monthly	Weekly	Daily or almost daily
How often during the last year have you found that you were not able to stop drinking once you had started?	Never	Less than monthly	Monthly	Weekly	Daily or almost daily
How often during the last year have you failed to do what was normally expected from you because of your drinking?	Never	Less than monthly	Monthly	Weekly	Daily or almost daily
How often during the last year have you needed an alcoholic drink in the morning to get yourself going after a heavy drinking session?	Never	Less than monthly	Monthly	Weekly	Daily or almost daily
How often during the last year have you had a feeling of guilt or remorse after drinking?	Never	Less than monthly	Monthly	Weekly	Daily or almost daily
How often during the last year have you been unable to remember what happened the night before because you had been drinking?	Never	Less than monthly	Monthly	Weekly	Daily or almost daily
Have you or somebody else been injured as a result of your drinking?	No		Yes, but not in the last year		Yes, during the last year
Has a relative or friend, doctor, or other health worker been concerned about your drinking or suggested that you cut down?	No		Yes, but not in the last year		Yes, during the last year

Table 14.4 Cage modified for substance abuse (CAGE-AID) (From Brown [12]. Approved with permission, Wisconsin Medical Journal)

1.	Have you ever felt you ought to *cut* down on your drinking or drug use?
2.	Have people *annoyed* you by criticizing your drinking or drug use?
3.	Have you felt bad or *guilty* about your drinking or drug use?
4.	Have you ever had a drink or used drugs first thing in the morning to steady your nerves or to get rid of a hangover (*eye-opener*)?

Table 14.5 The Drug Abuse Screening Test (DAST-10) (From Skinner [13]. Approved with permission, Addictive Behaviors)

1.	Have you used drugs other than those required for medical reasons?
2.	Do you abuse more than one drug at a time?
3.	Are you unable to stop using drugs when you want to?
4.	Have you ever had blackouts or flashbacks as a result of drug use?
5.	Do you ever feel bad or guilty about your drug use?
6.	Does your spouse (or parents) ever complain about your involvement with drugs?
7.	Have you neglected your family because of your use of drugs?
8.	Have you engaged in illegal activities in order to obtain drugs?
9.	Have you ever experienced withdrawal symptoms (felt sick) when you stopped taking drugs?
10.	Have you had medical problems as a result of your drug use (e.g., memory loss, hepatitis, convulsions, bleeding)?

A variety of findings may reveal psychological problems, such as insomnia, anxiety, depression, and suicide attempts or gestures. A social history should include questions about a patient's work, family, interpersonal relationship, and legal problems.

Substance dependence is notorious for causing sexual problems, especially impotence in men and menstrual irregularities and infertility in women. Decreased interest in sex may occur in either sex. Questions about sexual functioning should be part of every medical history [16].

Family history also may give physicians useful information. The tendency to become an alcoholic runs in families and is thought to be genetically transmitted. A male patient whose father was an alcoholic, for example, may have almost a fourfold increase in risk of becoming an alcoholic than someone in the general public [17]. Genetic transmission for other drugs has not been studied to the same extent as it has for alcoholism, but it seems certain, based on the studies that have been done, that a genetic tendency for dependence on these drugs exists as well [4].

Psychological and social findings that may indicate substance dependence are given in Table 14.6.

Patient Presentation

Addicts often try to get drugs from physicians. Certain behaviors are common among such patients, such as describing a dramatic and compelling but vague complaint; making subjective complaints not accompanied by the usual objective signs; offering a diagnosis and specifically requesting a certain drug, often claiming to be allergic to less potent ones; showing no interest in a diagnosis; failing to keep appointments for X-rays or laboratory tests or failing to see another physician for a consulting opinion; and rejecting all treatments that do not include psychoactive drugs.

Patient hustlers use many manipulative approaches. These include feigning physical problems. For example, those seeking narcotics often complain of renal colic, toothache, or tic douloureux. They generally can simulate symptoms exceptionally well. Those feigning renal colic may even prick their fingers to put drops of blood in their urine. Those feigning toothaches often claim to have an out-of-town dentist and to have left prescribed pain medication at home.

Hustlers also may feign psychological problems, such as anxiety, insomnia, or fatigue. Most such drug seekers want opioids, tranquilizers, sleeping pills, or stimulants. Often they are deceptive, complaining that their medication was lost, stolen, or accidentally dropped in the toilet. They may steal, alter, or forge prescriptions, request

Table 14.6 Psychological and social findings that may indicate substance dependence (From Milhorn [4]. Approved with permission, Springer)

Anxiety, insomnia, depression, suicide gestures or attempts
Any alcohol- or other drug-related arrests or driving under the influence
Binge drinking
Blackouts (not remembering what happened during a drinking or using spell)
Change in choice of friends or associates
Change in mood, including unpredictability and impulsivity
Child or spouse abuse
Children doing poorly in school, disturbed or runaway children
Complaints by family members about behavior related to the use of alcohol or other drugs
Continued drinking or using despite medical, psychological, or social contraindications
Decreased goal-directed drives (amotivational syndrome)
Decreased school performance
Divorce or separation
Drinking before a party (just in case there's not enough to drink at the party)
Frequent job changes
Frequent moves to new areas (geographic cure)
Gulping the first two or three drinks
History of increased tolerance to alcohol or other drugs; loss of tolerance in older individuals
Interpersonal problems at work or school
Loss of interest in nondrinking or nonusing activities
Loss of interest in personal hygiene or appearance
Other job or school problems (tardiness, calling in sick, absenteeism)
Preoccupation with recreational drinking or using
Repeated attempts to stop drinking or using (patients claim they can quit anytime)
Repeated requests for narcotics or stimulants
Self-medication, regular or prolonged use of sleeping pills or tranquilizers, or repeated requests for them
Social isolation
Underemployment for educational level
Use of alcohol before any office visit
Visiting many physicians or doctor shopping

refills in a shorter period of time than was prescribed, or phone physicians on call and claim to be a patient of his or her partner.

Patients may also pressure physicians to elicit sympathy or guilt. One way they do this is by suggesting that medical treatment caused their addiction. They may admit to being addicted and pressure physicians to detoxify them as outpatients, although they have no intention of giving up their drug use.

Alcoholics commonly seek prescriptions for minor tranquilizers either to help them quit drinking or to treat the anxiety and insomnia associated with alcoholism. Such outpatient detoxification is usually not advisable for many drugs and is illegal for narcotics. Patients may directly threaten physicians with physical, legal, or financial harm and may try to bribe them or may use the names of influential people, claiming them to be relatives or friends [18–20].

Physical Examination

Patients with substance use disorders may have a variety of physical signs that should prompt physicians to ask questions about alcohol or other drug use.

Alcoholism

All physicians are familiar with the signs and symptoms of late-stage alcoholism, such as cirrhosis of the liver, ascites, chronic pancreatitis, cardiomyopathy, and esophageal varicose, and they are experts at managing these conditions. The real challenge is to diagnose alcoholism in patients early in its course to prevent them from reaching advanced stages [8].

Physicians can find many clues to alcoholism in physical examinations. Acute intoxication causes sedation, confusion, disorientation, slurred speech, faulty judgment, and many other symptoms. Physicians may smell alcohol on a patient's breath. Chronic alcohol use leads to untidiness in personal habits and to depression.

Alcoholics may have slightly bloated and plethoric faces. They may even have parotid swelling and a cushingoid look. They may have small bruises in a variety of places and in a variety of colors, depending on how long ago the injuries were acquired. This is particularly true of women alcoholics, who tend to bump into furniture and doorknobs while doing housework. Cigarette burns on patients' fingers, chests, or legs may indicate alcoholism. Severe periodontal disease, despite an otherwise neat and clean appearance, is another clue.

Mild to moderate hypertension is very common among alcoholics. This usually disappears in a few days to a week after they stop drinking. Alcoholics are frequently admitted to treatment centers on hypertensive medications. Many are later discharged on no medications and with good blood pressure control. Cardiac arrhythmias, such as atrial fibrillation, as well as abnormal ST-T findings, are also common in alcoholics.

Elevated uric acid levels precipitate gouty attacks in some alcoholics. The attacks dissipate once patients stop drinking, and their uric acid levels return to normal. Gout may be particularly difficult to control in alcoholics.

Grand mal seizure in adults should make physicians think of alcoholism, especially if patients tell them they stopped drinking in the past 72 h. A seizure within a few days of a patient's being admitted to a hospital may be a clue to alcohol withdrawal.

Patients diagnosed with cancer of virtually any segment of the gastrointestinal tract should be questioned about drinking. Alcoholics have a higher incidence of cancers of the oral cavity, tongue, pharynx, larynx, esophagus, stomach, liver, pancreas, colon, and rectum than do nonalcoholics. Alcohol appears to act synergistically with cigarette smoking in this regard.

Multiple rib fractures that show different stages of healing on chest X-rays should be a tip-off to alcoholism. Fractured ribs are the most common abnormalities on chest X-rays in alcoholics. Alcohol use is frequently involved in motor vehicle accidents, drownings, accidental falls, beatings, shootings, and stabbings.

Gastrointestinal problems are the most common medical complaints of alcoholics. Alcohol irritates the gastric mucosa and can cause gastritis, ulcers, duodenitis, ileitis, irritable bowel syndrome, and pancreatitis. Alcoholics commonly show up at treatment centers on one or more stomach medications, some of which they have been on for years. These same patients are rarely discharged still needing these medications.

Some alcoholics' cushingoid appearance, along with the hypertension and glucose intolerance caused by alcohol, occasionally prompts physicians to do endocrine work-ups without first considering alcoholism. Similarly, physicians may confuse the combination of the mild tremors of minor alcohol withdrawal, hypertension, and occasional cardiac arrhythmias with hyperthyroidism [21, 22].

A number of physical findings may indicate alcoholism [4]. These are given in Table 14.7.

Other Drug Dependencies

Signs and symptoms can be very helpful in acquiring an idea of which substance a patient has been abusing.

Restlessness or agitated behavior most commonly suggests that patients are using stimulants or hallucinogens or are withdrawing from depressants or opioids. Marijuana use occasionally produces a similar response. Quiet, withdrawn behavior may indicate recent use of CNS depressants, opioids, or hallucinogens. Withdrawal from stimulants may be characterized by apathy, somnolence, and depression. Depression can also occur with chronic use of CNS depressants.

Disorientation most often occurs with the use of hallucinogens and phencyclidines but may also occur with the use of stimulants, CNS depressants, or cannabinoids. CNS depressants and stimulants are the drugs that most frequently cause psychotic reactions, although they may also occur with the use of hallucinogens, phencyclidine, or cannabinoids. Withdrawal from CNS depressants may precipitate psychotic episodes. Stimulant users may suffer paranoia.

Slurred speech is a characteristic of depressant intoxication, although any abused drug may alter speech patterns. Resting tremor may indicate stimulant or hallucinogen use or withdrawal from CNS depressants or opioids. Grand mal seizures may result from stimulant or opioid (meperidine) use or occur during withdrawal from CNS depressants. Seizures may not occur until 1 week after the last dose of a long-acting

Table 14.7 Physical findings that may indicate alcoholism (acute/chronic use) (From Milhorn [4]. Approved with Permission, Springer)

Nervous system: Sedation, confusion, disorientation, slurred speech, difficulty thinking, slowness of speech and comprehension, dizziness, poor memory, faulty judgment, narrowed range of attention, emotional lability, irritability, quarrelsomeness, hallucinosis, untidiness in personal habits, depression and suicide attempts, ataxia, impaired psychomotor performance, peripheral neuropathy, cerebellar degeneration, subdural hematoma, cerebral atrophy in a relatively young person, optic neuropathy, seizure disorder
Head, eyes, ears, nose, throat: Poor dentition, oropharyngeal lesions, hoarseness, plethoric faces, parotid enlargement, injected conjunctiva, flushed skin, head trauma, alcohol on breath
Chest: Repeated upper respiratory and bronchial infections, signs and symptoms of aspiration, pneumonia, appearance of lobar pneumonias particularly *Klebsiella* and *pneumococcus*, tuberculosis, fractured ribs
Cardiovascular system: Cardiac arrhythmias, sinus tachycardia, hypertension, cardiomyopathy
Abdomen and gastrointestinal system: Nausea, vomiting, ascites, large or small liver, caput medusa, palpable spleen, abdominal tenderness due to gastritis, ulcers, duodenitis, esophagitis, ileitis, irritable bowel syndrome or pancreatitis, findings compatible with advanced liver disease such as loss of secondary sex characteristics, hemorrhoids, spider angiomata, or gynecomastia, positive hemoccult stools
Musculoskeletal system: Gout, especially if it is difficult to control, trauma, avascular necrosis of the femoral head in a young adult, myopathy primarily in shoulders and hips
Dermatological system: Cigarette burns, bruises, seborrheic dermatitis, rosacea, palmar erythema
Genitourinary system: Impotence, menstrual disturbances, infertility, testicular atrophy, feminization in men, masculinization in women
Overdose
Stupor, respiratory depression, coma, death
Withdrawal
Insomnia, anxiety, tremor, nausea, vomiting, elevated blood pressure and pulse rate, agitation, sweating, hyperactive reflexes, grand mal seizures, delirium tremens

benzodiazepine, such as diazepam (Valium). They also may occur after overdose of hallucinogens or phencyclidine. Hyperreflexia occurs most often with stimulant use or withdrawal from CNS depressants or opioids.

Elevated blood pressure most commonly occurs with stimulant use, but it may also occur with phencyclidine or hallucinogen use or with withdrawal from CNS depressants or opioids. Pulse irregularities suggest the use of stimulants or inhalants. Tachycardia is present in most acute drug reactions and in withdrawal from CNS depressants or opioids.

Elevated temperature may occur with the use of stimulants or hallucinogens or in withdrawal from CNS depressants or opioids. It also may occur with phencyclidine overdose. Malignant hyperthermia may occur with stimulant overdose.

Sweating accompanies most acute drug reactions and can occur with withdrawal from CNS depressants and opioids. It is a common complaint of those on methadone. Piloerection (gooseflesh) is a classic sign of opioid (heroin) withdrawal and may also occur in acute LSD reactions. Needle tracks most commonly indicate the use of an opioid, although stimulants and CNS depressants also may be injected intravenously. Patients may wear long-sleeved clothing in warm weather to cover up needle tracks.

Excessive lacrimation, as well as rhinorrhea and dilated pupils, is a manifestation of opioid withdrawal. Opioid use, as a rule, constricts pupils. Stimulants, hallucinogens, cannabinoids, and sometimes meperidine (Demerol) dilate pupils. CNS depressants usually make pupils midpoint and slowly reactive. Horizontal or vertical nystagmus may occur with phencyclidine use. An exaggerated blink reflex is commonly associated with barbiturate withdrawal. Marijuana use produces conjunctival injection. Patients may wear sunglasses to hide this.

Respiratory depression may indicate the use of opioids or CNS depressants, particularly barbiturates. Pulmonary edema and pulmonary fibrosis may be caused by the use of intravenous heroin or some of its contaminants. Bronchial irritation may indicate recent heavy marijuana smoking.

The occurrence together with pinpoint pupils, depressed respiration, and coma strongly suggests opioid overdose. Opioids depress the cough reflex, and stuporous abusers may aspirate. A similar syndrome may be found in users of CNS depressants. Crampy abdominal pain and diarrhea occur with opioid withdrawal.

Phencyclidine use produces a combination of sympathetic (increased blood pressure, pulse rate, and reflexes) and cholinergic (sweating, drooling, flushing) overactivity. The combination of a coma-like state, open eyes, decreased perception of pain, periods of temporary excitation, and bodily rigidity should lead a physician to suspect phencyclidine overdose. Toxic reactions to phencyclidine are not only life threatening but tend to be the longest-lasting symptom caused by any abused drug.

Inhalant abuse may produce respiratory depression, cardiac arrhythmias, rapid loss of consciousness, and death. In typical reported cases, young people inhale a volatile hydrocarbon and feel an urge to run. After sprinting a short distance, they fall to the ground dead; usually, it is thought from a cardiac arrhythmia. Individuals who inhale drugs from plastic bags placed over their heads can die of suffocation. Inhalants sometimes cause rashes on the hands or around the mouth or nose and can irritate mucous membranes.

Traumas, such as head injuries, limb fractures, stab wounds, and gunshot wounds, are not uncommon in substance-dependent people. Weight loss and malnutrition may accompany chronic, heavy use of any drug.

Snorting stimulants (amphetamines, cocaine) can produce rhinitis, nasal bleeding, sinus problems, hyperemic nasal turbinates, abuse of nasal sprays, hoarseness, and difficulty swallowing. Snorting cocaine can lead to septal perforation.

Drug inhalation (cocaine, marijuana) can produce a variety of conditions, including decreased pulmonary function, wheezing, chronic cough, pharyngitis, uveitis, sinusitis, bronchitis, and hemoptysis [15, 23, 24].

Physical findings that may indicate addiction to other drugs are given in Table 14.8. A variety of physical signs may indicate subcutaneous, intramuscular, or intravenous drug injection. Signs of such injections include needle marks, local infections, and scars. Signs of systemic infection (hepatitis C, infective endocarditis, osteomyelitis, AIDS) may be present. Physical signs indicating that patients may be injecting drugs are given in Table 14.9.

Laboratory Tests

Abnormal laboratory values are not diagnostic of substance dependence; however, they should arouse suspicion and prompt further questioning. The absence of abnormal laboratory findings does not rule out substance dependence. Chest X-rays and EKGs are generally not helpful but should be done for patients over 40 years of age or for younger patients with a history of cardiac or pulmonary disease [15].

Alcoholism

Alcohol laboratory biomarkers are divided into direct and indirect biomarkers.

Direct Alcohol Biomarkers

Direct alcohol biomarkers include alcohol level and ethyl glucuronide (EtG). A blood alcohol level might be helpful in the office if the patient appears intoxicated but denies alcohol use. A blood alcohol level in the excess of 0.30 g/dL, a blood alcohol level of greater than 0.15 g/dL without gross evidence of intoxication, or a blood alcohol level of greater than 0.10 g/dL on routine examination indicates alcoholism with a high degree of reliability.

The short half-life of alcohol limits its use as a biomarker. Because the blood alcohol level detects alcohol intake for the previous few hours, it is not necessarily a good indicator of chronic excessive drinking.

EtG is a metabolite of alcohol that is formed by the conjugation of ethanol with activated glucuronic acid. Shortly after alcohol intake, even in small amounts, EtG becomes positive. After complete cessation of alcohol intake, EtG can be detected in urine for up to 5 days after heavy binge drinking, making EtG an important biomarker of relatively recent alcohol consumption [25].

Indirect Alcohol Biomarkers

Positive indirect biomarkers suggest heavy alcohol use by detecting the toxic effects that alcohol has had on organ systems or body chemistry. They include aspartate aminotransferase (AST), alanine aminotransferase (ALT), gamma glutam-

Table 14.8 Physical findings that may indicate other drug dependencies (From Milhorn [4]. Approved with permission, Springer)

CNS depressants	
Acute/chronic use	Sedation, confusion, disorientation, slurred speech, ataxia, difficulty thinking, slowness of speech and comprehension, dizziness, impaired psychomotor performance, poor memory, faulty judgment, narrowed range of attention, emotional lability, irritability, quarrelsome, untidiness in personal habits, depression, and suicidal gestures or attempts
Overdose	Shallow breathing, respiratory depression, hypotension, aspiration pneumonia, respiratory arrest and circulatory collapse, depressed sensorium to coma, death
Abstinence syndrome	Insomnia, anxiety, panic attacks, tremor, nausea, vomiting, elevated blood pressure and pulse rate, irritability, agitation, sweating, hyperactive reflexes, pleading for drugs, grand mal seizures, confusion, delirium, psychosis
Opioids	
Acute/chronic use	Decreased pain, sleepiness, euphoria, nausea, vomiting, pupillary constriction, constipation, decreased libido and altered menstrual cycle, generalized itching, suppression of cough reflex, grand mal seizures
Overdose	Drowsiness, hypothermia, pinpoint pupils (which may be dilated with meperidine), aspiration pneumonia, hypotension, respiratory depression, pulmonary edema, respiratory arrest, coma, death
Abstinence syndrome	Lacrimation, rhinorrhea, yawning, irritability, sweating, restlessness, tremor, insomnia, piloerection, abdominal cramps, nausea, vomiting, diarrhea, muscle and bone pain, increased pulse and blood pressure, drug craving with drug-seeking behavior
CNS stimulants	
Acute/chronic use	Euphoria with acute use and dysphoria with chronic use, increased energy with acute use and fatigue with chronic use, increased feelings of sexuality with acute use, decreased feelings of sexuality with chronic use, decreased appetite, insomnia, weight loss, excitement, tremor, pupillary dilation, increased blood pressure and pulse rate, indifference to pain, rhinitis, nasal bleeding, sinus problems, dull frontal headache, hyperemic nasal turbinates, nasal spray abuse, septal perforation, hoarseness, difficulty swallowing, personal neglect, delusions, suspiciousness, paranoid psychosis
Overdose	Headache, flushed skin, tactile sensations (coke bugs), hallucinations, acute anxiety, agitation, confusion, malignant hyperthermia, tachycardia and hypertension, stereotypical repetitious behavior, bruxism and face picking, toxic psychosis, chest pain with cardiac arrhythmias, myocardial infarction, grand mal seizures, cerebral hemorrhages, hypothermia, circulatory collapse, coma, death
Abstinence syndrome	Negativism, pessimism, lack of patience, irritability, depression, lack of energy, sleepiness, sleep disturbances, fear, paranoia, nervousness, diaphoresis, chills, hunger, drug craving
Cannabinoids	
Acute/chronic use	Euphoria, decreased psychomotor performance, increased pulse rate, decreased pulmonary function, exacerbation of asthma, conjunctival injection, uveitis, pharyngitis, bronchitis, stuffy nose, dry mouth, sinusitis, disruption of menstrual cycle, perceptual delusions, paranoid feelings, mood shifts (joy to sorrow, fear to elation), sleepiness, heightened sexual arousal, anxiety to panic, amotivational syndrome with chronic use, angina in those with preexisting heart trouble
Overdose	Tachycardia, hypertension, delusions, hallucinations, seizures in epileptics, acute toxic psychosis
Abstinence syndrome	Irritability, restlessness, nervousness, insomnia, mild tremor, mild body temperature elevation
Phencyclidines	
Acute/chronic use	Increased blood pressure and pulse rate, increased respiratory rate, dizziness, lack of coordination, ataxia, slurred speech, vertical and horizontal nystagmus, paranoid delusions, delusions of superhuman strength, agitation, unpredictable behavior, nudity in public
Overdose	Vertigo, skin flushing, nausea, vomiting, auditory and visual hallucinations, hyperreflexia, rhabdomyolysis and acute renal failure, tremor, bilateral ptosis, tachycardia, decreased respiration, grand mal seizures, acute toxic psychosis, fever, body rigidity, coma-like state with eyes open and temporary periods of excitation, decreased pain perception, respiratory depression, hypertensive crisis, death
Abstinence syndrome	Nervousness, anxiety, and depression may occur

(continued)

Table 14.8 (continued)

Hallucinogens	
Acute/chronic use	Visual hallucinations, flushed face, pupillary dilation, fine tremor, increased blood pressure and pulse rate, increased body temperature, hyperreflexia, muscle weakness, tremor, dizziness, weakness, nausea, vomiting, paresthesia, labile mood, anxiety, panic attacks, depression, flashbacks
Overdose	Toxic psychosis, tachycardia, hypertension, cardiac arrhythmias, hyperpyrexia, shock, convulsions
Abstinence syndrome	None known
Inhalants	
Acute/chronic use	Central nervous system effects (headache, euphoria, excitement, slurred speech, drowsiness, irritability, mental dullness, tremors, emotional lability, nystagmus, ataxia, polyneuropathies, permanent encephalopathies), intestinal effects (mucus membrane irritation, unpleasant breath odor, nausea, vomiting, gastric pain, anorexia, dyspepsia, chronic gastritis, hepatomegaly, weight loss), urinary dysfunction (renal tubular necrosis, renal failure), cardiovascular (irregular heartbeat, increased pulse rate), others (eye irritation, rash around mouth or nose, cough, chemical pneumonia, muscle weakness and atrophy)
Overdose	Confusion, disorientation, cardiac arrhythmias, respiratory depression, decreased sensorium, loss of consciousness, sudden death
Abstinence syndrome	Anxiety, irritability, difficulty concentrating, muscle spasms, depression, psychosis, seizures

Table 14.9 Physical findings related to drug injection (From Milhorn [4]. Approved with permission, Springer)

Skin tracks and related scars on the neck, axilla, forearm, wrist, foot, ankle, under the tongue, and penile veins; new lesions may be inflamed
Needle puncture marks located over veins
Pock mark-like scars from subcutaneous injections (especially in the deltoid, gluteal areas, abdomen, thigh, and shoulder)
Wheals or hives at injection site
Abscesses, infections, or ulcerations on the arm, thigh, shoulder, abdomen, chest, hand, or finger
Necrosis of the skin
Edema of the hand or irreducible finger flexion (camptodactyly); this occurs when drugs are injected into the veins of the fingers or the hands
Thrombophlebitis at possible injection sites
Accidental “tattoos” at injection sites; these result from carbon produced by heating needles to sterilize them
Dermatitis at injection sites
Allergic reactions (purpura, urticaria, pruritus)
Tourniquet pigmentation; this is a poorly defined linear mark above the antecubital space
Signs of hepatitis B (fever, jaundice, hepatomegaly, nausea, vomiting)
Signs of acute infective endocarditis (fever, mitral regurgitation murmur, septic pulmonary emboli, Roth’s spots, Janeway lesions, Osler’s nodes)
Signs of septic arthritis or osteomyelitis (fever, local joint, limb, or back pain)
Signs of AIDS (fatigue, anorexia, weight loss, fever, diarrhea, lymphadenopathy, *Pneumocystis carinii* pneumonia, pulmonary aspergillosis, candida esophagitis, tuberculosis, histoplasmosis, cryptococcal meningitis)

yltransferase (GGT), mean corpuscular volume (MCV), and carbohydrate-deficient transferrin (CDT). As a screen for alcohol dependence, the sensitivity and specificity of CDT are generally higher than AST, ALT, GGT, or MCV. CDT is less sensitive and specific in women than men.

The combination of GGT and CDT, compared with GGT or CDT alone, shows a higher diagnostic sensitivity, a higher diagnostic specificity, and a stronger correlation with the actual amounts of alcohol consumption.

The SGGT is generally thought to be the most sensitive enzyme test of liver disease, yet it is abnormal in only 31–70% of diagnosed alcoholics. The SGGT is a hepatic microsomal enzyme that is subject to induction; its elevation may, therefore, indicate either microsomal induction or hepatic injury. Alcoholism is the most common cause of its elevation; it is not elevated in social drinkers. Anticonvulsants that induce hepatic enzymes may be a nonalcoholic cause of elevated SGGT. An AST/ALT ratio greater than two is said to be suggestive of alcoholic liver disease.

Excessive consumption of alcohol is also the most common cause of an elevated MCV. Patients may or may not have anemia. Other causes of an elevated MCV include reticulocytosis, folic acid deficiency, vitamin B12 deficiency, and nonalcoholic liver disease. Prothrombin time (PT) may be prolonged by alcoholic liver disease, and patients occasionally have decreased platelet counts, along with decreased white blood cell counts secondary to bone marrow depression by alcohol. Serum magnesium, calcium, phosphorus, potassium, and BUN also may be decreased.

Alcoholics may have hypoglycemia or hyperglycemia. Alcohol impairs gluconeogenesis so that blood glucose levels may fall, especially in patients suffering from poor nutrition. Once the pancreas is damaged, it may not secrete enough insulin to respond to sugar loads, producing high blood sugar. Alcoholism should be considered in diabetic patients who have difficulty maintaining reasonable control of their diabetes [25].

Other Drug Dependencies

Laboratory tests are not nearly as helpful for the diagnosis of dependence on other drugs as they are for alcoholism. For the most part, they represent nonspecific findings or are the results of infections due to intravenous, subcutaneous, or intramuscular drug use. A urine drug screen may be helpful.

Inhalant use may initially cause leukocytosis and anemia, followed by pancytopenia or aplastic anemia. Myeloid leukemia has been reported. White blood cells, erythrocytes, and protein may be found in a patient's urine. Renal tubular necrosis may occur and lead to acute renal failure, with elevated BUN and creatinine. Liver toxicity may cause bilirubin, AST, ALT, LDH, and alkaline phosphatase to be elevated.

Opioid use may produce a depressed testosterone level, a high resting glucose level, an abnormal glucose tolerance test, and sometimes an eosinophilia. It may also cause false-positive serological tests for pregnancy or syphilis. Acute myoglobinemia and myoglobinuria may occur with heroin use or phencyclidine overdose. Abnormal arterial blood gases (elevated Pco_2, depressed Po_2 and pH) may result from the pulmonary edema associated with heroin injection or from overdoses of drugs (CNS depressants, opioids) that depress respiration.

Vomiting caused by drug use or withdrawal may produce electrolyte abnormalities (elevated $HCO3^-$ and pH, decreased K^+ and Cl^-).

Drug injection can lead to a number of findings. These include an increased white blood cell count and positive blood cultures from infection. The most common offending organisms with acute infective endocarditis are *Staphylococcus aureus*, *Enterococci*, gram-negative bacteria, and *Candida albicans*. The hemoglobin and hematocrit may be depressed with infective endocarditis secondary to hemolysis; an echocardiogram may be diagnostic.

Laboratory findings with hepatitis C include elevated bilirubin, AST, ALT, LDH, and alkaline phosphatase. X-rays or an MRI may be helpful for making the diagnosis of osteomyelitis. An elevated white blood cell count or positive culture on aspirated joint fluid may be helpful for diagnosing septic arthritis. Infection with the human immunodeficiency virus may produce a depressed lymphocyte count as well as a variety of abnormal tests resulting from infection with opportunistic organisms [15, 26].

Drug Screening

General Principles

Drug screening can be done on the urine, blood, hair, saliva, sweat, and nails. Urine is most often used for drug screening because it is easy to collect, collecting it is noninvasive, it is easier to analyze than blood or other fluids, and it can be refrigerated and stored. Drugs and their metabolites usually are found in higher concentrations in urine than in other body fluids because of the concentrating functions of the kidney.

Laboratory procedures for detecting drugs are divided into screening tests and confirmatory tests. Screening tests offer high sensitivity but sacrifice specificity; therefore, in screening, it is important to use tests that yield few false-negative results. Most screens detect drugs in 99% or more of specimens in which they are present at concentrations greater than a predetermined cutoff level. The number of false-positive results may be high. Confirmatory tests, on the other hand, are very specific and separate true positives from false positives with great accuracy.

Drug screen results do not give any indication of patients' patterns of drug use (how they administer drugs, how frequently they use them, when they last used them, the amount they used), whether patients are one-time users or are substance dependent, and they do not tell whether patients are impaired physically or mentally by the use of a drug.

Routine urine screening tests usually do not detect hallucinogens, many designer drugs, or alcohol. Specific requests must be made for tests of these substances, and such tests are usually fairly expensive. Alcohol is better tested for in a blood sample.

False-negative screens occur for several reasons. A mix-up of samples is an obvious cause, and it occasionally happens. A chain of custody should prevent this. False-negative screens may occur when patients have taken drugs so recently that they have not undergone sufficient renal excretion to be detectable in urine. Also, renal impairment may delay excretion. Patients afraid of testing positive for drug use may adulterate their urine samples with a variety of substances (salt, vinegar, bleach, lemon juice, water) or substitute a urine sample from drug-free individuals. Patients should be directly observed while collecting urine samples.

Also, drug users often ingest one drug, believing it to be another one. For example, a patient may use PCP thinking it is cocaine. A test for cocaine would, therefore, be negative.

The larger the dose, the longer a drug can be detected in the urine. If a patient is a chronic user, a drug may reach a steady state in the body, in which case the time needed to clear the drug from the body is longer than would be needed after an acute ingestion.

The half-life, volume of distribution, lipophilicity, and dissociation constant of a drug affect its rate of excretion. Drugs that are cleared by first-order kinetics (drugs for which the rate of clearance is proportional to serum concentration) are about 94% eliminated in four half-lives. Decreased cardiac output, as well as decreased liver or kidney function, can decrease the rate of excretion and, thereby, increase the half-life of a drug. Drugs with a small volume of distribution clear faster than those with a larger volume of distribution. Weak acids are excreted more rapidly in alkaline urine, and weak bases are excreted more rapidly in acidic urine [27–30].

Screening Tests

Two screening tests are currently in use—thin-layer chromatography and immunoassays. Thin-layer chromatography is based on the principle that drugs of different solubilities migrate at different rates and, thus, occupy different positions on a strip after a specified period of time. Migration is allowed to occur under acidic and basic conditions. The strips are then examined under ultraviolet light and combined with iodine. Under each of these four conditions (acidic, basic, ultraviolet light, iodine), a given drug has a characteristic pattern of migration and color. By comparison to controls, individual drugs can be identified. This test is, therefore, not quantitative but is read merely as positive or negative.

Immunoassays involve binding a drug (antigen) with an antibody from a test kit that has been generated to recognize and bind exclusively a specific drug. Two immunoassays are in common use—enzyme immunoassay and radioimmunoassay. The two methods differ in the way they measure the concentration of the resulting complex. The enzyme immunoassay determines the concentration of the antigen-antibody complex by measuring the activity of an enzyme attached to the antigen. The enzyme multiplied immunoassay technique (EMIT) is the most widely used test of this type. The radioimmunoassay determines the concentration of antigen-antibody complex by measuring the activity of a radioisotopically labeled antigen. Immunoassays give quantitative results. Immunoassay analysis is the most commonly used screening test of the two.

False-positive results in such tests sometimes occur because of a phenomenon known as cross-reactivity. Several drugs in the same substance class may give positive tests on assays intended to detect a specific drug. For instance, phenylpropanolamine, ephedrine, or pseudoephedrine may give positive results when physicians are testing for amphetamines. In such instances, false-positive tests can be identified by confirmatory tests [28, 31].

Screening Drug Panels

Routine screening drug panels usually consist of a five- or a ten-panel drug test. Other panels are available.

Five-Panel Drug Test Most standard drug screens are of the five-panel type. They test for the most common street drugs—marijuana, cocaine, phencyclidine, amphetamines, and opiates. Amphetamines include drugs such as methamphetamine and ecstasy. Opiates include heroin, opium, and codeine.

Ten-Panel Drug Test The ten-panel test screens for the five most common types of drugs that are in the five-panel drug test plus barbiturates, benzodiazepines, methadone, methaqualone, and propoxyphene [32].

Steps to Reduce Tampering in Urine Drug Screening

A number of steps can be taken to prevent tampering when collecting a urine drug screen sample [31]. These include:

- Requesting removal of any unnecessary outer clothing
- Removing anything in the collection area that could be used to adulterate or substitute a urine specimen
- Requesting the display and removal of any items in the patient's pockets, coat, hat, etc.
- Requiring all other personal belongings (briefcase, purse, etc.) to remain with the outer clothing
- Instructing the patient to wash and dry his or her hands (preferably with liquid soap) under direct observation and not to wash again until after delivering the specimen
- Placing a bluing agent in the commode and turning off the water supply to the testing site

Confirmatory Tests

Confirmatory techniques include gas chromatography/mass spectrometry (GC/MS) and high-pressure liquid chromatography. Both give highly specific results. Gas chromatology consists of a column, usually a glass tube, packed with an absorbent material and contained in a heated oven-like area. An inert gas continuously passes through the column. The mixture of drugs contained in an organic solvent is injected into one end of the column. The injected material is volatilized by the heat and carried through the column as a vapor. The components are separated as they pass through the column and pass out the other end one at a time.

A mass spectrometer is an instrument in which ions produced from a sample are separated by electric or magnetic fields according to their ratios of charge to mass. Gas chromatography/mass spectrometry combines the separating power of the gas chromatograph with the molecular-identifying power of the mass spectrometer. The gas chromatograph separates the compounds, and the mass spectrometer identifies them.

High-pressure liquid chromatography in principle works much like gas chromatography. A solvent mixture is pumped under high pressure through an absorbent material packed into a column, usually made of stainless steel. The mixture of drugs contained in an organic solvent is injected into one end of the column. Individual drugs are identified by their ultraviolet spectrum as they exit the other end.

Gas chromatography/mass spectrometry is the most commonly used confirmatory test of the two [28].

Cutoff Levels

The Department of Health and Human Services (DHHS) has established specific cutoff levels that define a positive result for the workplace as given in Table 14.10.

Length of Time Drugs Can Be Detected in the Urine

Several factors need to be considered to determine the length of time a drug can be detected in the urine. Pharmacokinetics, presence of metabolites, patient variability (body mass), short-term versus long-term use of a drug, pH of the urine, and time of last ingestion are some factors that influence detection times.

Table 14.10 Federal Workplace Cutoff Values (From Moeller [29]. Approved with permission, Mayo Clinic Proc)

Substance	Initial drug test level (immunoassay) (ng/mL)	Confirmatory drug test level (GC-MS) (ng/mL)
Marijuana metabolites	50	15
Cocaine metabolites	300	150
Opiate metabolites	2000	2000
Phencyclidine	25	25
Amphetamines	1000	500
Methamphetamine	Incomplete data	500

False-Positive Immunoassay Tests

A number of commonly prescribed medications can cause false-positive immunoassay tests [32, 33]. Some of these are given in Table 14.11.

Attempts to Cheat on the Urine Drug Screen

There are many ways for patients to circumvent drug testing; some of these include:

- Adding adulterants to urine at the time of testing
- Urine dilution through excessive water ingestion
- Diuretic use to dilute urine
- Consumption of substances that interfere with testing
- Substitution of a clean urine sample

Several chemicals can be added to a urine sample to interfere with urine drug testing. These include over-the-counter eye drops (containing tetrahydrozoline), bleach, vinegar, soap, ammonia, drain cleaner, and table salt.

Addicts may add a commercially available adulterant in vitro to the urine specimen after collection. Examples of these include Stealth (peroxidase and peroxide), Klear (nitrite), Clean ADD-IT-ive (glutaraldehyde), and Urine Luck (pyridinium chlorochromate).

Addicts also may use a commercially available product to flush out drugs, such as Absolute Detox XXL Drink, Absolute Carbo Drinks, Ready Clean Drug Detox Drink, Fast Flush Capsules, and Ready Clean Gel Capsules.

Many of these products contain caffeine or other diuretics to increase the output of urine as well as sugar and natural or artificial flavoring agents. The objective is to produce diluted urine so that concentrations of abused drugs and or metabolites fall below the recommended cutoff concentrations [34].

In situations where observed voiding is mandated, urinary substitution techniques and devices can be quite sophisticated and difficult to detect. An artificial penis with an electronic, temperature-controlled urine reservoir can be purchased online. Patients also may attempt to evade detection by voiding before testing and then refilling their bladder with clean urine using a catheter [31].

Findings suggestive of adulterated, diluted, or substituted urine specimens are given in Table 14.12.

Excessive dilute, adulterated, or any other rejected urine is reported as positive. Legally mandated drug testing requires a Certified Medical Review Officer (CMRO) who is a physician responsible for receiving, reviewing, and evaluating results generated by employers' drug testing programs [31].

Mixed Drug Dependencies

Few addicts use only one drug; however, virtually all can identify the drug they most prefer (drug of choice). Often, but not always, this drug produces the predominant signs and symptoms in the face of mixed drug use. Urine or serum drug screens can be of considerable help if they can be obtained rapidly.

Two CNS depressant drugs used simultaneously (e.g., alcohol and a barbiturate) act synergistically to depress the central nervous system and can lead to respiratory depression, coma, and

Table 14.11 Drugs that may cause false-positive results in immunoassay testing (From Standridge [31]. Approved with permission, Am Fam Physician)

Amphetamines	Amantadine (Symmetrel), bupropion (Wellbutrin), chlorpromazine (Thorazine), desipramine (Norpramin), fluoxetine (Prozac), L-methamphetamine (in nasal decongestants), labetalol (Normodyne), methylphenidate (Ritalin), phentermine (Ionamin), phenylephrine, phenylpropanolamine, promethazine (Phenergan), pseudoephedrine, ranitidine (Zantac), thioridazine (Mellaril), trazodone (Desyrel)
Benzodiazepines	Oxaprozin (Daypro), sertraline (Zoloft)
Cocaine	Topical anesthetics containing cocaine
Opiates	Dextromethorphan, diphenhydramine (Benadryl), fluoroquinolones, poppy seeds, quinine, rifampin (Rifadin), verapamil (Calan)
Phencyclidine	Dextromethorphan, diphenhydramine, ibuprofen, imipramine (Tofranil), ketamine (Ketalar), meperidine (Demerol), thioridazine (Mellaril), tramadol (Ultram), venlafaxine (Effexor)
Tetrahydrocannabinol	Dronabinol (Marinol), nonsteroidal anti-inflammatory drugs, proton pump inhibitors [pantoprazole (Protonix)]

Table 14.12 Findings suggestive of adulterated, diluted, or substituted specimens (From Standridge [31]. Approved with permission, Am Fam physician)

General	Temperature <90 °F or >100 °F Unusual appearance (e.g., bubbly, cloudy, clear, dark)
Adulterated	Nitrite concentration > 50 mg/dL (4.2 mmol/L) Urine pH < 3 or ≥11
Diluted	Creatinine concentration ≥2.0 mg/dL but <20 mg/dL Specific gravity >1.0010 but <1.0030
Substituted	Creatinine concentration <2.0 mg/dL Specific gravity ≤1.0010 or ≥1.0200

death. The simultaneous use of a depressant and an opioid acts much in the same manner.

Stimulants and depressants are often used together (alcohol to take the edge off cocaine or amphetamines to reduce the sleepiness from alcohol). Although some antagonism occurs at lower doses, at higher doses, the depressant tends to dominate. Stimulants and the chronic use of alcohol act synergistically to increase blood pressure.

Hallucinogens and stimulants act together to produce stimulatory side effects such as increased pulse rate and blood pressure.

Marijuana may increase the depressant effect of alcohol and other CNS depressants on the central nervous system. Patients showing signs of alcohol intoxication that do not correspond to their blood alcohol levels may have used other drugs as well, such as marijuana, other depressants, or opioids. When used together, marijuana and CNS stimulants synergistically increase pulse rate and blood pressure. Marijuana and alcohol or other depressant use decreases motor performance [4].

Criteria for Substance Dependence

The American Psychiatric Association's DSM-5, published in 2013, gives specific criteria for the diagnosis of substance dependence (discussed in Chap. 1). The term abuse is no longer used. Instead, DSM-5 combines substance abuse and substance dependence into a single substance dependence disorder measured on a continuum from mild to severe. Each specific substance is addressed as a separate use disorder, that is, alcohol use disorder, stimulant use disorder, hallucinogen use disorder, and so forth. In DSM-5, substance dependence includes 11 different criteria. A score of 2–3 indicates mild substance dependence (formerly called substance abuse), a score of 4–5 indicates moderate dependence, and a score of 6 or more indicates severe dependence [35].

Presenting the Diagnosis

Discussing the diagnosis of substance dependence with a patient is never easy. The major barrier is the patient's denial, which physicians should view as a symptom of the disease in the same way that thirst is a symptom of diabetes. By realizing that denial is primarily the result of unconscious psychological mechanisms and not of willful misrepresentation, physicians can maintain a sympathetic, nonjudgmental therapeutic stance. They should present the diagnosis as an expression of concern for a patient's health or safety. Moralization or threatening a patient is counterproductive.

Many drug users are unaware of the basic facts about drugs and substance dependence. Educating patients about these facts in a nonthreatening manner is appropriate. Discussing substance dependence as a disease legitimizes seeking care for the dependence itself, not just for the medical consequences of the drug use. Comparing substance dependence to other chronic diseases that require behavioral changes, such as hypertension or diabetes, reinforces the fact that abstinence from drugs is therapy, not punishment. Understanding substance dependence as a disease allows patients to address the problem with less guilt. Although recovery from substance dependence can take place only after patients accept the diagnosis, their refusal to call themselves drug addicts or alcoholics at this point needs not stand in the way of treatment. Getting patients into treatment is much more important than agreeing on a diagnostic label [6].

Summary

Many physicians underdiagnose substance dependence. Common problems that interfere with a physician's making the diagnosis of substance dependence include undereducation, false beliefs, denial, and feelings of inadequacy. A number of diagnostic tools are available to help physicians diagnose addiction to alcohol or other drugs. These include screening questionnaires, a patient's personal and family history, a physical examination, and laboratory tests.

Signs and symptoms can be very helpful in acquiring an idea of which substance a patient has been abusing.

Drug screening can be done on the urine, blood, hair, saliva, sweat, and nails. Urine is most often used for drug screening because it is easy to collect, collecting it is noninvasive, it is easier to analyze than blood or other fluids, and it can be refrigerated and stored.

Two screening tests are currently in use—thin-layer chromatography and immunoassays. Confirmatory techniques include chromatography/mass spectrometry (GC/MS) and high-pressure liquid chromatography. Addicts may add a commercially available adulterant in vitro to the urine specimen after collection.

The ultimate diagnosis of substance dependence depends on the criteria of DSM-5.

Few addicts use only one drug; however, virtually all can identify the drug they most prefer (drug of choice). Patient hustlers use many manipulative approaches to get drugs from physicians. Discussing the diagnosis of substance dependence with a patient is never easy. The major barrier is the patient's denial, which physicians should view as a symptom of the disease in the same way that thirst is a symptom of diabetes.

References

1. Curley B. Few medical students learn about addiction. Partnership for Drug-Free Kids website. http://www.drugfree.org/news-service/few-medical-students-learn-about-addiction. May 31, 2001.
2. Milhorn HT. Chemical dependency: is medical education falling short? Mississippi State Medical Association Impaired Physicians' Newsletter. April 1989.
3. Mulry JT, Brewer ML, Spencer DL. The effect of an inpatient chemical dependency rotation on residents' clinical behavior. Fam Med. 1987;19(4):276–80.
4. Milhorn HT. Chemical dependence: diagnosis, treatment, and prevention. New York: Springer; 1990.
5. Spickard A. Alcoholism: the missed diagnosis. South Med J. 1986;79:1489–92.
6. Barnes HN. Presenting the diagnosis: working with denial. In: Barnes HN, Aronson MD, Delbanco TL, editors. Alcoholism: a guide for the primary care physician. New York: Springer; 1987. p. 59–65.
7. Mooney AJ. Alcohol abuse and dependence. In: Taylor RB, editor. Family medicine. New York: Springer; 1983. p. 1631–62.

8. Milhorn HT. The diagnosis of alcoholism. Am Fam Physician. 1988;37:175–83.
9. Selzer ML, Vinokur A, VanRooijen L. A self-administered short version of the Michigan alcoholism screening test (SMAST). J Stud Alcohol. 1975;36:117–26.
10. Ewing JA. Detecting alcoholism: the CAGE questionnaire. JAMA. 1984;252:1905–7.
11. Babor TF, Higgins-Biddle JC, Saunders JB, Monteiro MG. The alcohol use disorders identification test: guidelines for use in primary care. 2nd ed. World Health Organization. Department of Mental Health and Substance Dependence; World Health Organization in Geneva Switzerland. 2016.
12. Brown RL, Rounds LA. Conjoint screening questionnaires for alcohol and drug abuse. Wis Med J. 1995;94:135–40.
13. Skinner HA. The drug abuse screening test. Addict Behav. 1982;7(4):363–71.
14. Van Cleave S, Byrd W, Revell K. Counseling for substance abuse and addiction. Waco: Word Books; 1987.
15. Milhorn HT. Screening, assessment, and diagnosis. In: Wilford BB, editor. Review course syllabus. New York: American Society of Addiction Medicine; 1990.
16. Liepman WR, Byrd W, Fisher JV, editors. Family medicine curriculum guide to substance abuse. Kansas City: Society of Teachers of Family Medicine; 1984.
17. Cloninger CR. Neurogenic adaptive mechanics in alcoholism. Science. 1987;236:410–6.
18. Hays JT, Spickard WA. Alcoholism: early diagnosis and intervention. J Intern Med. 1987;2:240–427.
19. Stamm D, Hansert E, Feuerlein W. Detection and exclusion of alcoholism in men on the basis of clinical laboratory findings. J Clin Chem Clin Biochem. 1984;22:79–98.
20. Wilford BB, editor. Review course syllabus. American Society on Alcoholism and Other Drug Dependencies; 1987.
21. Gitlow SE, Peyser HS. Alcoholism: a practical treatment guide. Orlando: Grune and Stratton; 1980.
22. Milhorn HT. Alcoholism: making the diagnosis in your practice. J Miss State Med Assoc. 1988;29(12):363–7.
23. Milhorn HT. Diagnosis and management of phencyclidine intoxication. Am Fam Physician. 1991;43(4):1293–30.
24. Schonberg SK, editor. Substance abuse: a guide for health professionals. Elk Grove Village: American Academy of Pediatrics; 1988. p. 48–66.
25. Thompson W. Alcoholism workup. Medscape website. http://emedicine.medscape.com/article/285913-overview. November 14, 2016.
26. Gold M, Dackis CA. Role of the laboratory in suspected drug abuse. J Clin Psychiatry. 1986;47:17–23.
27. Mersy DJ. Recognition of alcohol and substance abuse. Am Fam Physician. 2003;67(7):1529–32.
28. Mullen J, Bracha HS. Toxicology screening: how to assure accurate results. Postgrad Med. 1988;84:141–8.
29. Moeller KE, Lee KC, Kissak JC. Urine drug screening: practical guide for clinicians. Mayo Clin Proc. 2008;83(1):66–76.
30. Shapiro B, Coffa D, McCance-Katz EF. A primary care approach to substance misuse. Am Fam Physician. 2013;88(2):113–21.
31. Standridge JB, Adams SM, Zotos AP. Urine drug screening: a valuable office procedure. Am Fam Physician. 2010;81(5):635–40.
32. Drug screening services. Crimcheck website. https://www.crimcheck.com/services/drug-screening
33. Laino C. Drug tests often trigger false positives. WebMD website. http://www.webmd.com/news/20100528/drug-tests-often-trigger-false-positives. May 28, 2010.
34. Dasgupta A. How people try to beat drug testing. American Association for Clinical Chemistry. Clinical Laboratory News. February 1, 2015.
35. DSM-5. Arlington: American Psychiatric Association (APA); 2013.

15 Treatment

Key Chapter Points

- Steps in treating a substance-dependent person are (1) getting the addict into treatment, (2) the treatment itself, and (3) aftercare.
- Until an addict experiences some major crisis that causes emotional pain, he is usually not willing to seek help.
- Treatment options include support groups and various treatment program options (inpatient, partial hospitalization, and outpatient).
- Support groups are either non-12-step programs or 12-step programs.
- Treatment does not attempt to answer the question of why an addict drinks or uses drugs but instead takes a here-and-now approach. It takes the approach (1) let's see what we have (assessment) and (2) what needs to be done (rehabilitation).
- Behavioral therapy includes cognitive behavioral therapy, contingency management, and motivational enhancement therapy.
- Motivational enhancement therapy (MET) uses strategies to evoke rapid and internally motivated behavior change to stop drug use and facilitate treatment entry.
- Family therapy approaches a person's drug problems in the context of family interactions and dynamics that may contribute to drug use and other risky behaviors.
- Treatment program options include residential (inpatient) treatment, partial hospitalization, and outpatient treatment.
- Aftercare is follow-up care that patients receive after being in a substance use disorder rehabilitation program.
- A federal statue mandates confidentiality in the treatment of substance dependence.

Treatment simply means the combating of a disease or disorder. In our case, the disease or disorder is substance dependence [1].

History of Substance Dependence Treatment

Heninger and Sung [2] give an excellent review of the history of substance dependence treatment in the United States [2]. Treatment of substance use disorders in the United States, therefore, began with alcoholism.

Early Institutional Care

In the late eighteenth century and early nineteenth century, alcoholics were housed in local jails, almshouses (places for the poor, sick, or destitute), and asylums for the mentally ill. These places did not provide alcoholism treatment.

Benjamin Rush, a physician, in the latter half of the eighteenth century, proposed that "sober houses" be established to treat alcoholics using medical treatment and religious and moral instruction. Treatments of alcoholism used by

H.T. Milhorn, *Substance Use Disorders*, DOI 10.1007/978-3-319-63040-3_15

Rush included cold baths; aversion therapy, which caused vomiting; bleeding; blistering; and sweating the patient.

In 1849, the Swedish physician Magnus Huss described a disease resulting from chronic alcohol consumption and named it *Alcoholismus Chronicus*. This marked the introduction of the term alcoholism.

In 1864, the New York State Inebriate Asylum, the first in the country, opened in Binghamton, New York. In 1867, the opening of the Martha Washington Home in Chicago marked the first institution in America that specialized in the treatment of alcoholic women.

The most important feature of early institutional treatment was isolating the alcoholic from society so that he no longer faced the temptation of alcohol. Detoxification would either be done "cold turkey" or with the aid of medications to ease the withdrawal symptoms. Cannabis, cocaine, chloral hydrate, and belladonna were commonly used for this. Medical treatment, healthy meals, fluids, vitamins, and exercise followed. Massage therapy, sunlight, and electrotherapy also were used.

In the 1880s, cocaine was recommended by Sigmund Freud and a number of American physicians for the treatment of alcoholism and morphine addiction.

From 1891 to 1892, as inebriate homes and asylums began to close, alcoholics were once again relegated to city drunk tanks, cells in wards of public hospitals, and the back wards of aging insane asylums.

Private sanitaria were developed at the end of the nineteenth century to provide alcoholism treatment services to the wealthy.

Early Drug Treatment

Miracle cures abounded in the second half of the nineteenth century. These consisted of a short course of medication for alcoholism (Mickey Finn Powders, White Star Secret Liquor Cure), hangovers (Alka Nox, Sober Up), tobacco dependence (Tobacco Redeemer, Gustafson's Tobacco Remedy), cocaine dependence (Baldwin's Home Cure for Cocaine), morphine dependence (St. Anne's Morphine Cure), and opium dependence (Weatherby's Opium Antidote). Miracle cures could be purchased over the counter or through mail order services, and they were provided in inebriate houses.

Modern Alcoholism Treatment

With the end of prohibition by the 21st Amendment in 1933, a new phase in the treatment of alcoholism began. Alcoholism was again viewed as a disease rather than a moral weakness, and it was believed that alcoholism could be treated.

In 1944, Marty Mann founded the National Committee for Education on Alcoholism, now known as the National Council on Alcoholism and Drug Dependence. In 1949, International Doctors in AA was founded. In 1950, the National Institute of Mental Health established a special division on alcoholism. In addition, the halfway house movement culminated in the founding of the Association of Halfway House Alcoholism Programs of North America.

The Minnesota Model of addiction treatment began with the establishment of a new method of alcoholism treatment in three Minnesota centers in the late 1940s—Willmar State Hospital, Pioneer House, and Hazelden. One of the primary tenets of this model was respect.

Medical treatment was provided by physicians and nurses. Counseling was provided by psychologists and social workers, and spiritual guidance was provided by clergy. Standard treatment was 28 days, with the first few days being for detoxification. A counselor, who was usually a recovering addict, was assigned to each patient. Individual counseling was supplemented by group therapy, lectures, and working the 12 steps of AA. Patients received aftercare after returning home.

In 1970, Congress passed the "Comprehensive Alcohol Abuse and Alcoholism Prevention Treatment and Rehabilitation Act." In 1972, the Joint Commission on Accreditation of Hospitals developed accreditation standards for alcoholism treatment programs. In 1983, the National Association for Children of Alcoholics was founded.

Civil Commitments

By the late 1950s, addicts were viewed as people who were involved in a destructive lifestyle and who were not able or willing to change. It was believed that family and friends of addicts were in harm's way. In the early 1960s, involuntary civil commitment, the court-ordered institutionalization of the addict as a mentally ill person, came into existence. This replaced incarceration. Patients were typically committed for 1–3 years. After discharge, they returned to their communities for follow-up outpatient treatment.

Due to overcrowding of psychiatric facilities and continued relapse by the addicts, the Joint Commission of the American Bar Association and the American Medical Association recommended treating patients in community clinics.

In the early 1960s, the Supreme Court prohibited laws that made addiction a crime, framed addiction as a disease deserving treatment, and stated that civil commitments should be used sparingly.

Pharmacotherapy

Using opiates medically to maintain individuals suffering from opiate addiction was prohibited by the Harrison Narcotic Act of 1914. However, legislation in the 1960s called for research on using opioids to maintain heroin addicts.

Dr. Marie Nyswander and Dr. Vincent Dole successfully argued that methadone could be used to prevent craving and euphoria. During the 1970s, federally funded methadone programs were established in response to the return of heroin-addicted Vietnam veterans and a surge in urban crime.

Drug Courts

Drug courts in which drug treatment is an alternative to prison came into being in 1989.

Drug courts are specialized court docket programs that target criminal defendants and offenders, juvenile offenders, and parents with pending child welfare cases who have alcohol and other drug dependency problems.

Drug courts are usually managed by a non-adversarial and multidisciplinary team including judges, prosecutors, defense attorneys, community corrections, social workers, and treatment service professionals.

Getting the Addict into Treatment

The first step in treating substance dependence is to get an addict to agree to treatment. This is also the most difficult step. Until an addict experiences some major crisis that causes emotional pain, he is usually not willing to seek help. A crisis frequently occurs in one or more of the following areas.

Legal Problems

Many substance-dependent people eventually reach a point where they have to steal, sell drugs, or prostitute themselves to support their addiction. These activities often lead to trouble with legal authorities. Addicts also tend to be arrested for driving under the influence, for possessing drugs, or for disorderly conduct. Many judges now mandate treatment in place of sending addicts to prison [3].

Family Problems

Spouses frequently leave drug users because of the effects of their behavior on the family. This is a crisis for addicts because spouses may be the only emotional support they have. Addicts often agree to treatment not to get well but in hopes of getting their spouses back. At this point, this is a perfectly satisfactory reason for getting addicts into treatment and should not be discouraged [3].

Medical Problems

As their health deteriorates, addicts may realize that their drug use is killing them. They may become aware that their behavior is out of control or it may take a life-threatening event, such as a violent injury from a shooting, a stabbing, or an automobile accident, to make them aware that they have a serious problem. Serious medical problems may prompt addicts to seek help. Addicted people suffer from depression, not only from the effects of drugs on their brains but also from the effects of drugs on their lives. Suicide attempts are common among substance-dependent people [3] .

Work Problems

Substance-dependent people who are still drinking or using other drugs are poor employees because of their tardiness, absenteeism, and erratic job performance. They may eventually be threatened with loss of their jobs or may actually be fired. Many employers now require treatment as a condition for continued employment for drug users. This is particularly true of larger companies, many of which have established employee assistance programs to deal with such problems [3].

Court-Ordered Admission

In some states, suspected addicts can be admitted to treatment centers for evaluation of substance dependence by court order. Basically, a family member or close friend hires an attorney to present evidence to a chancery court judge. If the judge finds sufficient evidence to warrant further evaluation, he or she can order that the suspected addict be committed to a local treatment program for between 3 and 7 days of evaluation. At the end of this period, a patient has a right to appeal the judge's decision. If necessary, a representative of the treatment center may present evidence the center has gathered [4].

Tough Love and Intervention by Confrontation

If none of the above actions is successful in getting the addict into treatment, tough love or intervention by confrontation can be attempted.

Tough love is the practice of taking a stern attitude toward a spouse, a relative, or a friend suffering from an addiction. The purpose of tough love is to speed up the process of getting the addict to agree to being admitted to a treatment program.

Intervention is designed to precipitate a crisis to get an addict into treatment earlier than he might go otherwise. It is a planned confrontation between the addict and family members and other significant people. The purpose of the intervention is to convince an addict of the effects of his destructive behavior and to get the person into treatment. Tough love and intervention by confrontation are discussed further in Chap. 18.

Treatment options include support groups and various treatment program options (inpatient, partial hospitalization, and outpatient).

Support Groups

The first major treatment option for "treatment" is a support group. Support groups are either non-12-step programs or 12-step programs. When used as the initial treatment, they should be individuals with mild substance abuse problems. Twelve-step programs are by far more available.

Non-12-Step Programs

The main reasons people chose a non-12-step program is because they feel uncomfortable with the religious and spiritual components of the 12-step approach. In these programs, the addict is not required to believe in God or a higher power. They advertise that they use evidence-based, scientific approaches to treat addiction, which constantly evolve as scientific knowledge evolves.

Non-12-step drug and alcohol rehabilitation programs include inpatient and outpatient programs. Like 12-step programs, they design customized treatment plans that are flexible and based on the addicts' individual situation, including whether they have any co-occurring mental health disorders. They may use holistic treatments, such as yoga, massage, nutrition programs, vitamin therapy, and exercise programs.

Non-12-step addiction treatment centers do not view addiction as a lifelong disease, whereas 12-step programs do. The focus of non-12-step programs is said to be on self-empowerment and finding what motivates the addict to get clean and sober. These programs foster empowerment through encouragement and education.

Non-12 step programs include SMART Recovery (Self-Management for Addiction Recovery) and SOS (Secular Organizations for Sobriety), LSR (LifeRing Secular Recovery), and WFS (Women for Sobriety) [5].

Twelve-Step Programs

Twelve-step programs require that the addict complete a series of 12 steps based on powerlessness. Twelve-step programs promote the beliefs that addiction is a disease, addicts require the support of other recovering addicts, and reliance on a power greater than one's self is fundamental. They also feel that abstaining from the addictive behavior is the basis of recovery, recovery is a lifelong process, supporting others in recovery is necessary for lasting commitment and stability, and accepting the limitations of being human is essential.

The steps use the higher power concept in which the higher power is "God as we understood him." This is the major difference between non-12-step programs and 12-step programs. Because the majority of treatment programs by far are 12-step programs, we will devote the major part of our discussion to them. However, it should be noted that many of the processes are the same in both groups [6].

Treatment

Treatment does not attempt to answer the question of why an addict drinks or uses drugs but instead takes a here-and-now approach. It takes the approach (1) let's see what we have (assessment) and (2) what needs to be done (rehabilitation).

What Treatment Involves

Treatment involves changing deeply imbedded behaviors. The goals for patients in treatment include (1) learning factual information about alcohol and other drugs; (2) accepting the disease of addiction and understanding what it means to be substance dependent; (3) learning to identify feelings and deal with them appropriately; (4) learning to assume responsibility for their own behavior; (5) learning to deal appropriately with stress, insomnia, and depression; (6) eliminating maladaptive behaviors and substituting more adaptive ones; (7) becoming physically active; (8) becoming familiar with the twelve steps of Alcoholics Anonymous or various other support groups; (9) learning risk factors for relapse; and (10) learning how to prevent relapse [4].

Behavioral Treatment

To be successful, treatment must address the needs of the whole person. Behavioral treatments help. They modify addicts' attitudes and behaviors related to drug use, and they increase the addict's life skills to handle stressful circumstances and environmental cues that may trigger intense craving. They include cognitive behavioral therapy, contingency management, and motivational enhancement therapy.

Cognitive Behavioral Therapy

Cognitive-behavioral therapy (CBT) seeks to help patients recognize, avoid, and cope with the situations in which they are most likely to use drugs. Cognitive-behavioral strategies are based on the theory that in the development of maladaptive behavioral patterns, like substance abuse, learning processes play a critical role.

Individuals in CBT learn to identify and correct problematic behaviors by applying a range of different skills that can be used to stop drug abuse and to address a range of other problems that often co-occur with it.

A central element of CBT is anticipating likely problems and enhancing patients' self-control by helping them develop effective coping strategies.

Specific techniques include exploring the positive and negative consequences of continued drug use, self-monitoring to recognize cravings early and identify situations that might put one at risk for use, and developing strategies for coping with cravings and avoiding those high-risk situations [7].

Contingency Management

Contingency management uses positive reinforcement, such as providing rewards or privileges for remaining drug free, for attending and participating in counseling sessions, or for taking treatment medications as prescribed.

Contingency management principles involve giving patients tangible rewards to reinforce positive behaviors, such as abstinence. Incentive-based interventions are highly effective in increasing treatment retention and promoting abstinence from drugs. They consist of:

Voucher-Based Reinforcement Voucher-based reinforcement (VBR) augments other community-based treatments. In VBR, the patient receives a voucher for every drug-free urine sample provided. The voucher has monetary value that can be exchanged for food items, movie passes, or other goods or services that are consistent with a drug-free lifestyle.

Prize Incentives Contingency Management Prize incentives contingency management applies similar principles as VBR but uses chances to win cash prizes instead of vouchers. Over the course of the program (one or more times weekly), participants supplying drug-negative urine or breath tests draw from a bowl for the chance to win a prize worth a small amount of money [7].

Motivational Enhancement Therapy Motivational enhancement therapy (MET) uses strategies to evoke rapid and internally motivated behavior change to stop drug use and facilitate treatment entry. MET is a counseling approach that helps individuals resolve their ambivalence about engaging in treatment and stopping their drug use. This therapy consists of an initial assessment battery session, followed by two to four individual treatment sessions with a therapist.

In the first treatment session, the therapist provides feedback to the initial assessment, stimulating discussion about personal substance use and eliciting self-motivational statements.

Motivational interviewing principles are used to strengthen motivation and build a plan for change.

Coping strategies for high-risk situations are suggested and discussed with the patient.

In subsequent sessions, the therapist monitors change, reviews cessation strategies being used, and continues to encourage commitment to change or sustained abstinence [7].

Family Therapy

Family therapy approaches a person's drug problems in the context of family interactions and dynamics that may contribute to drug use and other risky behaviors. It is aimed at addressing not only substance use problems but other co-occurring problems in the family as well, such as conduct disorders, child mistreatment, depression, family conflict, and unemployment. It combines behavioral contracting with contingency management.

Therapists seek to engage families in applying the behavioral strategies taught in sessions and in acquiring new skills to improve the home environment.

Patients are encouraged to develop behavioral goals for preventing substance use.

During each session, the behavioral goals are reviewed, with rewards provided by significant others when goals are accomplished. Patients participate in treatment planning, choosing specific interventions from a menu of evidence-based treatment options [7].

Treatment Program Options

Treatment program options include residential (inpatient) treatment, partial hospitalization, and outpatient treatment. Outpatient treatment may be either intensive outpatient treatment or standard outpatient treatment. Other options are halfway houses, therapeutic communities, and support groups, such as AA (Alcoholics Anonymous), NA (Narcotics Anonymous), or CA (Cocaine Anonymous). Halfway houses and therapeutic communities are sometimes referred to as residential treatments.

ASAM Patient Placement Criteria for the Treatment of Substance-Related Disorders

The American Society of Addiction Medicine (ASAM) criteria help determine the appropriate level of treatment for a patient; that is, which one of the above treatment programs is most appropriate [8].

Categories that are rated are:

1. Acute intoxication and/or withdrawal potential
2. Biomedical conditions and complications
3. Emotional, behavioral, or cognitive (EBC) conditions and complications
4. Readiness to change
5. Relapse, continued use, or continued problem potential
6. Recovery environment

Each category is rated from zero to four based on given criteria:

0. No risk
1. Low risk
2. Moderate risk
3. High risk
4. Severe risk

Categories of treatment based on the ASAM criteria are:

- Level III residential treatment
- Level II partial hospitalization
- Level II intensive outpatient
- Level I standard outpatient

A detailed explanation of scoring is beyond the scope of this book. An explanation of the ASAM placement criteria can be found online [9].

Inpatient Treatment

Inpatient treatment takes place in a general medical-surgical hospital's substance dependency unit, a psychiatric hospital, or a freestanding facility. It is often referred to as primary treatment. A good inpatient program uses a multifactorial approach to treatment. Elements of such a program include medical assessment, detoxification, management of medical problems, psychosocial assessment, treatment plan development, rehabilitation, aftercare planning, and family treatment. Other possible components of an inpatient program include occupational therapy, vocational rehabilitation, and social services. On admission, each patient is assigned a counselor who guides his treatment. Inpatient treatment ideally lasts about a month but is usually less because lengths of stays are approved by insurance companies [10, 11]. Some inpatient treatment programs are still a standard 28 days, including state-run programs and private programs for people who can afford to pay their own expenses.

Medical Assessment Medical assessment consists of an initial drug history, a routine medical history, a physical examination, and laboratory studies. The initial drug history focuses on a patient's recent drug history rather than on that person's lifelong drug history. This is primarily for the purpose of planning detoxification.

The routine medical history includes questions about medical problems that substance-dependent people commonly encounter. Physicians ask patients about a history of blackouts, seizures, hallucinations, and delirium tremens. Because of the current AIDS epidemic, physicians may also ask patients about sharing needles or about homosexuality. If patients reveal a history of either of these, they may be offered HIV testing. Physicians obtain information about family history of substance dependence and question patients about previous treatment for substance dependence or for psychiatric problems. Because many substance-dependent people are depressed, physicians should ask patients about recent suicide thoughts or attempts. If patients have suicidal ideation, physicians should take precautions to prevent suicide and should arrange for psychiatric consultations for patients.

The physical examination focuses on physical abnormalities resulting from substance use, such as an enlarged liver, needle tracks, and abscesses formed from nonsterile injections.

Laboratory studies may include a comprehensive metabolic panel, complete blood count, urine analysis, and urine drug screen. If the patient is over 40 years old or has a history of a heart or pulmonary problem, an electrocardiogram and/or chest X-ray may be obtained [12].

Detoxification Based on information obtained in the medical assessment, physicians formulate a detoxification plan. In general, detoxification is required only for drugs that produce central nervous system depression, such as alcohol, barbiturates, benzodiazepines, and opioids. The dosing and scheduling of detoxification medication depend on several factors, such as a patient's age, sex, weight, health, and level of drug intake.

Because addicts may not be totally truthful about their use (minimization), they should be observed for withdrawal symptoms for at least 24 h. Nursing care is extremely important during this phase of treatment.

The American Society of Addiction Medicine lists three immediate goals for detoxification of alcohol and other substances: (1) to provide a safe withdrawal from the drugs of dependence and enable the patient to become drug free, (2) to provide a withdrawal that is humane and thus protect the patient's dignity, and (3) to prepare the patient for ongoing treatment of his dependence on alcohol or other drugs.

A problem in defining the duration of detoxification is the fact that some patients may have prolonged withdrawal signs or symptoms. Symptoms of prolonged withdrawal include disturbances of sleep, anxiety, irritability, and mood instability. Detoxification may take place in inpatient or outpatient settings [4, 13].

Inpatient detoxification has several advantages to outpatient detoxification. First, the inpatient detoxification restricts the patient's access to substances of abuse. Second, inpatient detoxification allows the clinician to monitor the patient closely for serious withdrawal symptoms and to adjust medications as indicated. Finally, detoxification in an inpatient facility can be accomplished more rapidly than in an outpatient setting.

Generally, inpatient detoxification is reserved for those expected to have severe withdrawal symptoms or a history of withdrawal seizures and who require a more intensive level of care. Monitoring is especially important if the patient is dependent on high doses of alcohol or other CNS depressant drugs or if they have significant medical problems [13, 14].

Outpatient detoxification has a number of advantages. First, it is much less expensive than inpatient detoxification. Second, the patient's life is not disrupted to the degree that it is during inpatient detoxification. Finally, the patient does not undergo the abrupt transition from a protected inpatient setting to an unprotected outpatient setting. Many individuals undergo detoxification more than once, and some do so many times [13, 14].

Detoxification of Patients with Medical Problems Patients with some medical conditions require special consideration in regard to detoxification.

Brain-injured patients are at risk for seizures. Slower medication tapers should be used in patients with seizure disorder. Doses of anticonvulsant medications should be stabilized before sedative-hypnotic withdrawal begins.

Patients with cardiac disease require continued clinical assessment and monitoring. Underlying cardiac disease may be worsened by the symptoms of autonomic arousal (elevated blood pressure, increased pulse) as seen in alcohol, sedative, and opioid withdrawal. Because of this, it may be necessary to withdraw the medication at a slower than usual rate.

Severe liver or renal disease can slow the metabolism of both the drug of abuse and the detoxification medication. Shorter acting detoxification drugs and a slower taper are appropriate for such patients [14].

Treatment of Health Problems Substance-dependent people have more health problems than other people. Although many health problems are drug-related, others are problems encountered in any general medical practice. Physicians address these early in treatment. Because drug dependence can produce some common medical problems (gastritis, hypertension, gout, depression, and insomnia), physicians can decide at admission which medications to discontinue and which to continue. Again, nursing care plays a major role. Physicians should request records from a patient's personal physician when they are pertinent [4].

Psychosocial Assessment Psychosocial assessment includes psychological assessment and sociological assessment.

Psychological assessment is used to measure attributes of the patient's personality, such as paranoia, depression, and hostility. These tests assess the strengths and weaknesses of those traits and how they relate to the patient's personality, behavior, and intelligence. They gauge the person's present functioning.

Two types of tests may be administered—intelligence and personality. Intelligence tests are the most common and help determine the patient's cognitive strengths and weaknesses. The Wechsler Adult Intelligence Scale–Fourth Edition (WAIS-IV) consists of a variety of questions that measure verbal, performance, and full-scale intelligence.

Personality assessments can help psychologists better diagnose and comprehend mental illness. Objective tests, like the Minnesota Multiphasic Personality Inventory (MMPI-2), are the most commonly used and helps identify dysfunction within a person's personality [15, 16].

Social assessment involves collecting data on the patients' social functioning from patients, members of their families, and employers. Information counselors gather includes educational level, employment history, leisure activities, marriage/divorce history, history of childhood abuse, legal history, and detailed drug history. In addition, counselors gather information about a patient's childhood role models and family life [4].

Treatment Plan

From medical and psychosocial assessments, the addictionist and counselors identify problems and list them on a master problem list. Individual problems may be dealt with in treatment, may be noted and merely monitored, may be dealt with after treatment, or may require no action. Problems to be dealt with in treatment might include such things as alcoholic gastritis, denial of substance dependence, or poor coping skills. For each problem to be addressed in treatment, the addictionist and counselors develop a treatment plan that sets forth specific objectives for resolving the problem and states how each objective is to be achieved and in what period of time. Each patient is assigned a treatment team that meets at least weekly to discuss the patient's progress on each identified problem and to update the treatment plan [4].

Rehabilitation

Next, the treatment plan is put into action. This is done using education, group therapy, individual therapy, peer assessment, recreational therapy, coping skills and relaxation training, support group participation, and spirituality [17].

Education Patients usually attend lectures or view films daily on such diverse subjects as (1) the disease concept of substance dependence; (2) medical, psychological, and social aspects of addiction to specific drugs; (3) cross-addiction; (4) various steps of Alcoholics Anonymous (if it is a 12-step program); (5) recovery; and (6) preventing relapse. Patients also may be given specific reading assignments dealing with substance dependence.

Group Therapy Involving 10–15 patients and a group leader who is usually a certified drug counselor and who moderates discussion, group therapy is an opportunity for patients to deal with a variety of issues, aided by other group members. Patients are more apt to accept insights or criticism when they come from fellow addicts.

Group therapy helps patients see themselves with the psychological camouflage stripped away. Denial of substance dependence and dishonesty are common problems patients deal with in group therapy. Many patients, if not all, have developed low self-esteem because of their drug use and its effects. As a result, over the years they build up a wall of defenses against anything that might threaten their self-esteem. They simply do not want to deal with such issues. Group therapy helps them to do this.

Many times patients' first group assignment will be to report their life story, focusing on their drug use and the effects it has had on their health, family, friends, and job. This helps them be honest with themselves and to let other group members get to know them.

Patients can also use group time to report family conferences and to deal with feelings, which are often intense, about what transpired in such conferences. Ideally, group therapy helps patients identify feelings, see how their addiction has hurt themselves and others, and begin to see the need for change.

Many treatment programs have specialized groups designed for specific patient categories—groups for men, women, adolescents, the elderly, and for patients prone to relapse. Some centers have groups for cocaine addicts. This is probably unwise, because having their own groups sets them apart from other patients. Many cocaine addicts already feel that they are members of an elite group because of the drug they use; having their own therapy groups only perpetuates this feeling [4].

Individual Therapy Problems inappropriate for group discussion or problems better dealt with in one-on-one situations can be addressed in individual therapy. Initially, therapy time is used to assess a patient's needs and to begin to plan treatment.

The concept of addiction as a disease is reinforced, specific character defects (self-centeredness, intolerance, procrastination, self-pity, impatience) are dealt with, and patients' undesirable behaviors in the treatment center are related to behaviors that have caused them problems in the past. Poor relationships with spouses, parents, or significant others are discussed, and plans are made for improving them.

Individual problems, such as irresponsibility and lack of trust, are addressed. Written assignments may be made and discussed when completed. Reading assignments, important to patient treatment, are made and later discussed in relation to how the material applies to a patient [4].

Peer Assessment A special type of group, peer assessment, allows patients an opportunity to contribute constructively to the treatment of another patient who is having difficulty understanding his behavior. Areas dealt with include dishonesty, defense mechanisms, and character defects. A patient's behavior in the treatment center may also be addressed, as may not participating in treatment, isolating, inappropriate behavior with the opposite sex, and playing counselor. A patient is not allowed to respond defensively to these discussions [4].

Recreational Therapy Substance-dependent individuals, as a rule, do not regularly exercise. Under supervision, patients are encouraged to participate in various physical activities, usually three times a week. These activities may include basketball, volleyball, racquetball, walking or running, or swimming. Exercise decreases depression, gives a person a sense of well-being, and promotes a good night's sleep without alcohol or sleeping pills [4].

Coping Skills and Relaxation Therapy Many substance-dependent people have used drugs for years to cope with stress, to get to sleep, or to relax. Without drugs, they have to learn new ways of doing these things. Role-playing specific situations that have led to stress and using drugs in the past teach patients appropriate ways of dealing with such situations.

Learning communication skills is also a major part of treatment. Instead of reaching for a bottle or a pill, patients with anxiety or insomnia learn to listen to tapes or to use other techniques to relax or to get to sleep [4].

Support Group Attendance Attendance and participation in support groups, such as Alcoholics Anonymous, Narcotics Anonymous, or Cocaine Anonymous, are important parts of most treatment programs. Initially, these meetings are held among patients in the treatment center. Later, as patients progress in treatment, they attend outside, local community meetings. Attendance at these meetings while in treatment is important because it introduces patients to support groups and familiarizes them with their function. After discharge from treatment, patients are expected to continue attending support groups in their hometowns for the rest of their lives [4].

Spirituality An elusive concept, spirituality is a term that is commonly associated with religion. However, in the treatment of substance dependence, it is used in a broader sense. One definition of spirituality is "a human quest to understand life's meaning." Another definition is "being in harmony with yourself, with those around you, and with a power greater than you." Alcoholics Anonymous, for example, is a deeply spiritual program. It is embraced by people of all faiths and by some with no religious preference or background. Working the AA program 1 day at a time is said to be a spiritual experience [18].

Discharge Planning Assessing the needs that individual patients will have following discharge from treatment is called discharge planning. From these needs, the patient and treatment staff jointly develop a personalized aftercare plan. If a treatment center has its own aftercare program, patients may be required to attend it. Patients are generally introduced to the aftercare program a week or so before discharge. They are also expected to attend local support groups once back at home. They may be given the names of contact people in support groups in their local areas and are referred back to their local physicians for specific care for individual needs, such as management of medical problems.

Patients who need further treatment for their substance dependence may be referred to halfway houses. A patient and an aftercare coordinator usually sign an aftercare contract [4].

Family Treatment Substance dependence is an illness that dramatically affects all members of the family. For successful recovery of an addict and other members of the family, treatment must include the family. Family treatment primarily involves education, group therapy, and support group participation. Family treatment is discussed in Chap. 18.

A typical daily patient schedule for inpatient treatment is given in Table 15.1.

Outpatient Treatment

Outpatient treatment takes place in mental health clinics, counselors' offices, hospital clinics, or local health department offices. Patients may move to outpatient treatment after a stay at an inpatient facility, or they may enter an outpatient program as their primary treatment. Unlike inpatient treatment, patients don't stay overnight so they are not provided with a safe, secure environment that isolates them from negative influences. Patients continue to face the usual problems at work and home.

Outpatient treatment attempts to build the skills patients need to deal with everyday problems. Unlike inpatient treatment, outpatient treatment does not address medical conditions and nutritional needs.

Outpatient programs have fewer components than inpatient programs. Common components of outpatient programs include psychosocial assessment, developing treatment plans, rehabilitation, discharge planning, and family treatment. Rehabilitation consists of group therapy, individual therapy, peer assessment, support group attendance, and spirituality.

Standard Outpatient Treatment With standard outpatient treatment, patients attend one or two group therapy sessions a week. Treatment may go on for a year or more. Sessions may be in the evening or on weekends.

Table 15.1 Typical daily schedule for an inpatient program (From Milhorn [4]. Approved with permission, Springer)

Morning	
7:00–8:00	Breakfast
8:00–8:30	Devotional
8:30–9:30	Lecture/film
9:30–10:00	Break
10:00–11:00	Group therapy (combined male and female groups)
11:00–12:00	Group therapy (separate male and female groups)
Afternoon	
12:00–1:00	Lunch
1:00–2:00	Peer
2:00–3:00	Coping skills/relaxation training
3:00–4:00	Recreational therapy
4:00–5:00	Free time/individual therapy
Evening	
5:00–6:00	Dinner
6:00–7:00	Free time
7:00–8:00	Support group attendance
8:00–11:00	Free time
11:00	Lights out

Table 15.2 Advantages and disadvantages of inpatient versus outpatient treatment (Based on Van Cleave [3])

Advantages	Disadvantages
Inpatient treatment	
24-h supervision by trained staff and therapists Impression on patient of gravity of situation More integrated healthcare More intense treatment No distractions of daily life activities No access to drugs Structured environment	Absence from work Arrangements for childcare may need to be made Away from home Higher costs Many insurers will only cover outpatient treatment Need to take a leave on the job
Outpatient treatment	
Can continue to work Can live at home Less expensive Lack of structured environment	Less impression on patient of gravity of situation Less integrated healthcare Less intense treatment More access to drugs

Intensive Outpatient Treatment With intensive outpatient treatment, patients attend 10–20 h of counseling or group therapy a week. Typically about 10 weeks in length, outpatient programs take place for 2–3 h in the evening, 3 days a week [19].

Because addicts have more access to drugs in outpatient programs, frequent random urine drug screening is important. Table 15.2 gives the advantages and disadvantages of inpatient versus outpatient treatment.

Therapeutic Communities and Halfway Houses

Two other forms of treatment that should be mentioned are therapeutic communities and halfway houses.

Therapeutic Communities

Stay in a therapeutic community usually lasts 3 months to 2 years. Therapeutic community programs share a number of common components with short-term programs. One feature that distinguishes therapeutic communities from short-term treatment, however, is their emphasis on a patient's resocialization. Some therapeutic community programs require that participants be forcibly separated from the outside world. Therapy is strongly confrontive. However, other therapeutic community programs are similar to short-term programs but extend treatment over a longer period of time and involve less confrontation and less separation from the outside world.

Therapeutic communities usually have dormitory-style living, daily chores, and family-style meals and require members to help maintain the facility. They may offer educational and vocational training. Therapeutic community treatment is best suited for adolescents [20].

Halfway Houses

A halfway house is a structured transitional living situation between inpatient treatment and returning home. Halfway houses are frequently referred to as secondary treatment or extended treatment. Halfway houses are best suited for those who have not made satisfactory progress in primary treatment or who should not return home because of an unresolved family situation, such as in the case of a female patient with an abusive spouse at home.

In halfway house programs, 10–20 patients live together, sharing responsibility for maintaining the house. They do their own grocery shopping, cook their own meals, do housework, and wash their own clothes. They are employed outside the house, which provides a supportive living environment, a low level of treatment, and a place to hold AA meetings or other support groups. Patients also attend other support meetings in the local community. The level of intensity in halfway house programs varies considerably.

Some halfway houses are little more than a group living situation, while others function almost as an inpatient treatment program. Halfway house treatment usually lasts 2 to 6 months but may last up to a year [21].

Support Groups as Primary Treatment

Support groups (Alcoholics Anonymous, Narcotics Anonymous, etc.) are used as primary treatment only when patients will not accept inpatient or outpatient treatment under any conditions or when public programs or funds for private programs are not available. Many times, patients who will not agree to formal treatment will agree to attend support group meetings. When this is the case, they should agree to attend a fixed number of meetings in a given time period. Traditionally, 90 meetings in 90 days, followed by less intensive but regular attendance, have been recommended. Patients should sign written contracts agreeing to enter treatment if they are not able to maintain sobriety by this method; physicians also sign the contracts [21].

Aftercare

Aftercare is follow-up care that patients receive after being in a rehabilitation program. Aftercare programs help prevent relapse by helping patients stay focused on their recovery. Each treatment program, inpatient and outpatient, usually has its own aftercare program. Most commonly, facilities conduct aftercare programs two evenings a week. Aftercare usually lasts for 1–3 months; however, some programs extend it to as long as 2 years. It should not be viewed as another kind of treatment but as a continuation of the initial treatment. It differs from outpatient treatment in that its goals are very limited, dealing with the problems of reentry while simultaneously attempting to consolidate the gains made during treatment. Each patient is assisted in making the transition from treatment to family, job, and community. The recovering addict is also expected to attend two to three support group meetings a week. Because substance dependence, like any chronic disease, requires lifelong care, recovering patients are expected to continue to attend support groups long after aftercare has ended [22].

Primary care physicians should be familiar with the types of programs available for referral for substance dependence treatment in the local community. A site visit to these facilities can be helpful when determining which programs to refer patients. The reward of seeing a patient who was impaired by substance abuse return to normal functioning in society is what makes the effort worthwhile [23].

Primary care physicians should have an understanding of what goes on in treatment so that they and their patients on discharge from a treatment facility will have common grounds for discussions about treatment, recovery, and aftercare.

Finally, when treatment is completed, physicians should be involved in the long-term recovery of patients. They should discuss attending support groups with patients at each office visit, be aware of prescribed medication that may lead to relapse, be alert for signs of relapse, and help patients get back into treatment should relapse occur (Chap. 17).

Confidentiality

A federal statue mandates confidentiality in the treatment of substance dependence. Specifically, the law applies to records of a patient's identity, diagnosis, prognosis, or treatment and records that are maintained for the purposes of education, training, treatment, rehabilitation, or research. The statute is applicable if the treatment facility receives any federal assistance, including registration to dispense a controlled substance that is used to treat substance dependence, tax-free exemptions, or Medicare. When not in use, written records must be maintained in a secure room, in a locked file cabinet, safe, or other similar container. Information in a patient's records cannot be used in making criminal charges or in investigating a patient.

The federal regulations do not apply to the Veteran's Administration or the Armed Forces. They also do not apply to communication within a treatment program or between a program and an agency with administrative control of the program. The statute also exempts crimes on program premises or against program personnel, situations involving serious risk of bodily harm to a third party, and reports of suspected child abuse and neglect. Information identifying patients may be disclosed to medical personnel in medical emergencies. The statute is not considered by most healthcare workers to prevent them from reporting venereal diseases to local health authorities. Identifying information also can be disclosed to qualified individuals for research purposes if the information will not be redisclosed and if the research has been approved by an independent group of three or more individuals who find that patient rights would be adequately protected and that the benefits of the research outweigh risks to patients' confidentiality.

A treatment center's acknowledgement of a patient's presence in its program requires the patient's written consent. Insurance information that a patient furnishes for admission constitutes permission for the treatment center to disclose information to the insurance company or its representative. Additionally, observations of patients by former patients attending support groups in the center or by visiting family members of other patients do not violate the statute. If the treatment facility is a unit of a general hospital, the acknowledgment that a person is a patient in the general hospital is not considered a breach of confidentiality.

In the case of an adult patient who has been judged to lack the capacity to manage his own affairs, consent may be given by a guardian or other person authorized under state law to act in the patient's behalf. The statute also addresses confidentiality of patients who have not yet reached the age of majority as specified in state law or, in the absence of a state law, are not yet 18 years of age. If the minor patient acting alone has the legal capacity under state law to apply for and obtain alcohol or drug abuse treatment, only then patient may give written consent for disclosure. Where state law requires consent of a parent or guardian, both the minor patient and his or her parent or guardian must give authorization for disclosure. When a minor patient is judged to lack the capacity for rational choice, because of extreme youth or a mental or physical condition, a parent or guardian may act in the minor's behalf.

A patient must be informed in writing at the time of admission, or as soon thereafter as the patient is capable of rational communication, of the confidentiality requirement. The statute provides for criminal penalties for those who violate its provisions [24].

The Primary Care Physician

Having made the diagnosis of substance dependence, primary care physicians should evaluate factors in a patient's life that might be used as leverage to get him to agree to treatment (legal problems, family problems, medical problems, work problems). If this does not prompt the addict to seek treatment, the family may wish to intervene (intervention is discussed in Chap. 18). The patient's physician can guide the family on intervention and may even wish to be a member of the intervention team. If the intervention fails or if the family does not want to use this approach, physicians can instruct family members on how to get a court order mandating treatment (depending on the law in the patient's state).

Primary care physicians should have an understanding of what goes on in treatment so that they and their patients on discharge from a treatment facility will have common grounds for discussions about treatment, recovery, and aftercare. Physicians should be aware that federal statute mandates confidentiality of patient records in a treatment facility.

Primary care physicians should be familiar with treatment programs available for referral for substance dependence treatment in the local community. A site visit to these programs can be helpful in determining which ones to refer patients for treatment [23].

Finally, when treatment is completed, physicians should be involved in the long-term recovery of patients. They should discuss attending support groups with patients at each office visit, be aware of prescribed medication that may lead to relapse, be alert for signs of relapse, and help patients get back into treatment should relapse occur (Chap. 17).

Summary

Modern treatment began with the Minnesota Model in the late 1940s—Willmar State Hospital, Pioneer House, and Hazelden. Steps in treating a substance-dependent person are (1) getting the addict into treatment, (2) the treatment itself, and (3) aftercare. Until an addict experiences some major crisis that causes emotional pain, he is usually not willing to seek help.

Treatment options include support groups and various treatment program options (inpatient, partial hospitalization, and outpatient). Support groups are either non-12-step programs or 12-step programs. Treatment does not attempt to answer the question of why an addict drinks or uses drugs but instead takes a here-and-now approach. It takes the approach (1) let's see what we have (assessment) and (2) what needs to be done (rehabilitation). Inpatient treatment takes place in a general medical-surgical hospital's substance dependency unit, a psychiatric hospital, or a freestanding facility.

Outpatient treatment takes place in mental health clinics, counselors' offices, hospital clinics, or local health department offices. Behavioral therapy includes cognitive behavioral therapy, contingency management, and motivational enhancement therapy.

Motivational enhancement therapy (MET) uses strategies to evoke rapid and internally motivated behavior change to stop drug use and facilitate treatment entry.

Family therapy approaches a person's drug problems in the context of family interactions and dynamics that may contribute to drug use and other risky behaviors. Treatment program options include residential (inpatient) treatment, partial hospitalization, and outpatient treatment.

Aftercare is follow-up care that patients receive after being in a rehabilitation program. A federal statue mandates confidentiality in the treatment of substance dependence.

References

1. Treatment. Farlex partner medical dictionary. Free dictionary website. http://medical-dictionary.thefreedictionary.com/treatment
2. Henninger A, Sung H. History of substance abuse treatment. In: Bruinsma G, Weisburd D, editors. Encyclopedia of criminology and criminal justice. New York: Springer; 2014. p. 2257–69.
3. Van Cleave SV, Byrd W, Revell K. What really works in treatment. In: Counseling for substance abuse and addiction. Waco: Word Book; 1987. p. 133–43.
4. Milhorn HT. Chemical dependence: diagnosis, treatment, and prevention. New York: Springer; 1990.
5. Non 12-step fellowships and programs. The Fix website. https://www.thefix.com/content/non-12-step-fellowships-and-programs
6. Addiction A–Z. Addiction website. https://www.addiction.com/a-z/12-step-program
7. Behavioral therapies. Principles of drug addiction treatment: a research-based guide. 3rd ed. Bethesda: National Institute on Drug Abuse (NIDA); 2012.
8. The ASAM Criteria. American Society of Addiction Medicine (ASAM) website. http://www.asam.org/quality-practice/guidelines-and-consensus-documents/the-asam-criteria/about
9. Mee-Lee D. Understanding and utilizing the ASAM placement criteria. The Association for Addiction Professionals website. http://www.naadac.org/assets/1959/2012-03-14_understanding_and_utilizing_asam_webinarslides.pdf. March 14, 2012.
10. Cook CC. The Minnesota model in the management of drug and alcohol dependency: miracle, method or myth? Part I. The philosophy and the programme. Br J Addict. 1988;83(6):625–34.
11. Shulman GD, O'Connor RD. The rehabilitation of the alcoholic. In: Gittow SE, Peyser HS, editors.

Alcoholism: a practical treatment guide. Orlando: Grune and Stratton; 1980. p. 103–29.
12. Milhorn HT. Screening, assessment, and diagnosis. In: Wilford BB, editor. Review course syllabus. New York: American Society of Addiction Medicine (ASAM); 1990.
13. Kasser C, Geller A, Howell E, Wartenberg A. Detoxification: principles and protocols. Am Soc Addict Med. 2004;20
14. Wesson DR. Detoxification from alcohol and other drugs: Treatment Improvement Protocol (TIP) Series 19. Rockville: Substance Abuse and Mental Health Services Administration (SAMHSA): Center for Substance Abuse Treatment; 1995. p. 95–3046.
15. Weschler Adult Intelligence Scale Fourth Edition (WAIS-IV). Psychological Resource Center website. http://www.psyresources.com/products/mentalabilitytests/waisiv
16. Framingham J. Minnesota Multiphasic Personality Inventory (MMPI). Psych Central website. https://psychcentral.com/lib/minnesota-multiphasic-personality-inventory-mmpi
17. Anderson RC, Fisher JV, Whitfield CL, Liepman MR. Substance abuse rehabilitation. In: Family medicine curriculum guide to substance abuse. Kansas: Society for Teachers of Family Medicine; 1984. p. 6-1–6-18.
18. King P. Spirituality. Adolescent Counselor. April/May 1989;16.
19. Where to find help: Outpatient vs. inpatient programs. Dual Diagnosis website. http://www.dualdiagnosis.org/dual-diagnosis-treatment/outpatient-vs-inpatient-programs/#out
20. What Are Therapeutic Communities? National Institute on Drug Abuse (NIDA) website. 2015. https://www.drugabuse.gov/publications/research-reports/therapeutic-communities/what-are-therapeutic-communities
21. Stoddart T. Halfway house tips for a better chance at recovery. Sober Nation website. https://sobernation.com/halfway-house-tips. August 10, 2011.
22. Beddoe J. Aftercare programs for people in addiction recovery. Recovery website. http://www.recovery.org/topics/aftercare-programs-for-people-in-addiction-recovery. December 2, 2015.
23. Weaver Michael F, Jarvis Margaret AE, Schnoll SH. Role of the primary care physician in problems of substance abuse. Arch Int Med. 1999;159:913.
24. Weger CD, Diehl RJ. The counselor's guide to confidentiality. Honolulu: Program Information Associates; 1987.

Recovery 16

Key Chapter Points

- Abstinence is not using addicting substances. It allows recovery to begin. Learning to live normally without alcohol or other drugs requires more than abstinence.
- Recovery from alcohol or other drug dependence is a process of change through which an individual achieves abstinence and improved health, wellness, and quality of life.
- Recovery has no time limit. It is a lifetime program.
- The recovery process moves from basic to more complex tasks.
- Recovery does not follow a progressive, straight line. Addicts reach and overcome plateaus, slip backwards occasionally, but usually move on.
- The longer the interval studied, the fewer alcoholics are able to sustain moderate problem-free drinking.
- Numerous drugs (legal, prescription, over the counter, illicit) may be hazardous to recovery.
- Alcoholics Anonymous was established in Akron, Ohio, in 1935 by two alcoholics, Bill Wilson (a stockbroker) and Dr. Bob Smith (a surgeon).
- Web-based recovery support can play an important role in sustained recovery.
- Medications used to aid recovery from alcohol dependence include disulfiram (Antabuse), acamprosate (Campral), and naltrexone (Revia, Vivitrol).
- Medications used to treat opioid dependence include naltrexone (Revia, Vivitrol), buprenorphine (Suboxone, Bunavail), and methadone (Dolophine).
- A form of outpatient treatment for heroin addiction, methadone maintenance, involves giving patients methadone (Dolophine) daily.

Abstinence is not using addicting substances. It allows recovery to begin. Learning to live normally without alcohol or other drugs requires more than abstinence. *Recovery* from alcohol or other drug dependence is a process of change through which an individual achieves abstinence and improved health, wellness, and quality of life. It is a process in which the physiological, psychological, and social damage caused by substance dependence is healed. Addicts learn to live healthy and productive lives without the need for alcohol or other drugs. Recovery is an individual process; no two people recover at exactly the same rate [1].

Recovery Dimensions

The Substance Abuse and Mental Health Services Administration (SAMHSA) defines recovery as a process of change whereby individuals work to improve their own health and wellness and to live a meaningful life in a community of their choice while striving to achieve their full potential.

H.T. Milhorn, *Substance Use Disorders*, DOI 10.1007/978-3-319-63040-3_16

SAMSHA has delineated four major dimensions that support a life in recovery [2]. These are:

1. *Health*. Overall well-being begins with addressing symptoms of addiction that complicate physical and emotional health. Abstinence from alcohol, non-prescribed medications, and illicit drug use is recommended so that any psychiatric disorders can be addressed and treated. This leads to more informed and healthier choices that will sustain ongoing recovery.
2. *Home*. Having a consistent, peaceful, and stable place to return to each day will help remove uncertainty and anxiety that can lead to a self-destructive behavior.
3. *Purpose*. Being productive, whether through volunteer work, employment, or going to school, provides meaning for every person, especially those who are rebuilding a life in recovery.
4. *Community*. An essential aspect of recovery from mental illness and addiction is the understanding that others have experienced similar difficulties and struggles. Having nonjudgmental support from friends, family members, and others in recovery can be just the thing to help an individual gain momentum in recovery.

Recovery has no time limit. It is a lifetime program. Primary care physicians must be prepared to enter into a lifelong relationship with recovering individuals and their families. Many crises—including relapse—may occur, especially in the first 2 years of recovery. By developing an open relationship with patients and their families, primary care physicians will be more likely to be consulted when such crises occur.

Recovery usually is anything but a straight line. It is typically a long path, with ups and downs, and often instances of slips or relapses. For an alcoholic, for example, one drink may only be a slip and he is able to get back into his recovery program. For others, that first drink is the start of a slide into total relapse. The addict may need to return to treatment to get properly grounded again and maintain sobriety. Some addicts go back to treatment multiple times before attaining a lasting recovery [1]. I had one friend, a general surgeon who went through treatment 13 times for alcoholism. For whatever reason, the light bulb came on the 13th attempt at recovery, and he remained sober for the rest of his life.

For a newly recovering addict, staying clean and sober for the rest of his life may seem a daunting task. A good piece of advice is to take recovery 1 day at a time. This way it seems more like an achievable task.

Tasks of Recovery

The first task of recovery is for addicts to recognize that they have a debilitating, life-threatening disease. Once they recognize this, the second task of recovery is total abstinence from psychoactive substances. The third task is to recognize the need for a program to give support and assistance in staying sober 1 day at a time [3].

The Recovery Process

The recovery process moves from basic to more complex tasks. The progression is from abstinence (learning to live without drugs) to sobriety (learning to cope with life without drugs), to comfortable living (learning how to live comfortably while abstinent), and to productive living (learning how to build a meaningful sober life) [3].

Three Stages of Recovery

Melemis [4] describes three stages of recovery: (1) abstinence, (2) repair, and (3) growth.

Abstinence Stage

The main focus of *abstinence stage* is dealing with cravings and not drinking or using. Some of the tasks for the recovering addicts in this stage are accepting that they have an addiction, practicing honesty, developing coping skills for dealing with cravings, becoming active in self-help groups, practicing self-care, saying no, and understanding the stages of relapse. Other tasks are getting rid of friends who are using, understanding the dangers of cross-addiction, dealing with post-acute withdrawal symptoms, developing healthy alternatives to using, and seeing themselves as a nondrinker or nonuser.

There are many risks to recovery at this stage, including cravings, having poor self-care, wanting to use just one more time, and struggling with whether one has an addiction. Individuals are often eager to make big external changes in early recovery, such as changing jobs or ending a relationship. It is generally felt that big changes (changing jobs, starting a new relationship) should be avoided in the first year until individuals have enough perspective use of good judgment in making these changes.

Post-acute withdrawal syndrome (PAWS) is a common cause of relapse. Unlike acute withdrawal, which has mostly physical symptoms, PAWS has mostly psychological and emotional symptoms. Its symptoms also tend to be similar for most addictions, unlike acute withdrawal, which tends to have specific symptoms for each addiction. Symptoms of PAWS include mood swings, anxiety, irritability, variable energy, low enthusiasm, variable concentration, and disturbed sleep. The symptoms tend to come and go. Symptoms gradually improve over time but can last up to 2 years.

Repair Stage

In the repair stage, the main task is to repair the damage caused by addiction. Addicts must confront the damage caused by addiction to their relationships, employment, finances, and self-esteem. They must also overcome the guilt and negative self-labeling that evolved during addiction. These are some of the developmental tasks of the repair stage of recovery. Common causes of relapse in this stage are poor self-care and not attending self-help groups. This stage usually lasts for 2–3 years.

Growth Stage

The growth stage is about developing skills that individuals may have never learned and that predisposed them to addiction. The growth stage is about moving forward. This also is the time to deal with family of origin issues or past emotional trauma. If tackled too soon, recovering addicts may not have the necessary coping skills to handle these issues, which may lead to relapse.

Some of the tasks of the growth stage are identifying and repairing negative thinking and self-destructive patterns; understanding how negative familial patterns have been passed down, which will help individuals let go of resentments and move forward; challenging fears with various techniques; setting healthy boundaries; beginning to give back and help others; and reevaluating one's lifestyle periodically to make sure the addict is on track in his recovery. This stage usually lasts 3–5 years.

Some of the causes of relapse in the growth stage of recovery are:

- Recovering addicts often want to put their addiction behind them and forget that they ever had an addiction. They feel they have lost part of their lives to addiction and don't want to spend the rest of their lives focused on recovery. They start to go to fewer support group meetings.
- As life improves, recovering addicts begin to focus less on self-care. They take on more responsibilities and try to make up for lost time. In a sense, they are trying to get back to their old life without using. They stop doing the things that contributed to their recovery.
- Recovering addicts feel they are not learning anything new at support group meetings and begin to attend less frequently. They fail to understand that one of the benefits of going to meetings is to be reminded of what addiction is like, because it is easy to forget.
- Recovering addicts feel that they should be beyond the basics. They think it is almost embarrassing to talk about the basics of recovery. They are embarrassed to mention that they still have occasional cravings or that they are no longer sure if they had an addiction.
- Recovering addicts think they have a better understanding of alcohol or other drugs and, therefore, think they should be able to control a relapse or avoid the negative consequences of relapses.

Six Developmental Periods of Recovery

Gorski and Miller divide the recovery process into six developmental periods: (1) pre-treatment, (2) stabilization, (3) early recovery, (4) middle recovery, (5) late recovery, and (6) maintenance [3].

1. *Pretreatment.* In pretreatment, addicts learn from the consequences of drug use that they cannot safely use psychoactive substances. As the consequences become more and more severe, addicts attempt to control their drug use. When this fails, they attempt periods of abstinence. Finally, they admit defeat and realize that they cannot control their drug use. Addicts are often forced into treatment before they recognize that substance dependence is a problem. The recognition of addiction that comes as a result of treatment is part of the pretreatment experience.
2. *Stabilization.* Stabilization is regaining control of thought processes, emotions, judgment, and behavior. It involves recovery from acute withdrawal and physical health problems. The major motivational life crisis that caused an addict to enter this period is stabilized.
3. *Early recovery.* Early recovery involves accepting the disease of addiction and learning to function without psychoactive substances. Addicts begin to recuperate from serious physiological, psychological, and social damage caused by substance dependence. This period relies heavily on structured recovery programs, which are often developed for addicts in treatment programs and later as aftercare plans. Early recovery creates an environment that educates addicts and their families about substance dependence and recovery. This period may be difficult for some because of the post-acute withdrawal symptoms.
4. *Middle recovery.* In the middle recovery period, the primary goal is to change lifestyles. Addicts work at developing normal, balanced lifestyles that are based on sobriety-centered values and activities. This involves living a recovery program that is active but less intense than that of early recovery. It includes work activities, family activities, social activities, self-development, recreation, exercise, and proper diet. Resisting the temptation to substitute another addiction, such as gambling, is an important issue in middle recovery. Sobriety can be maintained in this period with a less-restrictive recovery program than in the early recovery period.
5. *Late recovery.* The primary goal of the late recovery period is to develop self-esteem, the capacity for healthy intimacy, and the ability to live happily and productively. Personal beliefs, beliefs about self and others, self-defeating patterns of living, intimacy, and relationship skills are evaluated and, if necessary, restructured. For some recovering people—usually addicts who come from relatively functional families—the late recovery period poses no serious problems. From childhood they learned healthy beliefs and values, but their substance use interfered with their ability to live productively. For these people, recovery means rehabilitation—that is, returning to a previous level of health and well-being.

Other recovering individuals are not as fortunate. They have a great deal of work to do in the late recovery period, either because they grew up in dysfunctional families or because they began using alcohol or other drugs at such a young age that their emotional growth and development were arrested. They never learned normal, healthy beliefs and attitudes.

Participating in Adult Children of Alcoholics (ACOA) support groups may be helpful to those who grew up in alcoholic families. Those whose arrested emotional growth and development resulted from early use of psychoactive substances must undergo a long course of habilitation—that is, developing healthy beliefs and attitudes for the first time.

6. *Maintenance.* The primary goal of the maintenance period is for addicts to stay sober and live productively. This involves maintaining themselves on effective recovery programs, identifying warning signs of relapse, daily

problem-solving, maintaining honesty, and living productively. Addicts continue to avoid addictive chemicals. Recovery from substance dependence is a lifelong process; the disease of addiction never goes away.

The Five Rules of Recovery

Melemis [4] feels that preventing relapse is based on a few simple rules: (1) change your life, (2) be completely honest, (3) ask for help, (4) practice self-care, and (5) don't bend the rules.

Rule 1: Change Your Life The most important rule of recovery is that a person does not achieve recovery by just not using. Recovery involves creating a new life in which it is easier to not use. When individuals do not change their lives, then all the factors that contributed to their addiction will eventually catch up with them. But addicts and families often begin recovery by hoping that they don't have to change. They want their old lives back—without the using. Recovering individuals are often overwhelmed by the idea of change. However, if they make the necessary changes, they can go forward in their recovery process. They often aren't aware that only a small percent of their lives need to be changed.

Rule 2: Be Completely Honest Addiction requires lying. Addicts lie about getting their drug, hiding the drug, denying the consequences of using drugs, and planning their next relapse. Eventually, addicts end up lying to themselves. When recovering addicts feel they cannot be honest, it is a sign of emotional relapse. It is often said that recovering individuals are as sick as their secrets.

A common question about honesty is how honest should a person be when dealing with past lies. The general answer is that honesty is always preferable, except when it may harm others (AA Step 9).

Rule 3: Ask for Help Most people start recovery by trying to do it on their own. They want to prove that they have control over their addiction and that they are not as unhealthy as people think. Attending a self-help group has been shown to significantly increase the chances of long-term recovery. The way to get the most out of 12-step groups is to attend meetings regularly, have a sponsor, read 12-step materials, and have a goal of abstinence.

Some of the benefits of active participation in support groups include (1) individuals feel that they are not alone, (2) they learn what the voice of addiction sounds like by hearing it in others, (3) they learn how other people have done recovery and what coping skills have been successful, and (4) they have a safe place to go where they will not be judged.

Support groups help individuals overcome their guilt and shame of addiction by seeing that they are not alone.

Rule 4: Practice Self-Care To understand the importance of self-care, it helps to understand why most people use alcohol or other drugs—to escape, to relax, or to reward themselves. To acknowledge this helps to motivate them to find healthy alternatives.

Self-care is difficult because recovering individuals tend to be hard on themselves. They may feel that they don't deserve to be good to themselves or they tend to put themselves last. Self-care is especially difficult for adult children of addicts.

Poor self-care often precedes alcohol or other drug use. For example, individuals work hard to achieve a goal, and when it is achieved, they want to celebrate. Drinking or using was part of their normal way of celebrating in the past.

Rule 5: Don't Bend the Rules Recovering addicts should not insist that they do recovery their way. They should not look for loopholes in recovery. A warning sign is when they ask for professional help and consistently ignore the advice.

Recovering addicts can be divided into two categories: nonusers and denied users. *Nonusers* say that using was fun but acknowledged that it was not fun at the end. They want to start the next chapter of their lives. *Denied users* cannot imagine life without using. They make a secret deal with themselves that at some point they will try using again. Important milestones such as recovery anniversaries are often seen as reasons to use. Alternatively, once a milestone is reached, individuals feel they have recovered enough that they can determine when and how to use safely. A goal in recovery is to move from denied users to nonusers.

Partial Recovery

Recovery does not follow a progressive, straight line. Addicts reach and overcome plateaus, slip backwards occasionally, but usually move on. Many recovering people eventually achieve long-term and comfortable sobriety. Others, however, do not make it all the way through the recovery process.

Partial recovery begins when addicts confront a recovery task that they believe to be unmanageable or insurmountable. They get stuck at this level of recovery and only achieve a low-quality sobriety. Instead of taking productive steps to overcome their failure to progress, many deny that something is wrong. With help, many of these people overcome their denial and again begin to make progress. Unfortunately, in others, failure to progress causes relapse. Even then, some of them will become aware of what is happening to them and prevent the relapse episode before it actually occurs. Others go on to relapse. *The Big Book* of AA calls the failure to take the necessary steps to progress in recovery *half measures*. These individuals tend to believe that attendance at AA meetings alone will keep them sober [3].

Controlled Drinking

The controversy over whether alcoholics can learn to drink socially reached its peak with the publication of the Rand report in 1976. This study found that successful social drinking among men treated 18 months previously for alcoholism was not uncommon. Since that time, most studies have been less optimistic. In general, the longer the interval studied, the fewer alcoholics were found to be able to sustain moderate problem-free drinking. Thus far, the only factors identified as common to alcoholics who are able to drink moderately are that they have milder cases of alcoholism (fewer lifetime alcohol-related problems) and greater social support.

In a review of the literature, Taylor found that data from the majority of studies indicate that successful moderate drinking among treated alcoholics is uncommon [5]. Even if a small percentage of alcoholics are able to drink socially, there is currently no way to identify in advance who these will be. Therefore, an alcoholic attempting to drink moderately plays a form of Russian roulette. A realistic goal for the treatment of alcoholism is still abstinence.

Moderation Management is a nine-step, self-help program designed to assist individuals with mild to moderate levels of alcohol dependence to achieve either moderation or abstinence. The program views moderation as a sensible and natural first step to change harmful drinking. Problem drinkers give themselves 30 days of abstinence before testing whether moderation will work. If a moderation goal proves to be unattainable, a goal of abstinence is recommended.

Drugs That May Be Hazardous to Recovery

Numerous drugs (legal, prescription, over the counter, illicit) may be hazardous to recovery; some of these are listed in Table 16.1.

Recovering individuals are at particular risk for relapse when taking prescription drugs prescribed by well-meaning physicians who are not knowledgeable about substance dependence. It is not unusual for these physicians to become irritated when recovering patients tell them they cannot take a medication because it may be hazardous to their sobriety. Over-the-counter cough and cold preparations are particularly dangerous

Table 16.1 Drugs to avoid in recovery (Based on Milhorn [6])

Medication type	Examples
Any medication containing pseudoephedrine, diphenhydramine, or dextromethorphan	Sudafed, Dayquil, Theraflu, Benadryl, Robitussin DM, or any other DM cough syrups
Prescription opiates	Norco, Percocet, Vicodin, Ultram, (methadone in a maintenance program is an exception)
All benzodiazepines	Ativan, Xanax, Klonopin, Valium, Restoril, Valium, Dalmane, Xanax
Hypnotics	Sonata, Ambien, Lunesta
Stimulants such as diet pills or ADHD medications	Adderall, Ritalin, Concerta, phentermine
All preparations that have an alcohol base	Mouthwashes (Scope, Cepacol) and cough syrups (Alomine C, Ambenyl-D, Benylin, Formula 44 Cough)
OTC sleep agents	Tylenol PM, Advil PM
Muscle relaxants	Soma, Flexeril, Zanaflex
First-generation antihistamines	Dramamine, Chlor-Trimeton
First-generation antidepressants	Elavil, Norpramin, Vivactil
Beverage alcohol	Beer, wine, whisky
All illegal drugs	Cocaine, marijuana, LSD
Inhalants	Gasoline, glue, nitrous oxide

to recovering people; some have 30–40 proof alcohol concentrations.

Avoiding mood-altering substances in recovery is based on what is known in the treatment field as *cross-addiction*. The basic tenet of cross-addiction is that if a person has ever been addicted to a psychoactive substance, he can never again use any psychoactive substance without increasing the risk of relapse. It is not wise for a cocaine addict, for example, to begin drinking alcohol after treatment. The individual may become addicted to alcohol, or the alcohol may lead back to addiction to cocaine.

Treatment personnel usually tell recovering patients to avoid nonaddicting drugs that tend to cause sedation, such as classic antihistamines. There is little evidence to indicate that the use of these drugs leads to relapse. However, many recovering addicts will tell you that if they use them, they will abuse them. Since we now have newer nonsedating antihistamines, it is probably better to continue to tell recovering patients to avoid classic antihistamines. Other nonaddicting but sedating drugs (muscle relaxants, antidepressants) should be used only when absolutely necessary and then under the care of a knowledgeable physician. The least sedating ones should be used [6, 7].

Rational Use of Medications in Recovery

Recovering addicts should be upfront about their history of drug use when seeking medical treatment. They should tell their physician that they are recovering addicts and ask the physician to work with them to prevent relapse.

Recovering patients who must undergo surgery can have narcotics for postsurgical pain and can in fact have just as much of it as anyone else. However, some special rules apply. When possible, patients should be maintained in a hospital an extra few days if it means they can go home narcotic free. The use of some of the nonsteroidal drugs, such as ibuprofen (Motrin), for mild to moderate pain rather than narcotic preparations is very helpful. When an addict's pain is such that post-discharge narcotic medication is absolutely necessary, someone in his family or a close friend should keep the narcotic and dispense it as prescribed. The patient should never have direct access to it. It should be prescribed for as short time as possible. As soon as the recovering addict is physically able, he should temporarily increase their attendance at support groups. The same rules apply for dental procedures requiring pain medication or other medical procedures requiring psychoactive substances.

Patients with severe primary psychiatric disorders (unipolar or bipolar disorders, schizophrenia) and substance dependence may require drugs (antidepressants, lithium, antipsychotics) to control the psychiatric symptoms before their substance dependence can be treated. For lesser psychiatric illnesses, such as anxiety disorders, nonpharmacological approaches should be used first, followed by drugs with the least possible potential for abuse, such as SSRIs. Some patients with psychiatric disorders will require medication indefinitely. This sometimes presents as a problem in AA and NA meetings [7].

Support Groups

A support group consists of recovering addicts who voluntarily meet regularly to help one another maintain sobriety. Support groups are of two types—non-12-step and 12-step. Twelve-step support groups are by far the most common, so we will focus on them.

A 12-step program is any program modeled after the 12-step program used by Alcoholics Anonymous. Some other 12-step groups are Narcotics Anonymous, Cocaine Anonymous, and Nicotine Anonymous. Since AA was the first and is the most common 12-step program, we will discuss it [8].

History of AA

Alcoholics Anonymous was established in Akron, Ohio, in 1935 by two alcoholics, Bill Wilson (a stockbroker) and Dr. Bob Smith (a surgeon), who are affectionately referred to by AA members as Bill W and Doctor Bob. Unable to stay sober by themselves, they achieved sobriety through mutual support. They then directed their energies toward helping other alcoholics get and stay sober. They formulated their experiences into the 12 steps of AA in 1938. These steps provide guidelines for the personal growth necessary to achieve a stable recovery. The book Alcoholics Anonymous, known as *The Big Book*, was published in 1939.

As the organization grew, it developed, for its own preservation, a set of guidelines—the 12 Traditions. These traditions assured that AA would not affiliate with organizations, would espouse no other cause other than helping individuals achieve sobriety, and would never accept outside funding or charge fees. Anonymity was insisted on at all levels of the organization to prevent individuals from using AA for personal gain. With the exception of some paid secretarial help, AA is staffed entirely by recovering members who volunteer their time.

Each autonomous AA group sponsors meetings that take place on a regular schedule one or more times a week. There are now over 48,000 groups in at least 92 countries. AA has more than one million members in the United States alone [9].

Philosophy of AA

The single focus of AA is on staying sober, not analyzing why a person drank. Total abstinence is a basic tenet, which AA believes is the only way to stay sober. Sobriety is more than just abstinence; it involves a healthy, happy way of living without alcohol. The term "dry drunk" is used in AA to describe abstinent alcoholics who are living and behaving as if they were still drinking. AA considers alcoholism to be a disease, sort of an allergy to alcohol. It has no requirement for membership except a desire to stop drinking. There are no membership cards—people are members if they say so. It is free, supported only by voluntary contributions from members. Being anonymous, there are no membership lists [10].

The Twelve Suggested Steps of AA

The 12 steps of AA are a suggested model for the process of change and growth (Table 16.2). The

Table 16.2 The 12 suggested steps of AA (The 12 steps are reprinted with permission of Alcoholics Anonymous World Services, Inc. [10])

1. We admitted we were powerless over alcohol—that our lives had become unmanageable
2. We came to believe that a power greater than ourselves could restore us to sanity
3. We made a decision to turn our will and our lives over to the care of God as we understood him
4. We made a searching and fearless moral inventory of ourselves
5. We admitted to God, to ourselves, and to another human being the exact nature of our wrongs
6. We were entirely ready to have God remove all these defects of character
7. We humbly asked Him to remove our shortcomings
8. We made a list of all persons we had harmed and became willing to make amends to them all
9. We made direct amends to such people whenever possible, except when to do so would injure them or others
10. We continued to take personal inventory and when we were wrong promptly admitted it
11. We sought through prayer and meditation to improve our conscious contact with God, as we understood Him, praying only for knowledge of His will and the power to carry that out
12. Having had a spiritual awakening as the result of these steps, we tried to carry this message to alcoholics and to practice these principles in all our affairs

fact that the word alcohol appears in only the first step underscores AA's contention that the main work of sobriety is restructuring of an alcoholic's personality. Step 1 is admitting that one is an alcoholic and has lost control of his drinking. This sounds like an obvious and simple step to take, but because of the tremendous denial systems most alcoholics have built up, it is usually the most difficult one [10].

Having admitted powerlessness, Steps 2 and 3 give hope, that is, the recognition that something can lead the alcoholic on a path of sobriety. The phrase "God as we understood Him" is little less than a stroke of genius. It was an attempt to diffuse the religious language of the 12 steps. AA members usually refer to this "God as we understood Him" as their "higher power." For agnostic members of AA, their higher power may be AA itself or whatever they choose it to be. I had one patient who chose the large oak tree out back of the AA building as his higher power. It worked for him.

Steps 4 and 5 involve self-examination. The purpose of this self-examination is not to dwell on the past but to prevent relapse.

Steps 6 and 7 allow God to change the alcoholic. Steps 8, 9, and 10 have to do with accepting responsibility and being accountable, two traits which are lacking in the alcoholic lifestyle. Step 11 is for continued spiritual growth.

Step 12 is the keystone of the program, for it reinforces the work of the previous 11 steps. It involves helping drinking alcoholics in positive ways, such as accompanying them to meetings or helping them get medical care. By doing this work, recovering alcoholics not only help alcoholics who are still drinking but help develop an improved sense of their own self-worth [11–13].

AA Slogans

There are a multitude of slogans used by AA members worldwide. AA slogans for newly sober alcoholic members are purposely simple, direct, and catchy. They are designed to be comprehended by the recently detoxified brain [14]. Some AA slogans include:

- "Don't drink, go to meetings," which means immerse yourself in a network of recovering alcoholics.
- "Easy does it," which means avoid stress.
- "One day at a time," which means focus on not drinking today.
- "If I don't change, my sobriety date will!," which means the alcoholic will relapse.
- "It's always easier to take someone else's inventory," which means it's easier to tell someone else what to do than to do it yourself.
- "If you hang around a barber shop long enough, you'll get a haircut," which means that if you hang around those who drink, you will eventually drink.
- "First things first," sobriety comes ahead of everything else. Without sobriety there is nothing else.

The Twelve Traditions

The 12 Traditions of 12-step programs provide guidelines for relationships among the 12-step groups, members, other groups, the global fellowship, and the society at large. Questions of finance, public relations, donations, and purpose are addressed in the Traditions. They were originally written by Bill Wilson after the founding of the first 12-step group.

AA does not solicit members, promote any religion, provide social services, run hospitals or treatment services, follow up on its members, claim to be a help with any problem other than alcoholism, accept outside money for services or contributions, make medical or psychological diagnoses, prescribe or pay for treatment, or claim to be the only successful approach to alcoholism [10].

The Sponsor

Veteran AA members with at least 1 year of sobriety can serve as sponsors to offer guidance and support, including confrontation if a newcomer's behavior indicates he is ready to drink again. The most powerful influence sponsors exert may be as role models of people who have successfully achieved sobriety. Veteran AA members become a newcomer's sponsor by mutual agreement. Traditionally, to avoid development of intimate relationships, sponsors are of the same sex as their assigned newcomers [11].

The AA Meeting

There are two basic types of AA meetings—open and closed. Anyone can attend open meetings, whether or not he has had problems with alcohol. Only AA members and those wishing to stop drinking can attend closed meetings. Those who do not admit to have a problem with alcohol may be asked to leave. Unfortunately, at some meetings, this includes those who have problems with drugs other than alcohol. In general, however, AA is becoming more lenient and accepting of these nonalcoholic addicts. Closed meetings usually have a stable core of members and function more or less as leaderless support groups [11, 12].

Table 16.3 Typical agenda for an AA meeting (From Milhorn [6]. Approved with permission, Springer)

Moment of silence
Recital of the serenity prayer
Reading of "what AA is and is not"
Reading of "How It Works" (Alcoholics Anonymous, Chap. 5)
Program (one of the following)
The Big Book study
Step study
Topic discussion
Group discussion
Speaker meeting
Combination of these
Recital of the Lord's Prayer
Adjourn

Although they vary somewhat, AA meetings generally follow similar formats (Table 16.3). A meeting begins with a moment of silence. Members may use this time to say a personal prayer, reflect on the happenings of the day, or just to feel gratitude for being sober.

Next, the group, in unison, recites the serenity prayer. "God, grant me the serenity to accept the things I cannot change, the courage to change the things I can, and the wisdom to know the difference."

Someone is then asked to read a statement about what AA is and what it is not:

> Alcoholics Anonymous is a fellowship of men and women who share their experience, strength, and hope with each other that they may solve their common problem and help others to recover from alcoholism. The only requirement for membership is a desire to stop drinking. There are no dues or fees for AA membership; we are self-supporting through our own contributions. AA is not allied with any sect, denomination, politics, organization, or institution; does not wish to engage in any controversy; neither endorses nor opposes any causes. Our primary purpose is to stay sober and help other alcoholics to achieve sobriety. [15]

Next, someone is asked to read the first part of Chap. 5, "How It Works," from Alcoholics Anonymous [10].

> Our stories disclose in a general way what we used to be like, what happened, and what we are like now. If you have decided you want what we have and are willing to go to any length to get it—then you are ready to take certain steps. At some of these we balked. We thought we could find an easier, softer way. But we could not. With all the earnestness at our command, we beg of you to be fearless and thorough from the very start. Some of us have tried to hold on to our old ideas and the result was nil until we let go absolutely. Remember that we deal with alcohol—cunning, baffling, powerful! Without help it is too much for us. But there is One who has all power—that One is God. May you find Him now! Half measures availed us nothing. We stood at the turning point. We asked His protection and care with complete abandon. Here are the steps we took, which are suggested as a program of recovery.

The 12 suggested steps of AA are then read. Afterward, the reading continues from Chap. 5 of *The Big Book*:

> Many of us exclaimed, 'What an order! I can't go through with it.' Do not be discouraged. No one among us has been able to maintain anything like perfect adherence to these principles. We are not saints. The point is that we are willing to grow along spiritual lines. The principles we have set down are guides to progress. We claim spiritual progress rather than spiritual perfection. Our description of the alcoholic, the chapter to the agnostic, and our personal adventures before and after make clear three pertinent ideas: (a) That we were alcoholic and could not manage our own lives, (b) That probably no human power could have relieved our alcoholism, (c) That God could and would if He were sought. [10]

Next, the major portion of the meeting takes place—the program. It may take one of several forms. For instance, in *The Big Book* program, members read sections of Alcoholics Anonymous. After each section, members discuss how the particular passage relates to their experiences. In a step program, members discuss the various steps of AA. In a topic program, members discuss a topic such as gratitude, acceptance, honesty, or resentment. Each member relates what the topic means to him. A topic is usually selected by the chairperson prior to the meeting.

Some meetings are used to discuss personal problems related to the maintenance of sobriety, and in speaker meetings, recovering alcoholics, usually from different AA groups, tell their stories, which are called "drunkalogues." These are accounts of alcoholics' troubles with drinking and their recovery through AA. Many times they are humorous. In larger meetings, members may separate into smaller groups so that several of these types of programs may go on at the same time [6].

Finally the meeting ends with a group recital of the Lord's Prayer, usually with members holding hands:

> Our Father, which art in heaven, hallowed be Thy name. Thy kingdom come. Thy will be done, on Earth as it is in heaven. Give us this day our daily bread, and forgive us our debts, as we forgive our debtors. And lead us not into temptation, but deliver us from evil: For thine is the kingdom, and the power, and the glory, forever. Amen.

In addition to meetings, many local AA organizations operate clubhouses. These are open during the day and sometimes in the evening, and alcoholics can spend time there chatting with other recovering alcoholics. This setting provides a variety of benefits: It replaces the drinking environment and provides alcoholics a new social group and a supportive environment [16].

Web-Based Recovery Support

Web-based recovery support can play an important role in sustained recovery. The addict can connect with fellow recovering addicts 24 h a day 7 days a week. They can participate in discussions anonymously. Two of such support systems are Online Intergroup of Alcoholics Anonymous and SMART Recovery Online.

The *Online Intergroup of Alcoholics Anonymous* was formed to serve all online AA groups in the rapidly growing online fellowship. It offers links to international sites in several languages and sponsors real-time meetings, email meetings, event calendars, information, and links to other sites and groups. *SMART Recovery Online* offers donation-requested access to message boards, 24/7 live chat, and daily meetings in both type chat and voice chat formats [17].

Pharmacological Approaches

Several medications are available to aid the recovery from alcohol and opioid dependence.

Alcohol Dependence

Medications used to aid recovery from alcohol dependence include disulfiram (Antabuse), acamprosate (Campral), and naltrexone (Revia, Vivitrol).

Disulfiram

A chemical barrier to support abstinence, disulfiram is especially useful in the first year or two of sobriety. It is a safe medication with relatively few side effects. Disulfiram, by interfering with the action of aldehyde dehydrogenase, causes rapid accumulation of a toxic catabolite, acetaldehyde, after ethanol ingestion. Within 15 min after they consume alcohol, alcoholics' faces turn beet red, and they sweat and suffer palpitations, dyspnea, tachycardia, hypotension, syncope, chest pain, nausea, and vomiting. EKG changes of ST depression, T-wave flattening, and QT prolongation may occur. Disulfiram should always be prescribed with a patient's full knowledge and consent.

Although any substances that contain alcohol, including mouthwashes, aftershave lotions, food sauces, and cough medicine, can produce a reaction, the likelihood of them doing so has been exaggerated. When serious reactions occur, it usually means that alcoholics have deliberately consumed alcohol. However, patients should be given lists of common OTC products containing alcohol and be advised to avoid them. They should wear bracelets or carry cards to alert medical personnel that they are taking disulfiram.

Addicts take a 500 mg tablet of disulfiram at bedtime for 5 days and take 250 mg daily thereafter. They should have consumed no alcohol for at least 12 h before they begin taking disulfiram. The drug is slowly excreted. Therefore, reactions to alcohol usually continue to occur up to 5–7 days after patients stop taking the drug.

Side effects of disulfiram are usually mild and consist of a fatigue, somnolence, headache, dizziness, skin rash, gastrointestinal distress, and garlic-like taste and odor from the mouth. These side effects usually disappear in a week or two. If they are particularly troublesome, physicians can lower the drug's dosage for 2 weeks and then return to its previous level. A rare, idiosyncratic disulfiram-induced hepatitis, which is potentially fatal, has been reported. As a result, some doctors recommend that patients undergo tests of their liver function before they begin treatment and that these tests be repeated at 2-week intervals for the first 2 months of treatment and at 3–6 month intervals after that. If a patient's liver function tests become abnormal, the drug should be discontinued. Alcoholics can take disulfiram indefinitely if they need to.

There are few contraindications to the use of disulfiram. However, alcoholics with cardiac or other serious medical problems should not take the drug. Likewise, mentally impaired alcoholics should not take it because they tend to forget whether or not they have taken it. Disulfiram may intensify the effects of anesthetics, sedative-hypnotics, phenytoin, and Coumadin. When used by patients taking isoniazid, disulfiram occasionally causes confusion, changes in mental status, or unstable gait.

Many medications have been reported to produce a disulfiram-like reaction if patients ingest alcohol while taking them. These include oral hypoglycemic agents (chlorpropamide, tolbutamide), antibiotics (metronidazole, quinacrine, sulfonamides, chloramphenicol), some anti-inflammatory drugs (phenylbutazone, phenacetin), ethacrynic acid, and trinitroglycerin.

At AA meetings, some members who reject all drugs as crutches may criticize patients for taking disulfiram. Fortunately, most AA groups accept disulfiram today, and such criticism is declining.

Patients who do well on disulfiram are older, well-motivated people with long drinking histories; their social lives are stable, and they tend to be binge drinkers. Disulfiram therapy by itself is ineffective and should be coupled with appropriate counseling and attendance at AA meetings. Its use is controversial. A major Veterans

Administration study found no difference in sobriety between a group of patients treated with disulfiram and counseling and a control group treated with placebo and counseling.

Treating alcohol-induced reactions to disulfiram mainly involves restoring normal blood pressure and controlling shock if it should occur. Most reactions are mild and last 30 min to several hours. Intravenous diphenhydramine (50–100 mg) and ascorbic acid (1000 mg) may be beneficial [1, 18–23].

In recent years, disulfiram has fallen out of favor and is now a second-line drug.

Acamprosate

Acamprosate (Campral) is used along with counseling. It reduces symptoms of long-lasting withdrawal, such as insomnia, anxiety, restlessness, and dysphoria. Side effects include allergic reactions, irregular heartbeats, and low or high blood pressure, while less serious side effects include headaches, insomnia, and impotence. Diarrhea is the most common side effect. Its mechanism of action is unknown.

Acamprosate comes as 333 mg enteric-coated tablets. The dose is two tablets three times daily. Taking the medication with meals will help the alcoholic remember it.

The dosage should be reduced to one tablet three times per day in patients with moderate renal failure (creatinine clearance 30–50 mL/minute). It is contraindicated for a creatinine clearance less than 30 mL/minute. Acamprosate does not need to be discontinued in the event of a relapse [24, 25].

Naltrexone

Naltrexone is an opioid antagonist that has been approved by the FDA for the treatment of alcohol dependence since 1994. It is a synthetic congener of oxymorphone with no opioid agonist properties. Naltrexone prevents people from getting high from drugs like alcohol or heroin because it prevents the drugs from binding to the mu receptors in the brain.

The most common side effects reported with naltrexone are nonspecific complaints, such as mild gastrointestinal disturbances (nausea, vomiting), anxiety, and insomnia, which tend to disappear over a few days. It carries an FDA boxed warning for the rare side effect of liver damage.

Patients on naltrexone will not show a normal response to opioid pain medications. In a supervised medical setting, pain relief is possible but may require higher than usual doses, and the individual should be closely monitored for respiratory depression. All individuals taking naltrexone are encouraged to keep a card or a note in their wallet in case of an injury or another medical emergency. This is to let medical personnel know that special procedures are required if opiate-based painkillers are to be used.

Naltrexone should not be used by persons with acute hepatitis or liver failure or those with recent opioid use. They must be abstinent for 7–10 days [26, 27].

Naltrexone is supplied in a short-acting form, Revia, and a long-acting form, Vivitrol.

Revia

Revia comes in a pill form and is taken orally. It is available in scored film-coated tablets containing 50 mg of naltrexone hydrochloride. The dose of naltrexone for the treatment of alcohol dependence is 50 mg once daily, 100 mg every other day, or 150 mg every third day [28].

Vivitrol

Naltrexone is also available in an injectable suspension known as Vivitrol. The dosage is 380 mg injected intramuscularly every 4 weeks, given by a physician [29].

Opioid Dependence

Medications used to treat opioid dependence include naltrexone (Revia, Vivitrol), buprenorphine (Suboxone, Bunavail), and methadone (Dolophine).

Naltrexone

A useful adjunctive treatment for maintaining abstinence in detoxified opioid addicts, naltrexone reduces or eliminates the euphoria and drug-seeking behavior opioids produce. Physicians should not attempt to treat patients with naltrexone until they have stopped taking opioids for 7–10 days. If in doubt, physicians can perform a naloxone (Narcan) challenge test by administering 0.8 mg naloxone subcutaneously. The patient is then observed for 20 min for signs or symptoms of withdrawal. If the patient does not show withdrawal symptoms, the physician can start him on naltrexone therapy.

Patients may receive 50 mg of naltrexone hydrochloride tablets every weekday with a 100 mg dose on Saturday, 100 mg every other day, or 150 mg every third day. In doses higher than 300 mg per day, some patients show hepatic toxicity. Many patients drop out of treatment and stop taking the drug. When it is combined with family support and counseling, patients are more apt to remain opioid-free [30, 31].

Buprenorphine

Buprenorphine is a semisynthetic opioid derivative of thebaine. It is a mixed partial agonist opioid receptor modulator that is used to control moderate acute pain in nonopioid-tolerant individuals in lower dosages and to control moderate chronic pain in even smaller doses. It is used to treat opioid addiction in higher dosages in combination with naloxone (Suboxone) [32].

Suboxone

Naltrexone/naloxone (Suboxone) is supplied as 2 mg/0.5 mg, 4 mg/1 mg, 8 mg/2 mg, and 12 mg/3 mg sublingual films. On day 1, initially 2 mg/0.5 mg or 4 mg/1 mg is given. This may be increased in increments of 2 mg/0.5 mg or 4 mg/1 mg at 2-hr intervals up to 8 mg/2 mg based on response. On day 2 of maintenance, a single daily dose of up to 16 mg/4 mg may be given. Qualified physicians may dispense or prescribe buprenorphine products for up to 30 patients at a time.

Another naltrexone/naloxone combination (Bunavail) is supplied in three strengths: 2.1 mg/0.3 mg, 4.2 mg/0.7 mg, and 6.3 mg/1 mg.

Side effects include stomach pain, headache, constipation, vomiting, sweating, and difficulty falling asleep or staying asleep. More serious side effects include difficulty breathing or swallowing, unusual bleeding or bruising, extreme fatigue, abdominal pain, and jaundice.

Suboxone induction is only for patients dependent on short-acting opioids, such as heroin, and not for those dependent on long-acting opioids, such as methadone. Buprenorphine monotherapy is recommended for induction of long-acting opioids [33].

Methadone

A form of outpatient treatment for heroin addiction, methadone maintenance, involves giving patients methadone (Dolophine) daily. Since methadone is an opioid, methadone maintenance obviously does not have abstinence as its goal.

Methadone is a synthetic opioid that in large doses produces a degree of euphoria comparable to that of heroin (see Chap. 6). It has the advantage of having a longer half-life than heroin and of being effective in an oral form. Methadone often produces side effects, including sedation, constipation, excessive sweating, urine retention, and reduced sex drive. Intoxicated patients should not be given methadone because its effect with alcohol is synergistic.

The goals of methadone maintenance are to reduce illicit drug use, reduce criminal activity, increase productivity (as indicated by employment), increase self-esteem, and improve family and community functioning. In addition, because addicts take methadone orally, they reduce their risk of acquiring serious infectious complications of intravenous drug use, such as bacterial endocarditis, hepatitis B, and AIDS. Methadone maintenance helps a large number of people who are not motivated to become abstinent and who otherwise would return to criminal activity and illicit drug use. Patients on methadone maintenance commonly use cocaine, alcohol, and benzodiazepines.

Originally, physicians used large doses of methadone (100–200 mg/day) to block the effects of heroin. Daily doses in the range of 60–120 mg appear to achieve comparable results by reducing addicts' craving for opioids, indicating that the blocking ability of high doses is not as important as the relief of cravings for opioids.

A typical methadone maintenance clinic provides addicts daily doses of oral methadone, plus ancillary services such as vocational, legal, and social counseling. They usually also provide group therapy. Methadone maintenance programs periodically analyze addicts' urine for heroin and other drugs. Addicts take the medication in the presence of nurses or other responsible employees. After a few months of satisfactory cooperation with the program, programs may allow patients to take home a day's supply of methadone. As they continue to act reliably and responsibly, programs may permit them to take home a three-day supply.

Methadone maintenance programs are subject to stringent federal and state regulations. Some states do not allow this treatment. Federal regulations require that such programs be registered with the Drug Enforcement Administration (DEA) and comply with specific DEA reporting requirements. Further, regulations require detoxification, rather than maintenance, of patients who have been dependent on opioids for less than 1 year.

In recent years, there has been a movement to allow approved private practice physicians to prescribe methadone for maintenance outside the methadone maintenance clinics. This includes dispensing methadone through a general medical practice. In this circumstance, a physician provides methadone pharmacotherapy contingent on registration with the Drug Enforcement Administration, the US Food and Drug Administration, and the state methadone authority. Physicians and patients must comply with the requirements of methadone maintenance programs. This approach is a useful treatment option for patients who have limited access to specialized clinics, especially those who live in rural areas.

To practice office-based opioid therapy (OBOT) , physicians must have training in addiction medicine, be affiliated with a methadone clinic, or be monitored by the medical director of a methadone clinic. Physicians may incorporate up to 30 methadone-maintained patients into their practice. Eligible patients are referred exclusively from methadone clinics and must be stabilized, and they must have achieved 3 years of successful methadone maintenance. The burden of the federal and state requirements makes this option unpopular with physicians [34–36].

Levo-Alpha-Acetylmethadol

A long-acting formulation, levo-alpha-acetylmethadol (LAAM), at one time was used for opioid maintenance. The long duration of action enabled LAAM to be used on alternate days or three times a week. It had its use reduced in 2001 after it was found to be associated with a cardiac arrhythmia due to a prolonged QTc. The manufacturer ceased production of LAAM in 2004 [37].

Summary

Abstinence is not using addicting substances. It allows recovery to begin. Learning to live normally without alcohol or other drugs requires more than abstinence. *Recovery* from alcohol or other drug dependence is a process of change through which an individual achieves abstinence and improved health, wellness, and quality of life. Recovery has no time limit. It is a lifetime program. Primary care physicians must be prepared to enter into a lifelong relationship with recovering individuals and their families. Many crises—including relapse—may occur, especially in the first 2 years of recovery. The recovery process moves from basic to more complex tasks. Recovery does not follow a progressive, straight line. Addicts reach and overcome plateaus, slip backwards occasionally, but usually move on. The recovery process can be divided into six developmental periods: (1) pretreatment, (2) stabilization, (3) early recovery, (4) middle recovery, (5) late recovery, and (6) maintenance.

The longer the interval studied, the fewer alcoholics are able to sustain moderate problem-free drinking. Numerous drugs (legal, prescription, over the counter, illicit) may be hazardous to recovery. Alcoholics Anonymous was established in Akron, Ohio, in 1935 by two alcoholics, Bill Wilson (a stockbroker) and Dr. Bob Smith (a surgeon). Web-based recovery support can play an important role in sustained recovery.

Medications used to aid recovery from alcohol dependence include disulfiram (Antabuse), acamprosate (Campral), and naltrexone (Revia, Vivitrol). Medications used to treat opioid dependence include naltrexone (Revia, Vivitrol), buprenorphine (Suboxone, Bunavail), and methadone (Dolophine). A form of outpatient treatment for heroin addiction, methadone maintenance, involves giving patients methadone (Dolophine) daily.

References

1. Zuska JJ, Pursch JA. Long-term management. In: Gitlow SE, Peyser HS, editors. Alcoholism: a practical treatment guide. Orlando: Grune and Stratton; 1980. p. 131–64.
2. Del Vecchio. SAMHSA's working definition of recovery updated, Substance Abuse and Mental Health Services Administration (SAMHSA) website. https://blog.samhsa.gov/2012/03/23/defintion-of-recovery-updated/#.WL4PwoWcGZ8. March 23, 2012.
3. Gorski TL, Miller M. Staying sober: a guide for relapse prevention. Independence: Independence Press; 1986.
4. Melemis SM. Relapse prevention and the five rules of recovery. Yale J Biol Med. 2015;88:325–32.
5. Taylor JR, Helzer JE, Robins N. Moderate drinking in ex-alcoholics: recent studies. J Stud Alcohol. 1986;47:115–21.
6. Milhorn HT. Chemical dependence: diagnosis, treatment, and prevention. New York: Springer; 1990.
7. Bjork A. Medications in recovery. Hazelden Betty Ford Foundation website. http://www.hazelden.org/web/public/mar10medications.page. March 2010.
8. Walker L. Support groups and 12-Step programs. DrugAbuse.com website. http://drugabuse.com/library/support-groups-and-12-step-programs/#types-of-recovery-groups
9. History of Alcoholics Anonymous. The Alcoholics guide website. http://www.the-alcoholism-guide.org/history-of-alcoholics-anonymous.html
10. Alcoholics Anonymous. Alcoholics Anonymous world services. 4th ed. New York; 2001.
11. O'neil SF, Barnes N. Alcoholics Anonymous. In: Barnes H, Aronson MD, Delbanco TL, editors. Alcoholism: a guide for the primary care physician. New York: Springer; 1987. p. 93–101.
12. Royce JE. Alcoholics Anonymous. In: Alcohol problems and alcoholism. New York: Free Press; 1981. p. 242–55.
13. Van Cleave S, Byrd W, Revell K. What really works in treatment. In: Counseling for substance abuse and addiction. Waco: Word Book; 1987. p. 133–43.
14. Hundreds of AA Slogans and Quote's. AA Slogans and Quote's website. http://aaslogans.com
15. A newcomer asks. Recovery website. http://www.aa.org/assets/en_US/p-24_anewcomerask.pdf
16. Alfred GS. Psychoactive substance use disorders. In: Hsu LKG, Hersen M, editors. Recent developments of adolescent psychiatry. New York: Wiley; 1988. p. 309–31.
17. Hazelden study shows promise of web-based support for patients leaving addiction treatment. Hazelden Betty Ford website. http://www.hazelden.org/web/public/web_support_post_addiction_treatment.page
18. Barnes HN. The use of disulfiram. In: Barnes HN, Aronson MD, Delbanco TL, editors. Alcoholism: a guide for the primary care physician. New York: Springer; 1987. p. 73–7.
19. Cereda J, Bernuau J, Degott C, Rueff B, Benhamou J. Fatal liver failure due to disulfiram. J Clin Gastroenterol. 1989;11:98–100.
20. Methadone maintenance and patients in alcoholism treatment. Department of Health and Human Services. In Alcohol Alert. Rockville; August 1988.
21. Fuller RK, Branchey L, Brightwell DR, et al. Disulfiram treatment of alcoholism: a Veteran's Administration cooperative study. J Am Med Assoc. 1986;250:1449–55.
22. Hanbury R, Sturiano V, Cohen M, Stimmel B, Aguillaume C. Cocaine use in persons on methadone maintenance. Adv Alcohol Subst Abuse. 1986;6:97–106.
23. Wright C IV, Vafier JA, Lake CR. Disulfiram-induced fulminating hepatitis: guidelines for liver-panel monitoring. J Clin Psychiatry. 1988;49:430–4.
24. Williams SH. Medications for treating alcohol dependence. Am Fam Physician. 2005;72(9):1775–80.
25. Acamprosate dosage. Drugs.com website. https://www.drugs.com/dosage/acamprosate.html
26. Naltrexone (Revia). Office of Alcoholism and Substance Abuse Services (OASAS) website. https://www.oasas.ny.gov/AdMed/FYI/FYI-ReVia.cfm
27. Naltrexone dosage. Drugs.com website, https://www.drugs.com/dosage/naltrexone.html
28. Revia dosage. Drugs.com website. https://www.drugs.com/dosage/revia.html
29. Vivitrol dosing. Drugs.com website. https://www.drugs.com/vivitrol.html
30. Gonzalez JP, Brogden RN. Naltrexone: a review of its pharmacodynamic properties and therapeutic efficacy in the management of opioid dependence. Drugs. 1988;35:192–213.

31. Santos EF. Naltrexone: useful tool in the treatment of heroin users: a review of the literature. Bol Asoc Med P R. 1986 Mar;78(3):95–8.
32. Buprenorphine dosage. 2017. Drugs.com website. https://www.drugs.com/cdi/buprenorphine.html
33. Buprenorphine/naloxone(Rx).Medscapewebsite.http://reference.medscape.com/drug/suboxone-zubsolv-buprenorphine-naloxone-343334
34. Krambeer LL, Von McKnelly W Jr, Gabrielli WF Jr, Penick C. Methadone therapy for opioid dependence. Am Fam Physician. 2001;63(12):2404–11.
35. Forest GG. Antabuse treatment. In: Bratter TE, Forest GG, editors. Alcoholism and substance abuse. New York: The Free Press; 1985. p. 451–60.
36. Cohen S. Methadone maintenance. In: The substance abuse problems: volume one. New York: Haworth Press; 1981. p. 251–6.
37. Wieneke HH, Wolstein Conrads J, Breuckmann F, Gastpar M, Erbel R. Levo-α-acetylmethadol (LAAM) induced QTc-prolongation—results from a controlled clinical trial. Eur J Med Res. 2009;14:7.

Relapse

17

Key Chapter Points

- Relapse is not simply the act of taking a drink or using a drug. It is a process.
- Relapse progresses through stages.
- A number of factors contribute to relapse. There are a number of triggers for relapse.
- Women relapse less frequently than men, at least partly because women are more likely to engage in group counseling while in treatment and that this more intensive level of treatment engagement helps them to remain drug-free.
- A number of steps can be taken to prevent relapse.
- Relapse should be interrupted as soon as possible so that minimum damage is done to recovery.
- The chronic nature of substance dependence means that relapse at some point is not only possible, but likely.
- Primary care physicians, in the long-term management of substance-dependent individuals and their families, should follow a few simple rules.

Relapse is defined as a return to drinking or using other drugs following a period of abstinence. Relapse vulnerability is associated with cravings and urges to use. With addiction, relapses are a common part of the disease. A *slip*, also known as a lapse, is a situation where the addict drinks or uses but stops quickly afterward, avoiding a full relapse. Some addicts have a simple slip, but immediately return to recovery. It often strengthens their will to stay sober. Others allow a slip to turn into a full-blown relapse.

The Relapse Syndrome

Just as it is important for addicts to understand that recovery is more than abstinence, they need to recognize that relapse is not simply the act of taking a drink or using a drug. It, too, is a process. Addicts who believe that abstinence is synonymous with recovery also believe that not using alcohol or other drugs is their main task in recovery. As a result, when their behavior is dysfunctional, they become confused because their mistaken belief keeps them from identifying the real problem—their failure to progress in recovery. They believe that when they are abstinent, the only way to lose control is to use alcohol or other drugs.

A common mistaken belief about relapse is that it just suddenly occurs without warning. The truth is that many warning signs precede a relapse. Addicts who believe that relapse just suddenly occurs are unable to identify warning signs. They also forget that denial carries over into sobriety and can block their recognition of warning signs, which occur very late in the relapse process. By the time they develop, many addicts have already lost control of their judgment and behavior. As a result, they are unable to act to reverse the relapse process.

H.T. Milhorn, *Substance Use Disorders*, DOI 10.1007/978-3-319-63040-3_17

In the early days of AA, alcoholics were considered to relapse only when they began drinking again. As alcoholics started substituting other CNS depressant drugs, such as tranquilizers and sleeping pills, for alcohol it became obvious that they could not safely use any sedative. So relapse came to mean the use of any sedative, including alcohol. In the 1960s, physicians found that relapse was also associated with other drugs, such as marijuana, cocaine, amphetamines, and narcotics. As a result, relapse came to mean the use of any psychoactive substance.

The relapse process includes becoming dysfunctional in recovery. The dysfunction begins as a mental process that in AA is called "stinking thinking." This thinking leads to a change in behavior that AA calls a "setup for relapse." The dysfunctional behavior in AA is called a "dry drunk," which is sometimes thought of as an alcoholic's thinking and acting as if he or she were drinking despite being abstinent [1].

Women relapse less frequently than men, at least partly because women are more likely to engage in group counseling while in treatment and that this more intensive level of treatment engagement helps them to remain drug-free [2].

Major Kinds and Stages of Relapse

Three Kinds of Relapse

Melemis [3] identified three major phases of relapse: (1) emotional relapse, (2) mental relapse, and (3) physical relapse.

1. *Emotional Relapse.* With emotional relapse, recovering addicts are not thinking about using, but their emotions and behaviors are setting them up for relapse in the future. Denial is a big part of emotional relapse. Some of the signs of emotional relapse are (1) bottling up emotions, (2) isolating, (3) not going to meetings, (4) going to meetings but not sharing, (5) focusing on other people's problems or focusing on how other people affect them, and (6) having poor eating and sleeping habits. The common denominator of emotional relapse is poor self-care, including emotional, psychological, and physical care. Signs of emotional relapse are anxiety, intolerance, anger, defensiveness, mood swings, isolation, not asking for help, not going to meetings, poor eating habits, and poor sleep habits. The addict may lose interest in hobbies that he once loved.
2. *Mental Relapse.* In mental relapse part of the addict wants to use and part doesn't. In the early phase of mental relapse, the addict is just idly thinking about using. But in the later phase he is definitely thinking about using.

The signs of mental relapse are thinking about people, places, and things that involved using alcohol or other drugs; glamorizing past use; lying; hanging out with old using friends; fantasizing about using; thinking about relapsing; and planning the relapse.

3. *Physical Relapse.* Once the addict starts thinking about drinking or using, if he doesn't use some of the techniques mentioned later in this chapter, it doesn't take long to go from mental relapse to physical relapse. Trying to achieve abstinence through brute force is rarely successful. It's difficult to stop the process of relapse at this point.

Most physical relapses are relapses of opportunity. They occur when the recovering addict has a window in which he feels he will not get caught. Part of relapse prevention involves rehearsing these situations and developing healthy exit strategies.

Ten Stages of Relapse

Gorski and Miller [1] further divided relapse into the following ten phases:

1. *Return of denial.* During this phase, individuals in the relapse process become unable to recognize and honestly tell others what they are thinking or feeling. The most common symptom of this phase is a concern about well-being. Addicts feel uneasy, afraid, and anxious, but the uneasiness comes and goes, usually only lasting a short time. To tolerate

these periods of worry, fear, and anxiety, addicts ignore or deny these feelings in the same way they at one time denied addiction.

2. *Avoidance and defensive behavior*. During this phase, addicts begin to avoid anything or anybody who would force them to look at themselves. They believe that they will never drink or use drugs again, so that a daily recovery program seems unnecessary to them. They tend to worry about others instead of themselves; that is, judging others' recovery programs rather than their own. In AA this is called "working the other guy's program." Addicts in this phase tend to become defensive, defending themselves even when they do not need to.

Addicts become compulsive, or rigid, in the way they think and behave, tending to do the same things over and over again without good reasons. They also tend to control conversations either by talking too much or by not talking at all. They tend to work more than they need to, become involved in many activities, and may appear to be models of recovery because of their heavy work on AA's 12th step and their chairing of AA meetings. They are well-known by counselors for playing counselor. They avoid casual or informal involvement with people, however. They are impulsive, acting without thought or self-control, usually during times of high stress. As a result, they may make decisions that seriously damage their recovery program. Lastly, addicts in this phase are lonely—they begin to spend more time alone and usually have good reasons and excuses for staying away from other people.

3. *Crisis building*. During this phase, addicts have problems that result from denying personal feelings, isolating themselves, and neglecting their recovery programs. They commonly suffer tunnel vision—seeing only one small part of life rather than the big picture, which sometimes creates the illusion that everything is secure and going well. They blow small problems way out of proportion and come to believe that they are being treated unfairly and are powerless to do anything about it.

Addicts also often suffer minor depressions, the symptoms of which begin to appear and to persist. They are usually able to distract themselves from these moods by getting busy with other things, and they do not talk about depression. Addicts stop planning, often mistaking the AA slogan "1 day at a time" to mean that people shouldn't plan or think about what they are going to do tomorrow and beyond. They pay less and less attention to details and make plans more on wishful thinking than on reality. Finally, their plans begin to fail because they are unrealistic. As a result, addicts develop problems in their lives.

4. *Immobilization*. During this phase, addicts are unable to initiate action and merely go through the motions of living. Common symptoms of this phase include daydreaming and wishful thinking. Addicts have difficulty concentrating, and they frequently use the expression "if only" in conversation. They begin to have fantasies of escape and of being rescued by events that are unlikely to happen.

Addicts also begin to develop a sense of failure, which may be real or imagined. They blow small failures out of proportion. They also harbor an immature wish to be happy, without identifying what they need to be happy. They want things to get better without doing anything to make them better.

5. *Confusion and overreaction*. During this phase, addicts cannot think clearly. They become upset with themselves and those around them and are irritable, overreacting to small things. Periods of confusion steadily become more frequent, last longer, and cause more problems. Addicts often are angry with themselves because they cannot figure things out.

They become irritable, straining relationships with friends, family, and support group members. The conflicts continue to increase in spite of their efforts to resolve them. And addicts are easily angered, becoming frustrated, resentful, and irritable for no reason. They frequently overreact to small things and become increasingly stressed and anxious.

6. *Depression.* During this phase, addicts become so depressed that they have difficulty sticking to normal routines. At times they think of suicide, drinking, or using other drugs. Their depression may be severe and persistent. The most common symptoms are irregular sleeping habits, inability to take action, irregular eating habits, loss of daily structure, and periods of deep depression.
7. *Behavioral loss of control.* During this phase, addicts are unable to control their behavior and their daily schedules, but they deny being out of control. Their lives become chaotic. Their attendance at support group meetings becomes irregular, as they find excuses for missing meetings and don't recognize the importance of attendance. Other things seem more important to them. They develop an "I don't care" attitude, trying to act as if they are unconcerned about their problems. They use this attitude to hide feelings of helplessness and a growing lack of self-respect and self-confidence.

They reject help, cutting themselves off from those who could help with fits of anger, by criticizing or putting others down or by quietly withdrawing from others. They become dissatisfied with life, which seems to them to have become unmanageable since they stopped drinking or using other drugs. They begin to feel that they might as well start drinking or using other drugs again. Finally, they feel powerless and helpless. They have trouble getting started, thinking clearly, concentrating, and thinking abstractly. They begin to feel there is no way out.

8. *Recognition of loss of control.* During this phase, the addicts' denial breaks, and they realize how severe their problems really are, how unmanageable their lives have become, and how little power they have to solve any of their problems. By this time, they are so isolated that they have no one to turn to for help. They commonly begin to feel sorry for themselves and often use self-pity to get attention from family members and from support group members. They think about social drinking, imagining that alcohol or other drugs would make them feel better, and they begin to think that they can control their use. They recognize their lying, denial, and the excuses they make but are unable to do anything about them. They lose self-confidence and feel trapped and overwhelmed by the inability to think clearly and take action. This feeling of powerlessness leads them to believe that they are useless and incompetent.
9. *Option reduction.* During this phase, addicts feel trapped, with only three ways out—insanity, suicide, or drug use. They no longer believe that anyone or anything can help them. They feel an unreasonable resentment and anger because they cannot behave the way they want to. They stop attending all support group meetings and feel overwhelming loneliness, frustration, anger, and tension. They have intense fears of insanity and feelings of helplessness and desperation. Finally, they lose control over their behavior and have more and more difficulty controlling their thoughts, emotions, and judgment. They are unable to regain control.
10. *The relapse episode.* During this phase, addicts begin to use alcohol or other drugs again. Their failed struggle for abstinence leads to shame and guilt. Eventually, they lose all control and develop serious biopsychosocial problems. They begin using alcohol or other drugs in attempts to control their dysfunction. Their shame and guilt isolates them and makes them afraid their relapse will be discovered. They feel helpless and hopeless that they can do nothing to stop the relapse. They stop attempting to control their use of alcohol or other drugs and begin using them often, heavily, and destructively. The progressive relapse damages their physical, psychological, and social health. They become so ill that they cannot function. They either seek treatment, have a physical or

emotional collapse, commit suicide, or die from medical complications.

Factors Contributing to Relapse

There are a number of factors and triggers that contribute to relapse.

Factors

Talbott [4] identified 13 factors that contribute to relapse:

1. *Failure to understand and accept substance dependence as a disease.* This is the fundamental factor that can precipitate relapse. Addicts who do not believe addiction to be a disease tend to think that by willpower alone they can control their drinking and using.
2. *Denial of loss of control.* Addicts who don't believe in loss of control feel that they can drink or use as long as they do so carefully. They do not connect their abuse of psychoactive substances and the problems that follow. They continue with the same behavior but expect different results.
3. *Dishonesty.* For addicts, dishonesty usually means distorting reality and concealing emotions. It may include extensive rationalizations. Addicts may have extramarital affairs, which are likely to contribute to relapse.
4. *The dysfunctional family*. A family can contribute immeasurably to an addict's recovery. In the same way that the dysfunctional family contributed to the progression of the disease, however, it can also contribute to relapse.
5. *The lack of a spiritual program.* The lack of a spiritual program leads addicts to believe that no source of strength, other than themselves, is available to them. The concept of a higher power ceases to be important in their recovery.
6. *Stress.* The old way addicts handled stress was to use chemicals to get high. In recovery, they have to learn nonchemical coping skills. Emotional and physical traps that often are said to lead to relapse include getting too hungry, angry, lonely, or tired (HALT), as well as self-pity. Recognizing these traps and getting out of them is essential.
7. *Isolation.* Withdrawal from relationships to avoid conflict can also lead to relapse. Isolation in recovery can lead addicts to feel hopelessly different and worthless; addicts must combat it with the tools of recovery.
8. *Cross-addiction.* Recovering individuals may take over-the-counter or prescription medications without being aware of their mood-altering or addictive qualities. Addicts have relapsed while taking legitimately prescribed medication for pain, for anxiety, or for surgical procedures.
9. *Holiday syndrome.* The risk of relapse is high at special times of the year, such as Thanksgiving, Christmas, birthdays, or anniversaries, when memories of the past surface and increase the pain of the present. During such periods, addicts must go to more support group meetings, call their sponsors, and work the steps of the support group.
10. *Withdrawal.* Many people consider withdrawal from substance dependence to consist of the obvious acute physical signs—tremors, seizures, delirium—that occur when addicts stop using drugs. However, the physical and emotional effects of addiction may last up to a year or longer after addicts stop using drugs. This is sometimes referred to as the post-acute withdrawal syndrome.
11. *Overconfidence.* When in recovery, life's problems at last seem manageable to addicts. They can easily believe that things will continue to go well and can easily discard a sense of humility and dependence on a higher power. Such an attitude sets up an addict for relapse.
12. *Returning to drinking or drug-taking friends and to old habits*. When recovering individuals come to believe that they can handle the temptations they experience in such settings, the next step is for them to believe that they too can drink or use other drugs. The AA wisdom of avoiding old faces and old places is good advice.

13. *Guilt over the past.* To achieve sobriety with a measure of serenity, addicts must take a moral inventory (AA Step 4) and make amends for their past actions and attitudes (AA Step 9), thus acknowledging the past and making peace with it.

Triggers

Triggers for relapse [5–9] include:

- *Argumentativeness.* Arguing over small and insignificant points, indicating a need always to be right is sometimes seen as developing an excuse to drink.
- *Cockiness.* Feeling that they have "got it made." Compulsive behavior is no longer a problem. They start putting themselves in situations in which there are temptations to prove to others that they don't have a problem.
- *Complacency.* Everything is going so well that the addict begins to feel that he doesn't need to work his recovery program. More relapses occur when things are going well than when they are not.
- *Depression.* Depression can lead to the addict feeling sorry for himself, which can lead to relapse.
- *Dishonesty.* Dishonesty begins with a pattern of small, unnecessary lies to those the addict interacts with in family, social, and work situations. This is soon followed by lying to himself or rationalizing and making excuses for avoiding working his program.
- *Exhaustion.* Allowing himself to become overly tired can decrease willpower and increase craving and relapse risk.
- *Frustration.* When things may not seem to be going the addict's way, he should remind himself that things are not always going to be the way that he wants them to be, and that is perfectly normal.
- *Expecting too much from others.* "I've changed, why hasn't everyone else changed too?" The addict has his own problems to deal with. Everyone else (the family) has their problems to deal with. Developing trust in a recovering addict takes time. Addicts often don't understand this.
- *Impatience/frustration.* Things are not happening fast enough for the addict, or others are not doing what the addict wants them to do.
- *Letting up on discipline.* The addict can become bored with working his program (daily inventory, 12-step meetings, meditation, prayer). This can lead to letting up on the discipline it takes to maintain sobriety.
- *Self-pity.* Feeling like a victim and refusing to acknowledge that he has choices and is responsible for his own life and the quality of it. Self-pity is sometimes referred to as "sitting on the pity pot."
- *Use of mood-altering chemicals.* The addict may feel the desire to get away from things by having a few drinks or popping a few pills. The addict's unknowledgeable physician may think the addict will be responsible and not abuse prescribed medication.

Still other relapse triggers include:

- *Boredom.* Boredom means the addict has too much time on his hands—time to think about the good things about drinking or using.
- *Certain smells, tastes, or noises.* May remind the addict of his drug of choice.
- *Physical pain.* Physical pain, if significant enough, is a justifiable reason for an addict to be prescribed opioid pain medication provided other remedies have failed. Relapse occurs when sufficient precautions are not taken.
- *Romanticizing past drug use.* It can be easy to remember only the good times when the addict was drinking or using, the times when he was partying and having fun. In addition, it is easy to forget when alcohol or other drug use was no longer fun because of all the problems it caused. The addict should remember that he got sober for a reason. At some point, drug or alcohol use was no longer fun. In fact, it probably created a lot of harm to his health, personal life, professional life, financial situation, and perhaps even saddled him with legal issues.

Once the addict has learned to identify his triggers, he can take steps to deal with them effectively. For some, it helps to keep a list of coping techniques that have worked in the past, such as going for a run or calling a close friend or sponsor [8].

Preventing Relapse

Many addicts relapse because they do not understand relapse and what to do to prevent it. Gorski and Miller [1] identify nine steps in preventing relapse:

1. *Stabilization.* Before addicts in recovery can prevent relapse, they must be in control of themselves. Stabilization involves gaining control of thoughts, emotions, memories, judgment, and behavior. Addicts may need professional help.
2. *Assessment.* The past is the best teacher. Addicts should review previous relapses and learn from them. The information they gain should be included in their relapse prevention plans.
3. *Education.* To prevent relapse, addicts must understand it. The more information they have about addiction, recovery, and relapse, the more tools they have to maintain recovery. They should be familiar with the warning signs of relapse, as well as factors that contribute to it.
4. *Identifying warning signs.* Every addict has a unique set of personal warning signs that indicate he is relapsing. These may be health problems, thinking problems, emotional problems, memory problems, or problems with judgment and inappropriate behavior. Each addict should develop a list of personal warning signs.
5. *Managing warning signs.* For each warning sign that an addict identifies, he should develop a plan for coping with it. Listing several alternatives may be helpful.
6. *Inventory training.* A successful recovery program involves a daily inventory (AA Step 10), which helps identify warning signs of relapse. Two daily inventory rituals are recommended. First, each morning addicts should read the daily entry in the 24-hour-a-day book [10] and briefly outline plans for the day. Each evening, they should review the day's tasks, identifying what they handled well and what they need to improve.
7. *Review of the recovery program.* When addicts are not recovering, they are in danger of relapsing. They should periodically review their personal recovery program to identify strengths and weaknesses and correct the weaknesses.
8. *Involvement of significant others.* Recovery cannot take place in isolation. It involves the help and support of others. Since relapse is often totally unconscious, family members, coworkers, and fellow support group members can be extremely helpful in recognizing warning signs. For them to help, they must know an addict's personal warning signs, information the addict should share with significant individuals in his or her life.
9. *Follow-up and reinforcement.* Like recovery, preventing relapse should be a way of life. Addicts should practice it until it becomes a habit. Addicts should periodically revise and update the relapse prevention plan as they grow and change in recovery.

What to Do When Relapse Occurs

It is not uncommon for people who have had a period of recovery to relapse. The relapse should be interrupted as soon as possible so that minimum damage is done to recovery. The experience should be used to build a stronger recovery. When relapse occurs, according to Talbott, addicts should be instructed to do the following [4]:

1. *Call their sponsors.* Recovering addicts should have sponsors in their support groups. This is especially important in the first few months of recovery. Addicts will then, it is hoped, call their sponsors before using psychoactive substances.
2. *Go to a support group meeting.* Addicts should be instructed to go to a meeting imme-

diately and at least daily thereafter to resolve the conflict that resulted in the relapse.
3. *Call support group friends*. Addicts should share honestly with their support group and friends their psychoactive substance use or the urge to drink or use other drugs.
4. *Discuss the relapse with their physicians*. Addicts should discuss their relapse with their primary care physicians. In many cases, addicts can also talk to their treatment program physicians for advice.
5. *Pick up a white chip*. In AA a white chip denotes the desire to become abstinent and to begin a recovery program. Addicts who have relapsed should be instructed to pick up white chips at support group meetings and to begin again with the first step of AA.
6. *Talk with their spouses, families, or significant others*. Although it may be difficult for addicts' spouses, families, or significant others to accept the relapse. Addicts should share the experience with these people.

Addicts should not view relapse as the ultimate failure. They should reach out to others and seek help. They should begin working their recovery program again. They should process the events and emotions that led to relapse so that they will not be repeated.

Does Relapse Mean Treatment Has Failed?

The chronic nature of substance dependence means that relapse at some point is not only possible, but likely. Relapse rates for people with substance use disorders are similar to those for other chronic medical illnesses, such as diabetes, hypertension, and asthma. Treatment of chronic diseases, including substance dependence, involves changing deeply imbedded behaviors, and relapse does not mean treatment has failed. For a person recovering from addiction, lapsing back to drug use indicates that treatment needs to be reinstated or adjusted or that another treatment should be tried [11].

Primary Care Physician's Role in Preventing Relapse

Primary care physicians, in the long-term management of substance-dependent individuals and their families, should follow a few simple rules. They should not assume responsibility for keeping patients sober. That is the responsibility of the patient. They should be careful with their prescription pads, and they should not try to treat patients alone; in times of crisis, such as relapse, they should get help from appropriate professionals. Physicians should monitor patients' recovery by watching for warning signs of relapse, inquiring about their families, jobs, friends, and support group attendance, and by giving them general support.

Many recovering addicts have had negative experiences with health care professionals. Some negative experiences may be attributable to problems in physicians' attitudes, behaviors, or expertise in addiction medicine. Another possibility is inadvertent harm, such as relapse precipitated by a prescribed medication that altered the patient's vigilance and judgment.

Physicians must be cautious, sensitive, and nonjudgmental when caring for addicted patients. The patient should observe the formal recording of his sobriety date in the medical chart. This demonstrates the importance of recovery and the joint commitment of the physician and patient to success. At every patient visit, the sobriety date should be confirmed. If the sobriety date changes, the physician should remain nonjudgmental, record the new sobriety date, and discuss the details of the relapse.

When planning for renewed recovery, the physician should inquire about and document the patient's use of support groups and ask if the patient's spouse, friends, and significant others are supportive of recovery or are themselves using alcohol or other drugs.

At every visit the physician should review all of the medications, including nonprescription drugs and herbal supplements, that the patient is currently taking. Patients with chronic illnesses should be reminded that maintaining sobriety helps with the successful treatment of other medical and psychological conditions.

Recovering patients may be reluctant to use medications, fearing that they will precipitate relapse. If appropriate, physicians should recommend nonpharmacologic treatment (lifestyle changes) as initial therapy. Patients may require referrals to learn stress reduction and relaxation techniques and healthy eating and exercise habits. When medications are necessary, mood-altering or addictive drugs should be avoided whenever possible. Even nonaddictive, nonprescription medications may alter the patient's judgment, triggering relapse behavior [12].

General guidelines for caring for patients recovering from substance dependence are given in Table 17.1.

Jones et al. suggested some alternative medication for use with recovering addicts [12]:

Insomnia Acute and post-acute drug withdrawal can affect sleep in recovering addicts. Patients may have problems initiating sleep, staying asleep, or both. Treatment of patients with insomnia should include avoidance of stimulants, development of appropriate sleep hygiene, and use of relaxation techniques. When pharmacotherapy is necessary, a sedating antidepressant like trazodone (Desyrel) may be used judiciously and for the shortest time possible.

Table 17.1 General guidelines for caring for a patient recovering from substance dependence (From Jones [12]. Approved with permission, Am Fam Physician)

Physician attributes	Sensitive Nonjudgmental Supportive Open Aware
Charting guidelines	Record sobriety date in the patient chart Confirm sobriety date at every visit Record support or 12-step groups regularly attended Record current prescription and over-the-counter medications Update the medication list at every visit
Prescribing guidelines	Use nonpharmacologic treatment as the first line of therapy Refer to physical therapy, counseling, or nutrition support as appropriate Avoid mood-altering or addictive medications, including those that alter judgment Provide patient education regarding specific medications

Diphenhydramine (Benadryl) should be avoided, as should benzodiazepines [triazolam (Halcion), estazolam (ProSom), temazepam (Restoril)] and the Z drugs [zolpidem (Ambien), zaleplon (Sonata), eszopiclone (Lunesta)].

Upper Respiratory Problems Patient education about the self-limited nature of most upper respiratory infections allows the recovering patient to accept non-mood-altering medications for to control symptoms. Instead of sedating antihistamines [diphenhydramine (Benadryl), chlorpheniramine maleate (Chlor-Trimeton)] which may cause fatigue, sedation, and impaired judgment, substitute nonsedating antihistamines [loratadine (Claritin), cetirizine (Zyrtec)]. Nasal steroids, azelastine nasal spray, and ipratropium bromide nasal spray are safe to use. Be careful of prescribing nasal sprays to addicts who snorted their drug of choice.

Decongestants may be stimulating and trigger relapse in CNS stimulant addicts. Saline nasal spray and sinus irrigation are okay. Dextromethorphan and other opioid cough medications (codeine, hydrocodone) should be avoided. Benzonatate (Tessalon Perles) and guaifenesin (Humibid L.A.) are okay.

Gastrointestinal Conditions Instead of diphenoxylate-atropine (Lomotil) for diarrhea, prescribe over-the-counter loperamide (Imodium) or bismuth compounds (Pepto-Bismol, Kaopectate).

Instead of chlordiazepoxide/clidinium bromide (Librax) or belladonna alkaloids/phenobarbital (Donnatal) for hyperactive bowels, prescribe dicyclomine (Bentyl) or hyoscyamine sulfate (Levsin).

Obesity Instead of stimulant drugs [phentermine (Fastin), sibutramine (Meridia)], prescribe Orlistat (Xenical).

Pain Disorders Pain management in the recovering addict is challenging. Most physicians generally avoid prescribing narcotics, but unrelieved pain also may lead to relapse. Heat, ice, rest, and elevation are the first line of therapy for pain. If symptoms are not relieved, physical therapy may be tried. When possible, instead of opioid medications prescribe acetaminophen (Tylenol) or an NSAID [ibuprofen (Motrin), naproxen (Aleve)]. When opioid therapy is necessary to manage pain, one physician in the practice should be responsible for prescribing all pain medications to avoid confusion and exploitation.

If opiates are necessary for the management of chronic pain in recovering addicts, frequent office visits should be required. Safeguards, including a signed treatment contract for pain management, can lower the risk of relapse. Physicians should prescribe opiates sufficient to last only until the next appointment. Early refills should not be provided under any circumstances. Physicians may need to educate patients who are fearful of opioids use about the relapse risk associated with untreated pain. A physician who is considering the use of opioids for the management of chronic pain in a patient recovering from substance dependency should collaborate with physicians who specialize in addiction medicine and pain management.

For headaches, instead of acetaminophen/dichloralphenazone/isometheptene (Midrin) and migraine treatments containing butalbital [butalbital/aspirin/caffeine (Fiorinal), butalbital/acetaminophen/caffeine (Fioricet)], prescribe a triptan [sumatriptan (Imitrex), rizatriptan (Maxalt)].

Muscle Spasm Instead of carisoprodol (Soma), prescribe orphenadrine (Norflex) or metaxalone (Skelaxin).

The last thing a physician wants to do in regard to a recovering patient is to be responsible for the patient's relapse because of inappropriate prescribing practices.

Summary

Just as it is important for addicts to understand that recovery is more than abstinence, they need to recognize that relapse is not simply the act of taking a drink or using a drug. It is a process. Relapse progresses through stages. A number of factors contribute to relapse. There are a number of triggers for relapse.

Women relapse less frequently than men, at least partly because women are more likely to engage in group counseling while in treatment and that this more intensive level of treatment engagement helps them to remain drug-free.

A number of steps can be taken to prevent relapse. Relapse should be interrupted as soon as possible so that minimum damage is done to recovery. The chronic nature of substance dependence means that relapse at some point is not only possible, but likely.

Primary care physicians, in the long-term management of substance-dependent individuals and their families, should follow a few simple rules and guidelines to help their patients avoid relapse.

References

1. Gorski TL, Miller M. Staying sober: a guide for relapse prevention. Independence: Independence Press; 1986.
2. Stocker S. Men and women in drug abuse treatment relapse at different rates and for different reasons. National Institute on Drug Abuse (NIDA) website. 13(4). https://archives.drugabuse.gov/NIDA_Notes/NNVol13N4/Relapse.html. November 1998.
3. Melemis SM. Relapse prevention and the five rules of recovery. Yale J Biol Med. 2015;88:325–32.
4. Talbott GD. Elements of the impaired physician's program. J Med Assoc Ga. 1984;73:749–51.
5. 12 triggers to relapse. PsychPage website. www.psychpage.com/learning/library/assess/relapse.htm
6. Bennett C. The 4 most common causes of addiction relapse. Huffington Post. December 1, 2011.
7. Recognizing drug and alcohol relapse warning signs for you and your loved ones. Reccovery.org website. http://www.recovery.org/topics/alcohol-or-drug-relapse-warning-signals. October 7, 2016.
8. Warning signs of an alcohol or drug relapse: recognizing the steps leading to a relapse. VeryWell website. https://www.verywell.com/warning-signs-of-an-alcohol-or-drug-relapse-67895. June 8, 2016.
9. Weiss R. Understanding "triggers" for addiction. PsychCentral website. https://blogs.psychcentral.com/sex/2013/07/understanding-triggers-for-addiction
10. Walker R. Twenty-four hours a day: a meditation book and journal for daily reflection. Center City: Hazelden Publishing; 2001.
11. Drugs, brains, and behavior: the science of addiction. National Institute on Drug Abuse (NIDA) website. https://www.drugabuse.gov/publications/drugs-brains-behavior-science-addiction/treatment-recovery. July 2014.
12. Jones EM, Knudson D, Haines D. Common problems in patients recovering from chemical dependency. Am Fam Physician. 2003;68(10):1971–9.

The Family

18

Key Chapter Points

- A family is a group of people related by blood or marriage or a strong common bond, such as those descended from a common ancestor or a husband, a wife, and their children. Other types of families are single-parent families, gay families, and extended families.
- A codependent is a person who lets another person's behavior (the addict) adversely affect him or her and who is obsessed with controlling that person's behavior.
- Most families are basically healthy, and family members are usually happy, working, contributing members of society.
- In response to addiction, a family develops a denial system and specific rules, and members tend to assume specific, unhealthy roles.
- Denial is a characteristic distortion in thinking experienced by family members of someone addicted to alcohol or other drugs.
- Families with a member who is addicted to alcohol or other drugs often grieve the loss of the loved one they once knew.
- The person who holds the power in the family—the addict—makes the rules.
- The process of getting the addict into treatment can be speeded up by the use of two concepts: Tough love and intervention by confrontation.
- Treatment of the family is important for several reasons.
- In recovering families, members develop flexible roles, and they depend on one another. Recovering families develop a sense of purpose and grow over time toward their optimal level of functioning.
- Children of alcoholics may carry into adult life certain dysfunctional characteristics.

A family is a group of people related by blood or marriage or a strong common bond, such as those descended from a common ancestor or a husband, a wife, and their children. Other types of families are single-parent families, gay families, and extended families. An extended family is a family that extends beyond the nuclear family, consisting of aunts, uncles, and cousins all living nearby or in the same household. Other types of families include foster relationships, grandparents raising grandchildren, stepfamilies, and elected families. An elected family is one joined by choice and not by the usual ties of blood, marriage, and law. In this chapter, I will consider a family to consist of a husband, a wife, and their children (the traditional family).

The effects of substance abuse on the family are profound. If one accepts 12 million as the number of adult alcoholics in the United States, probably 48 million people are codependent for alcoholism. A *codependent* is a person who lets another person's behavior (the addict) adversely affect him or her and who is obsessed with controlling that person's behavior. How many people

H.T. Milhorn, *Substance Use Disorders*, DOI 10.1007/978-3-319-63040-3_18

are addicted to other drugs or codependent with those who are is not known, but it is thought to be a substantial number [1, 2].

Addicts may have young, teenage, or grown-up children; they may have wives or husbands; they may have brothers or sisters; and they have parents or other relatives. An addict can totally disrupt family life and cause harmful effects that can last a lifetime for all of these people.

Living with an addict can put family members under significant stress. Normal routines are constantly interrupted by unexpected and sometimes frightening experiences. What is said often does not match with what family members sense or feel beneath the surface. The addict, as well as other family members, may deny reality in their attempt to maintain family order. The entire family slowly seems to be spinning out of control [3].

Each member of the family may be affected by alcohol differently. Female alcoholism may affect the fetus even before a child is born by the development of fetal alcohol syndrome or congenital defects produced by other drugs.

Because crime and violence are associated with addiction, incest and battering are common in these families. Almost 30% of father-daughter incest cases and 75% of domestic violence cases involve a family member who is an addict [4].

Although we will primarily discuss alcohol in this chapter, the principles outlined apply to any family that has a chemically dependent member, regardless of the drug that person uses.

The Healthy Family

Most families are basically healthy, and family members are usually happy, working, contributing members of society. A healthy family, however, is not necessarily perfect. Members go through the illnesses, career crises, accidents, and losses that are part of normal living. Healthy families remain intact when faced with stressors because they adjust to changes in a healthy manner. Curran [5] has identified 15 traits of a healthy family:

1. *The healthy family communicates and listens*. Children in healthy families are able to observe open and honest communication between their parents. Members are encouraged to share feelings, to think independently, and to support each other. They have the freedom to challenge each other in discussions because all members' opinions are valued. It is acceptable to disagree.
2. *Healthy family members affirm and support one another*. When the wives have jobs outside of the house, other family members accept additional responsibilities at home and support her efforts. As sons and daughters become busy with jobs and school, parents support their efforts. Responsibilities change and adjustments are made when a parents' job requires travel outside the community. One family member's goals are as important as another's. Parents model self-esteem and set a positive mood within the family.
3. *The healthy family teaches respect for others*. Members of a healthy family respect each other's differences and opinions. Self-respect is taught. Each member is encouraged to develop strengths and talents. Respect for minority groups, other cultures, neighbors, and their property is taught through role modeling.
4. *A healthy family develops a sense of trust*. Husband and wife role model trust toward each other and provide opportunities for the children to earn trust. The parents model dependability and thoughtfulness. When trust is broken, a healthy family uses the experience to teach that trust can be restored
5. *The healthy family has a sense of play and humor*. All work and no play truly does make Jack a dull boy. Healthy families laugh together. Members don't take themselves too seriously. As a result, when the children are grown, they will have fond memories of growing up.
6. *A healthy family shares responsibility*. In a healthy family, children learn that their responsible actions create self-esteem. Family members recognize that responsible behavior includes recognizing other member's emotional needs. The parents

understand their children's capabilities and set their expectation levels accordingly. Recognition is given for accomplishments, and consequences are given for failure to act responsibly.

7. *A healthy family teaches a sense of right and wrong*. Parents agree on important values and set clear, specific guidelines for their enforcement. They help the children distinguish between appropriate and inappropriate behavior. The children are expected to be responsible for their own moral behavior. The family has a strong moral base.
8. *Rituals and traditions abound in the healthy family*. A healthy family has rituals and traditions that are carried over from one generation to the next; it treasures its stories and memories.
9. *A healthy family has a balance of interactions*. Children readily observe that parents are equal partners in family relationships. Separate coalitions of family members are not condoned. Work and activities are not routinely allowed to infringe on family activities.
10. *A healthy family has a shared religious core*. Healthy families integrate faith into daily family life. Faith is passed on to the children in healthy ways. The religious core of the family nourishes and strengthens the family support system.
11. *Members of a healthy family respect each other's privacy*. Members of a healthy family respect each other's choice of friends, time alone, and personal tastes. Each family member is accepted and respected regardless of age, sex, talents, skills, or any other personal characteristic. The healthy family looks forward to their children reaching their teenage years when rules can be negotiated rather than set by parents. Healthy families gradually let go of their children both physically and emotionally as they grow up and leave home.
12. *A healthy family values service to others*. Members of a healthy family demonstrate their value of service to others by such activities as car pooling, involvement in school functions, and service on community committees and task forces. They accept a simpler lifestyle, so that time is created for service to others. Volunteerism, however, is kept under control so that members have time for each other.
13. *Shared meals and conversation are valued*. Unfortunately, outside demands, such as team practices and committee meetings, along with the ever-present television, computers, and video games, are making unhealthy intrusions on family dinner table conversation. Mealtime is a time when family members can share achievements and frustrations, discuss their day, and teach values.
14. *The healthy family shares leisure time*. Balance is the key to sharing leisure time. To find balance, a healthy family prioritizes its activities, plans how it will use its time, and controls television watching, etc. Members spend time with each other individually as well as within the family group.
15. *A healthy family admits to and seeks help with problems*. Healthy families don't seek perfection. They do admit their problems and seek help. They realize it is normal to have problems and teach their members coping skills and problem-solving strategies. Healthy families understand that having problems and solving them is a way to experience growth.

No one family is presumed to embody all the traits; there is no such thing as the perfect family. However, individuals can identify some of the traits that are present and become aware of the areas in which they can strengthen others.

Every family has problems, some of them major and some of them minor. The healthy family develops techniques to deal with its difficulties. Communication is vital—between husband and wife—to identify a marital problem and to isolate the cause and find the roots of a child's problem.

The healthy family with a major problem is not ashamed to go outside the family for help. An older relative or a good friend or neighbor may have been in a similar situation and can offer advice and support [5].

There are support groups and professionals available for almost every family problem—abused children, battered wives, single parents, children with learning disabilities, attempted suicides, alcohol and drug addictions, and so forth.

The Addicted Family

Addiction to alcohol or other drugs exacts a tremendous emotional toll on a family and its individual members. As a result, a family develops a denial system and specific rules, and members tend to assume specific, unhealthy roles. The addicted person becomes the central figure around which family members organize their behaviors and reactions. This family system becomes unpredictable, chaotic, and frightening. Traumatized family members develop their own symptoms as a result [6].

A Family Disease

Everyone whose life touches the alcoholic's is, in one way or another, affected by the disease, but its most direct consequences fall on family members. A boss can dismiss the alcoholic, employees can quit, and friends can drift away. Family members, however, cannot so easily turn their backs on the alcoholic and that person's problem. To do so would mean totally disrupting their own lives as well as deserting someone they love. So they often choose to stay and adapt to the alcoholic's illness. Unfortunately, there is no healthy way to adapt to alcoholism. It is in the family environment, therefore, that alcoholics find their greatest allies. Here, the people who suffer the most from the alcoholic's behavior become the people who nurture that addiction [7].

Some of the most common ways addiction affects the family include [8]:

Conflict Among Family Members Addiction can lead to negativism, where all the communication taking place among the addict and their family members is negative. Anger and resentment can cause family members to lash out at one another. Complaints, criticism, and put-downs may become the norm, which leaves everyone in the situation feeling bad.

Financial Distress Addiction can lead to problems at work, including decreased productivity, missed work, and job loss. Addiction creates a financial burden that may cause families to lose their home or have difficulty providing basic needs, such as food and health care for their children. The addict may rely on financial support from other family members, which further strains relationships.

Instability Within the Family System People suffering from addiction are often unreliable and cannot be counted on to do what they say they will do. Other family members are left to pick up the slack when the addict does not attend to his responsibilities. This causes conflict and instability within families as family members are continuously let down or can never predict the addict's behavior.

Mistrust, Lying, and Stealing Once addiction has taken hold, addicts may turn to lying and stealing to hide and support their drug use. This behavior creates resentment, mistrust, and turmoil within relationships in the family.

Shame and Denial When one member experiences addiction, often the whole family will suffer from shame and denial. Families may work hard to hide the consequences of addiction from outsiders and develop elaborate systems of denial to make it appear that there is no problem at all. Deep feelings of shame may lead other family members to use psychoactive substances as a way to cope.

The enabling relationships that develop follow a predictable pattern and cause alcoholism to be accurately labeled "a family disease [7]."

Family Denial

Denial is a characteristic distortion in thinking experienced by family members of someone addicted to alcohol or other drugs. They are convinced that the addict's problem is something other than addiction—weak health, bad luck, depression, tendency to be preoccupied and worried, mean temper, or countless other possible problems—but not addiction. Many adults have experienced a shock of recognition when they look back over their childhoods and realize that their mother or father was an alcoholic or opioid addict.

Some family members don't put pressure on the addict because they don't want to be abandoned. They would rather keep the addict in their lives than take a chance on losing him. Rather than talk about drug rehabilitation or tell the addict their true feelings about the problem, they play it safe and avoid the truth.

If one person tries to speak the truth about an addict and put up boundaries, that person quickly can become the outcast. It takes courage to stand up to an entire family, and many people aren't sure they have it.

Some people may believe they are helping their loved one by rescuing him. They give money, shelter, food, or whatever the alcoholic needs at the moment. It may make the family feel better that the alcoholic isn't suffering as much because of their help. However, it's suffering that can make an alcoholic realize how much he needs to turn his life around [9].

The Grief Process

Families with a member who is addicted to alcohol often grieve the loss of the loved one they once knew. They may go through the five stages of grief—denial, anger, bargaining, depression, and acceptance. Denial of the problem is often the longest of these stages and may prevent the chemically dependent member from receiving help for years [10].

One of the most baffling aspects of alcoholism is the inability of the people closest to an alcoholic to recognize the reality of the addiction. Even more puzzling, many family members continue to deny the alcoholic's addiction long after he has died from an alcohol-related disease or accident. Enabling plays a major role in family denial. Enabling is a process whereby well-meaning family members unwittingly allow and even encourage irresponsible and self-destructive behavior by shielding the alcoholic from the consequences of his actions. They simply ignore evidence of alcohol abuse.

Spickard and Thomson [7] identified three important factors that contribute to the family's distorted perception of reality: (1) Isolation, (2) emotional turmoil, and (3) centricity.

1. *Isolation*. It is rare to find a family that talks together about an alcoholic in its midst. Shame and embarrassment build a wall of silence around each individual member and gradually cut off all but superficial communication. Family members increase their isolation by gradually separating themselves from outside friends and interests. The world of the family gradually narrows until it includes only those essential for its survival.
2. *Emotional turmoil*. Family members eventually become trapped in much the same emotional turmoil that afflicts the alcoholic. They wrongfully feel guilty for causing the alcoholic to drink and for hating or resenting someone they know they should love. They are ashamed and embarrassed by the alcoholic's actions, and they are angry at their own helplessness. They seldom share their emotions with one another. Instead, they suppress them and allow them to fester into despair and self-hatred. The alcoholic's unpredictable behavior leads to fear and anxiety about the future; increasing isolation leads to loneliness and depression.
3. *Centricity*. In a healthy family, no one person is always the center of attention. However, in a family with an alcoholic, that person is the primary focus of everyone's attention. The family is always on guard, trying to predict the unpredictable and hoping to keep a bad situation from becoming worse. Because of the stresses on individual family members, they often internalize the rationalizations and projections of the alcoholic, and like the alcoholic they deny the addiction, even while they pay an extraordinarily high price for it.

As alcoholics gradually lose control over their own lives and behavior, they wield more and more power over those close to them. Although they are increasingly dependent on those people for emotional, social, and financial support, they play dictator to them. Addicts control what family members say, what they do, and even what they think. Soon everyone displays the psychological symptoms of the disease [10].

Rules in the Alcoholic Family

The person who holds the power in the family—the alcoholic—makes the rules. Thus, the most powerful person in terms of rule making is also the most dysfunctional. These rules are never openly stated, but everyone in the family understands them and lives by them. Wegscheider-Wegscheider-Cruise [11] has identified six such rules:

Rule 1 An alcoholic's use of alcohol is the most important thing in a family's life. The alcoholic is obsessed with maintaining a supply of alcohol, and the rest of the family is obsessed with cutting it off. The family plans its day around the alcoholic's drinking hours. The alcoholic's drinking is the concern everything else in the family revolves around.

Rule 2 Someone or something else caused the alcoholic dependence. The alcoholic is not to blame, and that person's increasing tendency to blame something or someone else for his situation develops into a rule that is imposed on the rest of the family.

Rule 3 The status quo must be maintained at all costs. Alcoholics are afraid to quit drinking, for without alcohol they are afraid they cannot survive. So, as the rule makers, they make sure that their families remain rigid enough to protect them from change.

Rule 4 Everyone in the family must be an enabler. Family members, if asked, will very quickly say that they would do anything to get an alcoholic to quit drinking. But all the while they unconsciously help, or enable, that person to keep drinking. They make up alibis for him, cover up, take over his responsibilities, and accept his rules. They defend these actions on the basis of love, loyalty, or family honor, but the actions effectively preserve the status quo.

Rule 5 No one may discuss what is really going on in the family, either with one another or with outsiders. Feeling threatened, the rule maker tries to avoid letting people outside know about family affairs, specifically his degree of dependence and the magnitude of its impact on the rest of the family. An alcoholic also avoids letting family members have access to new information and advice from outside that might undermine their willingness to enable.

Rule 6 No one may say what he or she is really feeling. The rule maker is in so much emotional pain that he cannot handle the painful feelings of the family. So that person requires everyone to hide his or her feelings. As a result, communication among family members is severely hampered.

Family Members

The Alcoholic

The alcoholic's life is motivated largely by shame, inadequacy, and guilt—shame over using a chemical crutch, inadequacy in not finding another way to cope with the pressures of life and the world, and guilt about the effects of his drinking on the family. Alcoholics are protected from the painful results of their drinking by the chemical effect of alcohol on their judgment and memory, their sophisticated denial systems, and the well-intentioned efforts of the people closest to them.

The alcoholics' behavior is addiction, and their defense mechanism is denial of their alcoholism. Their payoff from addiction is temporary relief from emotional pain. The price they pay is personal destruction [11].

Addiction often creates interpersonal problems for all family members. According to Lameman [12], it may cause:

Cheating The addict may become distant from his spouse and seek satisfaction through pornography, Internet sex, prostitution, or someone else in his life who he feels understands him.

Conflict with Partner The addict may have arguments, get or give the silent treatment, or grow apart by putting his addiction first. The addict may argue with his children, and they may disregard his authority or become afraid of him.

Emotional Trauma The addict may create emotional hardships for his spouse and children by yelling, talking down to them, or being insulting or manipulating.

Financial Problems The addict may struggle economically because of losing his job, taking time off from his job, making poor financial choices, or putting the family's money into his addiction.

Jealousy and Resentment The addict can grow jealous of the spouse's friends, his partner, other family members, or other people in his life. The spouse may be resentful of the addict because of the pain he inflicts on other family members.

Violence The addict may become violent with family members by slapping, hitting, smashing walls, or throwing objects.

Patterns The addict's life example influences his partner, his children, and other family members. There is a high likelihood that his children will become addicted to alcohol or other drugs.

Separation The addict's behavior due to his addiction may cause separation, divorce, and/or isolation from other family members, particularly children, either because they've been taken from him or because they don't want to be around him.

The Spouse of an Alcoholic

When a family member is addicted to alcohol or another drug, every family activity comes to a halt. The ability to communicate or make plans for the family endeavors becomes more difficult if the addict ends up drinking or using at those occasions—or doesn't show up at all.

The focus, rather than being on each other or the children, becomes addiction and the problems it causes, including legal issues, debt and bankruptcy, and marital problems. The nonaddicted spouse (often known as "the chief enabler") usually ends up enabling the addicted partner by cleaning up the mistakes the addict makes with neighbors, the children, extended family members, and at his job. This allows the addict to remain comfortable and to continue drinking or using.

Addiction has negative effects on the spouse. The spouse may have feelings of hatred and self-pity. She may avoid social contacts, suffer exhaustion, and become physically or mentally ill.

Often the spouse has to perform the roles of both parents. As a result, she may be inconsistent, demanding, and neglectful of the children. Financial difficulty is another issue that families of addicts have to deal with. Addiction is one of the major reasons for divorce.

The spouse of an alcoholic often becomes codependent. A codependent is someone who has a psychological condition in which he or she has an unhappy and unhealthy relationship that involves living with and providing care for another person, such as an alcoholic. It also describes a relationship that enables the other person to maintain his irresponsible, addictive behavior. Codependent symptoms get worse if left untreated [7, 11, 13, 14].

Choices

The spouse of an addict has three choices. She can leave, she can stay and do nothing, or she can stay and take steps to make things better [15].

Leave Most spouses don't see leaving as an option, but at some point it may become the only choice to protect herself and the children. Leaving may be temporary or permanent.

Stay and Do Nothing The spouse can stay and do nothing and wait for the addiction to ruin further her life and the lives of other family members.

Stay and Take Steps The spouse of an addict can stay and take some steps to help herself and other members of the family. She can educate herself about addiction. She can take the attitude of putting herself first. The spouse of an addict should learn to separate her own personal growth and happiness from the addict's alcohol or other drug use. She should attend Al-Anon or other support meetings.

It is important for the spouse to share her concerns with the addict. She should let the addict know that she is concerned about him and that she wants him to seek help. She should set boundaries. If the addict continues to drink or use, she may tell him that she doesn't want him around her if he continues to use alcohol or another drugs. In addition, she can tell him that if he continues to drink and drive, she will call the police next time before he harms her, the children, or someone else.

If the spouse defines a boundary, she should define a clear consequence and be ready to follow through. The consequence may be that she won't bail the addict out the next time he get in trouble, or it may even be necessary to kick him out of the house.

If all else fails, she may need to organize a formal intervention, which is discussed later in this chapter [16].

Things the Spouse Can Do to Help Her Children

The spouse of an addict can do a number of things to help her children [17]. She can:

Give Children Hope That Things Will Get Better She should tell the children that things will get better. If the addict is not already in treatment, she should tell the children that she is trying to get help for him. If the addict is in treatment, she should tell the children that things won't be perfect, but they will be better than they were before he left.

Keep Children Safe Substance dependence can lead to unpredictable behavior and even violence. Safety should always be the spouse's main concern. She should teach the children that if there is trouble, they should call a neighbor or family member. If there is a physical crisis, they should get help from the police, a shelter, professionals, family, or friends. The spouse should try to keep children away from people who are under the influence of alcohol or other drugs.

Keep Things Normal as Possible at Home The family should try to eat together and celebrate special events together. Rules and limits, like homework and bedtime, provide structure. If the addict is under the influence or disruptive during a family activity, the spouse should stop the activity. She shouldn't pretend that the unacceptable behavior is not happening or that it is acceptable behavior.

Look for Problems A child may have problems as the result of the addict's alcohol or other drug use or his behavior. The spouse should not try to place blame on anyone. She does need to know how to tell if a child is stressed or having problems.

Teach Them Addiction Is a Disease The spouse should teach the children that addiction is a disease. They should be told that it isn't their fault. They shouldn't blame themselves. They can't stop the disease or make it go away.

Know When to Get Help Some children act out at school or in the community. Some have emotional problems, such as anxiety, depression, mood swings, feeling hopeless, or talking about suicide. If the child exhibits behavioral or emotional problems, the spouse should get help. The spouse can ask the school counselor, the family doctor, or a minister priest for help.

The spouse also can see to it that the children become engaged in support groups, such as Alateen.

The Children

Addicted Parent

One in four children in the United States is exposed to alcoholism or other drug addiction in the family. An estimated 6.6 million children under the age of 18 live in households with at least one alcoholic parent. These children are at risk for a range of cognitive, emotional, and behavioral problems.

Children who grow up in homes where one or both parents are addicts end up struggling with issues that follow them the rest of their lives. Neglect, and even abuse, of children are often the result when a parent has an alcohol or other drug addiction. The children often end up fending for themselves, feeling emotionally abandoned. They tend to develop self-esteem issues that cause them to make poor choices, including unprotected sex at an early age, skipping school, and substance use.

The children learn to lie to cover up for a parent's behavior. Physical abuse, emotional abuse, and neglect occur in some alcoholic homes.

Having a parent that they can depend on helps children grow up to be happy and healthy adults. Unfortunately, children of alcoholics have to endure a particularly unstable childhood. Depending on the age of the child, different response may occur. Older children may experience low self-esteem, depression, fear, and guilt that they are to blame and may keep to themselves. They may take on parental responsibilities that the chemically dependent parent has given up, such as providing care for younger siblings by cooking for them, getting them ready for school, putting them to bed, doing laundry, and so on. These children may do well in academic and athletic pursuits.

Another child may be rebellious, perhaps even antisocial. He or she may be involved in fights, theft, or trouble at school or in the community; they are often labeled juvenile delinquents.

Another child may seek to avoid conflict at all costs. Such children tend to feel powerless and may be very quiet, emotionally disturbed, depressed, isolated, or withdrawn. They may be shy, be followers, or engage in much fantasy.

Other children may act silly and make jokes, even at their own expense. The clownish behavior acts as a defense against feelings of anxiety and inadequacy.

The stress at home causes some children to have difficulty concentrating and performing well in school. The school problems may include lack of motivation, difficulty relating to friends or teachers, and truancy [11, 13].

In America, 40–80% of all child abuse cases are within families where addiction is present. As well, parents with a substance dependence problem will often put their addiction first, leaving their children to fend for themselves, which lead to cases of neglect of varied severity [18].

Even if severe neglect and abuse are not present, alcohol and drug addiction can lead to inconsistent parenting, including erratic rules and inconsistent consequences. In these situations, children may experience confusion about what is right and wrong as they receive mixed signals from parents about acceptable behavior.

Growing up with parents who use drugs and alcohol creates an environment of chaos and instability. Children from homes where one or both parents are struggling with addiction can experience shame, guilt, confusion, fear, and insecurity as their emotional development is not nurtured or made a priority within the family.

Addicted Adolescent

When an adolescent begins using alcohol or other drugs, it can turn the dynamics of the relationships between everyone else in the house upside down. Parents often argue, blaming each other for their adolescent's addiction, and disagree on how to help the child. Other siblings may resent the problems caused by the addicted adolescent. Little occurs in the way of family bonding when one member is an addict. The substance-using adolescent is discussed in Chap. 20.

Getting the Addict Sober

Pain—emotional, physical, spiritual—is the dominant feeling in the alcoholic's life. This pain may result from loss of a job, being arrested, severe illness, self-disgust, shame, separation from spouse and children, or rejection by family and friends. Addicts can temporarily cover up pain with more alcohol, but sooner or later they will hit rock bottom and have to come to grips with it. The process can be speeded up by the use of two concepts: Tough love and intervention by confrontation.

Tough Love

The application of tough love consists of five steps: (1) Open acceptance, (2) education, (3) joining support groups, (4) assigning responsibility, and (5) allowing the consequences [13].

1. *Open acceptance*. Open acceptance is based on an alcoholic's need for a relationship with a significant other—a relationship he values and does not want to lose. This person is usually the spouse, and that person's objective is to openly accept the alcoholic as a person worthy of love. This love is based on the alcoholic's needs, not on his behavior, which the spouse should not condone.
2. *Education*. Family members should learn as much as they can about alcoholism and codependency. As they learn the hard facts of addiction, they will acquire the emotional detachment necessary to overcome their fear and their dependence on the alcoholic. This objectivity will allow them to think and behave rationally enough to implement the remaining steps of tough love.
3. *Support groups*. Families should find local support groups, such as Al-Anon and Alateen, and should attend the meetings. Alcoholics are threatened by anything that undermines their ability to control the people around them and will go to great lengths to prevent their families from attending these meetings. Family members should attend regardless of the addicts' resistance. They should inform alcoholics that they are attending the meetings for themselves to learn more about the disease that is making their entire family ill.
4. *Assigning responsibility*. In this step, the family quits making excuses for an alcoholic's behavior and actions and no longer accept that person's rationalizations and excuses. The alcoholic is expected to take responsibility and to be accountable for his behavior.
5. *Allowing the consequences*. As an alcoholic's pain increases from being forced to face the consequences of his actions, he may plead to be rescued. The family must take a loving but firm stand. As a result, the alcoholic may eventually reach a point where he is ready for treatment. If not, the family may need to intervene and confront the addict.

Intervention by Confrontation

Intervention by confrontation consists of two steps: (1) Preparing for the confrontation and (2) the actual event itself.

Preparing for the Confrontation

The purpose of direct confrontation is to convince alcoholics of the effects of their destructive behavior and insist that they get treatment. During confrontations, alcoholics are told the harmful effects of their behavior on themselves and on the people close to them, are told the consequences of continuing an alcoholic lifestyle, and are offered a way to avoid the consequences—treatment.

A family prepares for a confrontation by taking six steps: (1) consulting a professional, (2) choosing members of the team, (3) choosing the confrontation date, (4) choosing its time, (5) holding a practice confrontation, and (6) investigating treatment options [13].

Step 1: Consult a professional. The first step in preparing for the confrontation is for the family to consult a professional. Every intervention team should have a substance dependence counselor or a physician familiar with the process to supervise the preparation and direct the actual confrontation. Families can usually find such a person by calling a local treatment center.

Step 2: Choose members of the team. Families should select members of the intervention team on the basis of their close relationships with the alcoholic and their willingness to participate in a confrontation. Not all family members will be appropriate for the team. The most strategically important members of the intervention team are the spouse, an employer, and the alcoholic's physician, if he or she is knowledgeable about addiction. Individuals that should be excluded include those whose psychological state is too fragile to withstand the emotional impact of the confrontation, anyone likely to berate the alcoholic or preach moralistically, and family members too angry or full of hate to perceive the alcoholic as a sick person in need of help.

Step 3: Choose the data. With the help of the professional, each team member selects three or four examples of the alcoholic's inappropriate behavior. These should be as detailed and as current as possible. Team members should focus on facts and observations rather than feelings and judgments. They should not use the data to humiliate the alcoholic but to help him see the seriousness of addictive behavior. Angry, hostile remarks will only activate the alcoholic's defense mechanisms.

Step 4: Choose the time. A team should confront the alcoholic when he is sober or at least as sober as possible. If the alcoholic is drunk at the scheduled confrontation time, the meeting should be postponed. It may be necessary to schedule the meeting early in the morning before the alcoholic has had time to do much drinking.

Step 5: Hold a practice confrontation. Members of the intervention team need to meet at least once, and preferably twice, to rehearse the confrontation. During these meetings, the professional plays the role of the alcoholic, and team members practice giving their evidence in a detached, nonjudgmental manner. They also practice how they will respond to the alcoholic's manipulation, evasion, or anger.

Step 6: Investigate treatment options. Team members by now should have investigated local treatment options for types of programs offered, the costs of each, and their appropriateness for the particular alcoholic. They should have taken care of financial matters, such as insurance clearance. And a suitcase should have been packed. If the intervention is successful, there should be no delay in getting the alcoholic into treatment. The treatment program is waiting on the alcoholic's arrival [7].

The Confrontation

Family members, the professional, and significant others assemble at a planned time. Once the alcoholic arrives, the facilitator speaks first, explaining to the alcoholic why they have gathered and asking him to listen without speaking for a while. When everyone else is finished speaking, the alcoholic will have a turn.

As rehearsed, each person then speaks directly to the alcoholic, sharing facts, events, and personal reactions to that person's behavior, telling how it has adversely affected him or her. Members then share options for help.

The group should be prepared for the alcoholic's tearful acceptance, anger, hostility, counter accusations, or bolting from the room. If the alcoholic agrees to enter treatment, he should not be allowed to bargain with the group or postpone it, which only gives him time to develop new excuses and rationalizations for his behavior, allowing him to deny the facts members present in the intervention. Once the group makes a decision, the alcoholic should enter treatment without delay [13].

If the intervention is unsuccessful, the family has three options. They can secure the alcoholic's word to stop drinking, having him sign a contract agreeing to enter treatment if he drinks again. They can continue to live with the actively drinking alcoholic, in which case they should continue to work on their own recovery by attending Al-Anon and Alateen meetings. And, in many states, the family can obtain a court order to commit the alcoholic to treatment against his will.

Getting the Family Well

Once the alcoholic enters treatment, all too often family members believe their problems are over. In reality they are not, and in some cases when the alcoholic gets better, without treatment the family gets worse. Therefore, it is imperative that the entire family go through a treatment process just as the alcoholic does.

Family recovery passes through a number of key stages. In the first stage, the family member is still abusing alcohol or other drugs. In the second stage, a transition from substance dependence to sobriety takes place. Early recovery is the third stage; this can be a difficult time for the family as everyone is adjusting to the new situation. The final stage is ongoing recovery. By this time, the family usually has adapted to the new conditions [13].

Importance of Family Treatment

Treatment of the family is important for several reasons. Most family members do not realize the extent to which their responses to the alcoholic—isolation, enabling, depression, anxiety, physical illness—have resulted in dysfunctional behavior. Also, without a better understanding of alcoholism and its effects on the family, spouses of alcoholics commonly remarry alcoholics, and their sons and daughters often marry alcoholics or become alcoholics. Treatment of the family helps to set the groundwork for leading a normal family life during the alcoholic's recovery.

A couple facing a sober marriage after many years of alcoholism may have unrealistic expectations. Recovering alcoholics may throw themselves so heavily in Alcoholics Anonymous that their spouses may sense competition from new partners.

Recovering alcoholics must be given responsibility for roles that they relinquished due to their drinking; spouses may find it difficult to relinquish such roles. And, finally, the children of alcoholic parents are more likely to be healthy in the long run if the whole family participates in treatment [19, 20].

Family Treatment Resources

Three useful treatment resources are available for the family: (1) family therapy, (2) codependent treatment, and (3) self-help groups.

Family Therapy Programs

Family therapy is based on the principle that the family is a system, and that all parts of the system are related and thus have an effect on each other. When one part of the system changes, it causes changes in other parts of the system. Addiction destroys families as much as it destroys individuals. Family members are torn between how to help the addict and how to avoid being sucked into the addict's world. Family therapy involves sessions with various members of the family or the family as a whole.

Approaches to family therapy include individual treatment of couples or group treatment with several couples. In some programs, families join alcoholics for up to a week at a treatment center, with follow-up group therapy for couples after alcoholics return home. A typical family week at a treatment center would include interviews with all family members to assess their understanding of alcoholism. Presentation on the pharmacology of alcohol, its medical complications, and the concept of alcoholism as a disease follow.

Group sessions with members of several families are helpful for sharing experiences, for recognizing that an alcoholic's problem is truly a family problem, and for breaking down defenses family members have developed. Properly supervised confrontations between an alcoholic and family members are helpful in releasing long-standing anger and resentment. They help reestablish communication and lead both parties to better insights into each other's needs.

Commonly, weekly group sessions involving several couples are conducted for up to 6 months after an alcoholic has returned home from a treatment center [21–23].

The three Cs of dealing with an addict are as follows: (1) you didn't cause the addiction, (2) you can't control the addiction, and (3) you can't cure the addiction by yourself [24].

Codependent Treatment

Treatment for family members and close friends who have been adversely affected by an alcoholic's drinking is available in many programs. The spouse of the alcoholic, who is very often codependent, is often referred to as the "chief enabler."

The majority of codependent treatment programs are outpatient, although more inpatient programs are becoming available. A typical outpatient program lasts about a month and meets for 2–3 h, usually in the evening, 3 days a week.

Treatment is directed at breaking through codependents' denial about their role in the disease of alcoholism, educating them about codependency, and giving them an opportunity to express an idea with feelings in a group setting. They are introduced to a 12-step program adapted from that of Alcoholics Anonymous, and they are encouraged to join support groups such as Al-Anon and Alateen. The treatment's premise is that codependents can get well whether an alcoholic does or not [2, 25].

Support Groups

Al-Anon is a fellowship of men and women whose lives have been adversely affected by an alcoholic family member or close friend. It developed as an outgrowth of AA in the 1940s because family members of early AA groups learned from experience that they needed to apply the AA principles to their own affairs. As a result, they began to work together in their own groups. Today Al-Anon groups are found virtually everywhere, generally meeting at the same time that AA meetings take place. So closely did the 12 steps of AA meet their needs that they changed only one word. The word "alcoholics" was changed to "others" in step 12:

Step 12. "Having had a spiritual awakening as a result of these steps, we tried to carry this message to others, and to practice these principles in all our affairs."

In essence, they admit they cannot control the excessive drinking of their spouse, parent, or close friend. They learn that an alcoholic is sick, not weak-willed or malicious. This shifts their focus from the alcoholic to learning how to manage their own lives more effectively. No longer can they blame an alcoholic's drinking for their shortcomings. They learn that shielding an alcoholic by lying to his boss, paying bail, and all other such behavior only helps an alcoholic keep drinking.

Members learn to detach from the problem, not the person. Denial plays a big role in the family as it does in an alcoholic's thinking. The group helps to penetrate this denial by sharing insights [26, 27]. Like AA, Al-Anon is compatible with all religions and offends none. It is a spiritual program that lets members conceive of God in their own way. The fellowship of Al-Anon lets people know they are not alone, that others have the same fears and frustrations and have made the same mistakes. It also gives them the opportunity to help others, a source of great personal satisfaction to them [27].

Al-Anon's primary purpose is not to try to stop alcoholics from drinking but to help those who have been affected by that drinking lead saner, happier, and more productive lives. Among Al-Anon members are the relatives and close friends of AA members who are leading sober lives, alcoholics who are still drinking sporadically but who are trying to overcome their compulsion, alcoholics who continue to drink and refuse help from any source, and alcoholics who are divorced or separated from their families or have died [26].

Codependents Anonymous, when available, is also an excellent source of help for the codependent spouse. It is a program based on the 12 steps of AA. Only the first and 12th steps changed:

Step 1. "We admitted we were powerless over others – that our lives had become unmanageable. The other steps are identical to those of AA."

Step 12. "Having had a spiritual awakening as the result of these steps, we try to carry this message to other co-dependents, and to practice these principles in all our affairs."

Alateen was begun in 1957 by a teenager whose parents were in AA to have a group for people his own age. Alateen meetings, too, are widely available [19]. *Nar-Anon* is a 12-step support program designed to help relatives and friends of addicts recover from the effects of living with and or knowing addicted relatives or friends. Nar-Anon's 12 steps are adapted from Narcotics Anonymous' 12 steps. Non-AA-related support groups may be preferred by some if such programs are available locally [28].

The Family in Recovery

In recovering families, members develop flexible roles, and they depend on one another. Families develop a sense of purpose and grow over time toward their optimal level of functioning. Recovering members should gauge their progress by their sense of stability, adaptability, and flexibility in relationships rather than by comparing their evolving families with an idealistic normal family. Families should begin to feel free to talk about anything, to think any thoughts, to ask for what each member wants, to express any emotion, and to pursue any goal. Indicators of family recovery are clear communication; cooperation; empowerment rather than subjugation; enhancement of individual uniqueness; using authority to guide rather than forcing compliance, love, valuing, and respect among members; personal and social responsibility; and an ability to use problems as challenges. Families begin to take on many of the traits of the healthy family discussed earlier in this chapter. Support groups such as Al-Anon and Alateen continue to play important roles in recovery [29].

Stages of Family Recovery

When an addicted family member finally enters recovery, the rest of the family often breathes a collective sigh of relief. With the addict's sobriety, the family members sense that the nightmare is over, the painful feelings are in the past, and their loved one will rejoin the family as a fully participating member. However, the void created by removing the problematic substance is not automatically filled with healthy feelings and behaviors.

Families need to recognize that recovery is a process, not an event. It moves through three stages…early recovery, middle recovery, and ongoing recovery [30].

Early Recovery

The primary task of early recovery is for each family member to individually heal from the past and develop the skills to enhance his or her own well-being. Family members now need to attend to their own individual growth—to become reacquainted with themselves and their own needs. Without developing healthy self-care and communication practices in the early stages of recovery, family members will find it more difficult to address the inevitable recovery challenges they will face in the future.

The primary tasks of early recovery are (1) learning about and accepting alcoholism or other addictions as a disease, (2) understanding the impact of alcoholism and other addictions on the family system, (3) learning to accept responsibility for one's own actions and feelings, (4) developing a support network of others with similar experiences, (5) learning coping skills to address life issues without alcohol or other drugs, and (6) learning to ask for help.

Middle Recovery

The goal of middle recovery is for family members to integrate progressively healthy change into each of their lives, building a foundation for change within the entire family system. There will be continued periodic individual and family tensions and disruptions, some related to recovery and some not.

The primary tasks of the middle stages of recovery are developing the ability to openly discuss past hurts and grievances, developing a willingness and ability to share concerns and fears about recovery, learning to recognize and respectfully communicate individual needs, developing sensitivity to the impact of one's actions on others, learning to respect the recovery needs of other family members, developing a positive vision of a life in recovery, and continuing to develop resources that support other family members.

Using the new tools and skills acquired, families in recovery will be able to meet and manage life's challenges without reverting to old unhealthy behaviors and unproductive emotional responses.

Ongoing Recovery

The tasks of ongoing recovery include understanding and respecting the power of addiction;

recognizing individual and family recovery as a lifelong process; appreciating the need to focus on one's own recovery, rather than that of others; having the courage and willingness to let go of resentments; and maintaining a consistent commitment to physical and emotional self-care.

Adult Children of Alcoholics

Between 20 and 34 million adults in the United States grew up in alcoholic homes, and around seven million children live in such environments [12, 21].

Consequences of Growing Up in an Alcoholic Home

The tremendous emotional scars inflicted on children growing up in alcoholic families lead directly to marital discord, emotional depression, vocational instability, and job dissatisfaction when they become adults. Being a child of an alcoholic increases the likelihood of growing up to be an alcoholic, marrying an alcoholic, or both, thereby perpetuating the cycle. Adult children of alcoholics (ACOAs) often don't relate their problems to having grown-up in a family with an alcoholic parent. Many of them have problems of depression, aggression, or impulsive behavior [31].

Dysfunctional Characteristics of ACOAs

Children of alcoholics may carry into adult life certain dysfunctional characteristics, ones not only ACOAs possess but many adults who grew up in other types of dysfunctional families, regardless of the cause of their dysfunction. Woititz [32] has identified 12 characteristics of ACOAs called The Laundry List:

1. *ACOAs guess what normal is.* ACOAs grew up in homes that, because of alcoholism, were not normal. They simply have no experience with what is normal. They often bring a fantasized concept of the perfect family into a marriage, thus, making life very difficult.
2. *ACOAs have trouble following a project through from beginning to end.* In the typical alcoholic family, there are a lot of promises. The great job was always just around the corner, the big deal was almost always about to be made, and the work that needed to be done around the house would be done. But these things never happened. Thus, ACOAs had role models for their procrastination. Not only that, they really never had anyone to show them how to carry a project through from beginning to end, which they then have difficulty doing in later life.
3. *ACOAs lie when it would be just as easy to tell the truth.* Lying is basic to an alcoholic family. The first and most basic lie is the family's denial of the problem, so the pretense that everything at home is in order is a lie. The nonalcoholic parent lies to cover up for the alcoholic and makes excuses for that person's not fulfilling an obligation, not being on time, or not showing up for an appointment. Alcoholics make a lot of promises that turn out to be lies. Because lying is a habit in an alcoholic's household, it is not surprising that the children carry this habit over into adulthood.
4. *ACOAs judge themselves without mercy.* When they were children, ACOAs never felt they were good enough. They were constantly criticized. Because they were never able to meet the standards of perfection expected of them in childhood, they carry the feeling into adulthood that whatever they do, it is not quite good enough. They have trouble accepting compliments, and they do not judge others nearly as harshly as they judge themselves.
5. *ACOAs have difficulty having fun.* The childhoods of ACOAs were probably not much fun. They seldom heard their parents laughing or joking. Life was a very serious business, and they grew up with the same attitude. They tend not to join in games because they

are afraid of looking foolish or making mistakes; that is, they are afraid of not playing the game perfectly. They have difficulty having fun and take themselves very seriously.

6. *ACOAs have difficulty with intimate relationships.* ACOAs have trouble developing healthy, intimate relationships because they don't have a frame of reference for such relationships because they did not grow up in one. They grew up with inconsistent parent-child relationships—where loved one day and rejected the next. They have developed a fear of being close, yet have a need for it, and develop a fear of abandonment that causes them to lack confidence in relationships.
7. *ACOAs overreact to changes they have no control over.* Growing up, ACOAs were not in charge of their lives. Alcoholics inflicted their lives on them. As a result, they fear that when a change is made without them participating in it, they will lose control of their lives. Therefore, they tend to overreact—they simply don't adjust to change well. They are often accused of being controlling, rigid, and unspontaneous.
8. *ACOAs constantly seek approval and confirmation.* Children begin to believe who they are from the messages they get from their parents. As they get older, they internalize these messages, which then contribute significantly to their self-images. These messages were confusing to them, so that they grew up lacking self-confidence. They feel that anyone who would care about them must not be worth very much and constantly seek approval and confirmation of their self-worth.
9. *ACOAs usually feel different from other people.* ACOAs assume that in any group of people, everyone else feels comfortable and that they are the only ones who feel awkward. They feel different from other people. When growing up, they become isolated and so did not develop the social skills necessary to feel comfortable as part of a group. It is difficult for ACOAs to believe that they can be accepted because of who they are and that they do not have to earn the acceptance.
10. *ACOAs are super responsible or super irresponsible.* ACOAs tried unsuccessfully as children to please their parents by doing more and more. Some continue this characteristic into adulthood, while others reach the point where they realize it doesn't really matter and begin doing as little as they can. Those that continue to strive feel that if they are not perfect, they will be rejected, so they tend to be super responsible. They subject themselves to enormous pressure trying to be perfect spouses, perfect parents, perfect friends, and perfect employees. Those who are super irresponsible tend to procrastinate and have trouble getting started.
11. *ACOAs are extremely loyal.* Family members of alcoholics are extremely loyal and remain in bad situations long after reason dictates they should leave. They do not walk away just because the going gets tough. This leads ACOAs to remain in relationships that they would be better off leaving. Because making friends or developing relationships is so difficult for them, the relationships and friendships they make tend to be permanent. The fact that they may be treated poorly doesn't matter; they can rationalize that.
12. *ACOAs are impulsive.* ACOAs grew up in homes in which impulsive behavior by alcoholics was the norm. The alcoholic never seriously considered what happened the last time or what the consequences would be this time. The reality in the alcoholic home was that if something were not done immediately, it never got done. ACOAs tend to be impulsive, which leads them to be confused, to loathe themselves, and to lose control over their environment. They spend an excessive amount of time cleaning up the mess.

The Other Laundry List

Not all children of alcoholics are affected by their experiences the same way. Although many live their lives victimized by the abuse and neglect of their alcoholic parent, others have the opposite reaction and become victimizers. The "*Other*

Laundry List," from Adult Children of Alcoholics World Services Organization, outlines characteristics of ACOAs who compensate for their childhood experiences by becoming aggressive and defensive [33].

1. To cover our fear of people and our dread of isolation, we tragically become the very authority figures who frighten others and cause them to withdraw.
2. To avoid becoming enmeshed and entangled with other people and losing ourselves in the process, we become rigidly self-sufficient. We disdain the approval of others.
3. We frighten people with our anger and threat of belittling criticism.
4. We dominate others and abandon them before they can abandon us or we avoid relationships with dependent people altogether. To avoid being hurt, we isolate and dissociate and thereby abandon ourselves.
5. We live life from the standpoint of a victimizer and are attracted to people we can manipulate and control in our important relationships.
6. We are irresponsible and self-centered. Our inflated sense of self-worth and self-importance prevents us from seeing our deficiencies and shortcomings.
7. We make others feel guilty when they attempt to assert themselves.
8. We inhibit our fear by staying deadened and numb.
9. We hate people who "play" the victim and beg to be rescued.
10. We deny that we've been hurt and are suppressing our emotions by the dramatic expression of "pseudo" feelings.
11. To protect ourselves from self-punishment for failing to "save" the family, we project our self-hate onto others and punish them instead.
12. We "manage" the massive amount of deprivation we feel, coming from abandonment within the home, by quickly letting go of relationships that threaten our "independence" (not too close).
13. We refuse to admit we've been affected by family dysfunction or that there was dysfunction in the home or that we have internalized any of the family's destructive attitudes and behaviors.
14. We act as if we are nothing like the dependent people who raised us.

There are many adult children of alcoholics that do not become aware of how much they were affected by their childhood experience until a problem in their life becomes so overwhelming that they seek help for that specific situation. One adult child tendency is to become an alcoholic, marry one, or both. If so, many adult children will end up experiencing serious problems—either with their own substance dependence or in their business or personal relationships.

Research has shown that adult children of other substance-addicted parents behave in similar manners to ACOAs.

Support Groups for ACOAs

Because of the needs of ACOAs, much like the needs of alcoholics for AA, a support organization for ACOAs evolved, which adapted the 12 steps of AA. The 12 steps of ACOAs are based on those of AA. Only Steps 1 and 12 are changed:

Step 1. "We admitted we were powerless over the effects of alcoholism or other family dysfunction, that our lives had become unmanageable."

Step 12. "Having had a spiritual awakening as a result of these steps, we tried to carry this message to others who still suffer, and to practice these principles in all our affairs [34]."

Summary

A family is a group of people related by blood or marriage or a strong common bond, such as those descended from a common ancestor or a husband, a wife, and their children. Other types of families are single-parent families, gay families, and extended families. A codependent is a person who lets another person's behavior (the addict) adversely affect him and who is obsessed with controlling that person's behavior.

Most families are basically healthy, and family members are usually happy, working, contributing members of society. A healthy family, however, is not necessarily perfect. Members go through the illnesses, career crises, accidents, and losses that are part of normal living. In response to addiction, a family develops a denial system and specific rules, and members tend to assume specific, unhealthy roles. Denial is a characteristic distortion in thinking experienced by family members of someone addicted to alcohol or other drugs.

Families with a member who is addicted to alcohol often grieve the loss of the loved one they once knew. The person who holds the power in the family—the addict—makes the rules.

The process of getting the addict into treatment can be speeded up by the use of two concepts: Tough love and intervention by confrontation. Treatment of the family is important for several reasons. There are support groups and professionals available for almost every family problem—abused children, battered wives, single parents, children with learning disabilities, attempted suicides, alcohol and drug addictions, and so forth.

In recovering families, members develop flexible roles, and they depend on one another. Recovering families develop a sense of purpose and grow over time toward their optimal level of functioning. Children of alcoholics may carry into adult life certain dysfunctional characteristics.

References

1. Mulry JT. Codependency: a family addiction. Am Fam Physician. 1987;35(4):215–9.
2. Beattie M. Codependent no more. Center City: Hazelden; 1986.
3. Family disease. National Council on Alcoholism and Drug Addiction (NCADD). https://www.ncadd.org/family-friends/there-is-help/family-disease. February 24, 2016.
4. Heffner CL. Alcoholism and its effect on the family. All Psych. https://allpsych.com/journal/alcoholism. December 14, 2003.
5. Curran D. Traits of a healthy family. Minneapolis: Winston Press; 1983.
6. Milhorn HT. The alcoholic family: part I. Mississippi State Medical Association Newsletter. 1990 Dec.
7. Spickard A, Thompson BR. The family trap. Dying for a drink: what you should know about alcoholism. Waco: Word Books; 1985. p. 68–75.
8. Mai C. Alcohol and drug abuse affects the whole family. The Cabin. https://www.thecabinchiangmai.com/alcohol-and-drug-abuse-affects-the-whole-family. July 20, 2015.
9. Krull E. When family members protect alcoholics. Psych Central. https://psychcentral.com/lib/when-family-members-protect-alcoholics. May 17, 2016.
10. Wegscheider-Cruse S. The family disease. In: Another chance. Palo Alto: Science and Behavioral Books Inc; 1981. p. 76–103.
11. Lamping RA, McAdams-Mahoud V. Families in recovery. Insight. 1989;10:28–31.
12. Van Cleave S, Byrd W, Revell K. Addiction is a family affair. In: Counseling for substance abuse and addiction. Waco: Word Books; 1987. p. 76–88.
13. Lancer D. Symptoms of codependency. Psych Central. http://psychcentral.com/lib/symptoms-of-codependency. 2016.
14. Lameman BA. Effects of substance abuse on families. Chicago Tribune. http://www.chicagotribune.com/sns-health-addiction-families-story.html. 2016.
15. How to deal with an alcoholic husband. Clean and Sober Live. http://www.cleanandsoberlive.com/how-to-deal-with-an-alcoholic-husband
16. What can you do to help an alcoholic family member? Clean and Sober Live. http://www.cleanandsoberlive.com/what-can-you-do-to-help-an-alcoholic-family-member
17. Substance abuse and the family: helping your children. University of Pittsburgh Schools of the Health Sciences (UPMC). http://www.upmc.com/patients-visitors/education/behavioral-health/Pages/substance-abuse-family.aspx. 2016.
18. Parental substance abuse a major factor in child abuse and neglect. National Council on Child Abuse and Family Violence. http://nccafv.org/parentalsubstance-abuse.htm
19. Griner ME, Griner PF. Alcoholism and the family. In: Barnes HN, Aronson MD, Debanco TL, editors. Alcoholism: a guide for the primary care physician. New York: Springer-Verlag; 1987. p. 159–66.
20. Kaufman E. The family of the alcoholic patient. Psychosomatics. 1986;27(5):347–349, 352, 356–360.
21. Anderson RC, Liepman MR. Chemical dependency in the family. In: Liepman MR, Anderson RC, Fisher JV, editors. Family medicine curriculum guide to substance abuse. Kansas City: Society of Teachers of Family Medicine; 1984. p. 8-1 to 8-34.
22. Usher ML, Jay J, Glass DR. Family therapy as a treatment modality for alcoholism. J Stud Alcohol. 1982;43(9):927–38.

23. Milhorn HT. The alcoholic family: part II. Mississippi State Medical Association Newsletter. 1991 Mar.
24. Help for families with addictions. Addictions and Recovery. https://www.addictionsandrecovery.org/families-and-addiction.htm. February 28, 2017.
25. Cermak TL. Diagnosing and treating co-dependence. Minneapolis: Johnson Institute Books; 1986.
26. Al-Anon Family Groups. Al-Anon Family Group Headquarters Inc. New York: 1987.
27. Al-Anon Family Group. Al-Anon's twelve steps and twelve traditions. New York: Al-Anon Family Group Headquarters Inc; 1988.
28. Royce JE. Alcoholics anonymous. In: Alcohol problems and alcoholism. London: Free Press; 1981. p. 242–55.
29. What is Nar-Anon? Nar-Anon. http://www.nar-anon.org/what-is-nar-anon
30. Friel J, Friel L. Adult children: the secrets of dysfunctional families. Deerfield Beach: Health Communications Inc; 1988.
31. Querin DS, Querin KB. Substance abuse as a family disease. Part II: the family in recovery. American Mental Health Alliance (AMHA): Oregon Metro. http://or.americanmentalhealth.com/media/pdf/2-recovery-substanceabusefa.pdf
32. Woititz JG. Adult children of alcoholics. Pompano Beach: Health Communications; 1983.
33. The laundry list. Adult Children of Alcoholics World Service Organization. http://www.adultchildren.org/lit-Laundry_List
34. The steps. Adult Children of Alcoholics World Service Organization. http://www.adultchildren.org/lit/Steps.s

Part IV

Special Groups

19 Women

Key Chapter Points

- Equality for women has included greater freedom to drink.
- Women are particularly at risk for becoming dependent on prescription drugs.
- The T-ACE questionnaire was the first validated screen for pregnancy-risk drinking (defined as alcohol consumption of 1 oz or more per day) developed for use in obstetric-gynecologic practices.
- The TWEAK questionnaire is used to screen for pregnancy-risk drinking, defined as the consumption of 1 oz or more of alcohol per day while pregnant.
- Women, like men, are at risk for developing alcoholism, prescription drug addiction, and addiction to illicit drugs. Women, however, can directly affect other human beings, their unborn fetuses, by their drug use.
- Gestational abuse of any mood-altering substance can cause serious maternal and perinatal problems.
- Detoxification of pregnant women should be individualized according to the primary drug used and the stage of gestation.
- Because approximately 85% of drug-addicted women are of childbearing age, there is a corresponding increase in the number of infants at risk for a complicated prenatal and postnatal course, including congenital defects and withdrawal symptoms.
- The type and severity of an infant's withdrawal symptoms depend on the drug(s) used, how long and how often the birth mother used them, how her body breaks the drug down, and whether the infant was born full term or premature.

In the 1970s and 1980s, the fact that little was known about providing appropriate care for women with substance abuse problems began to be addressed. At that time, programs were ill equipped to help women, and research to that point had focused on how men fared in substance dependence treatment [1].

In response, government organizations began to support research and treatment for women. The focus was on understanding and addressing gender differences in treatment access, treatment provision, and outcomes. Social circumstances of women with substance dependence problems began to be addressed, as were the barriers that prevented women from entering treatment. Also addressed were gender-specific issues related to women's success in treatment.

Many treatment programs also began to pay greater attention to the special needs of the women in their programs. Some began to offer gender-specific services, such as gender matching with counselors, mixed-gender treatment groups led by male and female coleaders, gender-specific treatment groups, and gender-specific treatment content. Some programs also began to provide services, such as childcare and parenting education [2].

H.T. Milhorn, *Substance Use Disorders*, DOI 10.1007/978-3-319-63040-3_19

Gender Differences

Women drinkers tend to drink less alcohol less often than men. When they develop substance abuse problems, they report problems of greater severity and experience more health-related consequences. Women's problems related to substance abuse interfere with functioning in more areas of life than men's do. Women are older than men when they begin drinking to intoxication, but once they develop a pattern of regular intoxication, they encounter drinking-related problems more quickly than men. They also lose control over their drinking more quickly than men.

Women's and men's substance use patterns have become more similar in the past few years. Women make up about one-third of the population with alcohol problems and slightly less than half of those who have problems with other drugs.

Women are less likely than men to use almost all types of illicit drugs, and illicit drug use is more likely to result in emergency department visits or overdose deaths for men than for women. However, women are just as likely as men to become addicted [3].

Women can become addicted quickly to certain drugs, such as crack cocaine; therefore, by the time they seek help, their addiction may be advanced and more difficult to treat. They often suffer from other serious health problems, such as sexually transmitted diseases and mental health problems like depression. Almost 70% of AIDS cases in women are related to either injecting drugs or having sex with a man who injects drugs. Many women who use drugs have had troubled lives. Studies have found that at least 70% of women drug users had been sexually abused by the age of 16. Most of these women had at least one parent who abused alcohol or other drugs. Often, women who use drugs have low self-esteem, little self-confidence, and feel powerless. They often feel lonely and are isolated from support networks [4].

The unique issues women face when it comes to substance use in part are influenced by sex (differences based on biology) and gender (differences based on culturally defined roles for men and women). Sex and gender also can interact with each other to create even more complex differences between men and women. As an example of the sex and gender differences related to drugs, consider nicotine [5]:

Sex Difference: Women metabolize nicotine faster than men. Differences in metabolism may help explain why nicotine replacement therapies, like patches and gum, work better in men than in women. Men appear to be more sensitive to nicotine's pharmacological effects related to addiction.

Gender Difference: Although men are more sensitive than women to nicotine's addiction-related effects, women may be more susceptible than men to non-nicotine factors, such as the sensory and social stimuli associated with smoking.

For most age groups, women have lower rates of use or dependence on illicit drugs and alcohol than do men; however, women are just as likely as men to become addicted to the drugs they use. In addition, women may be more susceptible to craving and relapse.

Prevalence of Use

Almost half of all women age 15–44 have used illicit drugs other than alcohol at least once in their lives. Of these women, nearly 2 million have used cocaine, and more than 6 million have used marijuana within the past year. Most women drug abusers use more than one drug [4].

Men are twice as likely as women to have a substance use disorder (13.8% of men versus 7.1% of women). Twelve-month prevalence rates of alcohol abuse are almost three times as high among men as they are among women (6.9% of men versus 2.6% of women). In contrast, prescription drug dependence in women closely approaches that of men.

The rates of dependence for nonmedical use of pain relievers were 1.4% for men and 1.1% for women 18–25 years old and 0.5% for men and 0.4% for women 26 years and older. Only slightly more men than women report tobacco use (13.5% men versus 10.2% women) [6].

The Drugs

Alcohol

Equality for women has included greater freedom to drink. As a result, heavy drinking is on the rise among young, employed women. In the United States, the number of people who drink alcohol has increased from 45 to 66% over the past 40 years, and community surveys indicate that 5% of women are heavy drinkers. Because society considers it less acceptable for a woman to be a heavy drinker than a man, family, friends, and employers often hide or ignore a woman's drinking problem. This attitude delays or prevents women from receiving treatment.

Alcohol-related ulcer surgery, gastrointestinal hemorrhage, fatty liver, hypertension, anemia, and malnutrition occur at significantly higher rates in women, who also seem to be more susceptible to the hypertensive and cirrhotic effects of alcohol. For comparative ages, the death rate for alcoholic women is greater than the death rate for nonalcoholic women. Their unique physiologies (menopause, postpartum depression, premenstrual mood changes) have been mentioned as possible contributors to alcohol abuse in women, but there is no clear documentation of this.

In the early days of ancient Rome, drinking wine by women was an offense punishable by death. This law, which prohibited women from drinking alcohol, was linked to the prohibition against adultery by women. Thus, drinking women were considered to be "loose" early in Western culture. In contemporary US society, women who drink excessively are triply stigmatized. First, they are included in society's negative attitude toward all alcoholics. Second, they are subjected to the special disgust focused on intoxicated women. And third, the idea that drunkenness and sexual promiscuity are linked adds to the burden of disapproval. As a result, alcoholic women drink alone more commonly than alcoholic men, so that female alcoholics are often referred to as "hidden alcoholics."

The negative attitude of society in general influences not only the behavior of the alcoholic woman herself, her family, and her friends but also affects the attitudes and expectations of those in the helping professions (physicians, nurses, psychologists, social workers). Rather than diagnosing alcoholism, a physician all too often prescribes tranquilizers for anxiety with the result that many alcoholic women become cross-addicted to prescription drugs.

Divorce rates for alcoholic women are much higher than for alcoholic men. Nonalcoholic wives are far more likely to remain with their alcoholic husbands than nonalcoholic husbands with their alcoholic wives.

When women drink at a rate comparable to that of men, their smaller size and smaller proportion of body water causes higher blood alcohol levels. Whereas men are inclined to snack while drinking, women often diet, so they drink on empty stomachs, which results in quick absorption of alcohol into the bloodstream. Women taking oral contraceptives metabolize alcohol significantly more slowly than women who do not take them. Furthermore, in the premenstrual phase, women absorb alcohol significantly more quickly and completely than do women in the postmenstrual phase. Women tend to begin using alcohol at a later age than men and to progress more rapidly into middle- and late-stage alcoholism, a phenomenon known as *telescoping* [7].

Drinking over the long term is more likely to damage a woman's health than a man's, even if the woman has been drinking less alcohol or drinking for a shorter length of time. Comparing people with alcohol use disorders, women have death rates 50–100% higher than men, including deaths from suicides, alcohol-related accidents, heart disease, stroke, and liver disease. In addition, there are some health risks that are unique to female drinkers. For example, heavy drinking is associated with increased risk of having unprotected sex, resulting in pregnancy or sexually transmitted disease, and an increased risk of becoming a victim of violence or sexual assault. In addition, drinking as little as one drink per day can slightly raise the risk of breast cancer in some women, especially those who are postmenopausal or have a family history of breast cancer [8].

In addition, men and women metabolize alcohol at different rates. After drinking comparable amounts of alcohol, women have higher blood ethanol concentrations. As a result, women become intoxicated from smaller quantities of alcohol than men.

Psychoactive substances disrupt neuroendocrine and gonadal functions with sufficient magnitude to cause infertility in some patients. Normal individuals may only experience subtle changes in sexual function. However, women with compromised reproductive function may have major problems. The disruptive effects of these drugs are usually completely reversible after patients stop using them. Most protocols for evaluating unexplained infertility now include drug abuse history [9].

Other Drugs

Women are particularly at risk for becoming dependent on prescription drugs. They make visits to physicians more frequently than men and tend to complain of nonspecific anxiety. As a result, physicians often prescribe minor tranquilizers, such as diazepam (Valium), alprazolam (Xanax), or lorazepam (Ativan). They thus learn that the use of chemicals is a quick and easy way to cope with stress. It is not as easy for many women to unwind with a few drinks in a bar as it is for men, so they are more likely to seek medical relief from stress.

Women are at risk for addiction to the same illicit drugs as men; however, some differences do exist. Female cocaine addicts, for example, have a greater incidence of major depression than men. Furthermore, abstinent women do not appear to recover from their depression as rapidly as men. Women also tend to become addicted to cocaine more readily than men [10].

Marijuana Fewer females than males use marijuana. For females who do use marijuana, however, the effects can be different than for male users. Marijuana impairs spatial memory in women more than it does in men. Men who are addicted to marijuana tend to have higher rates of other substance use problems as well as antisocial personality disorder and more severe addiction. By contrast, women who are addicted to marijuana have more panic attacks and anxiety disorders and develop cannabis use disorder more quickly. Although the severity of cannabis use disorders is generally higher for men, women tend to develop these disorders more quickly [11].

Stimulants Women may be more vulnerable to the reinforcing (rewarding) effects of stimulants, with estrogen possibly being one factor causing this increased sensitivity. Women may also be more sensitive than men to cocaine's effects on the heart and blood vessels. In contrast, female and male cocaine users show similar deficits in learning, concentration, and academic achievement as a result of cocaine use, even if women have been using it longer. Female cocaine users are also less likely than male users to exhibit abnormalities of blood flow in the brain's frontal regions. These findings suggest a sex-related mechanism that may protect women from some of the damage cocaine inflicts on the brain.

Women tend to begin using methamphetamine at an earlier age than men, with female users typically becoming more dependent on methamphetamine compared to male users. Women are also less likely to switch to another drug when they lack access to methamphetamine. Women who use methamphetamine also have high rates of co-occurring depression. In addition, women tend to be more receptive than men to methamphetamine treatment [11].

MDMA MDMA produces stronger hallucinatory effects in women compared to men, although men show higher MDMA-induced blood pressure increases. Both men and women show similar increases in aggression a few days after they stop using MDMA.

MDMA can interfere with the body's ability to eliminate water and decreases sodium levels in the blood, causing a person to drink large amounts of fluid. In rare cases, this can lead to increased water in the intercellular space, which may eventually produce swelling of the brain and even death. Young women are more likely than men to die from this reaction, with most reported cases of death occurring in young females between the ages of 15 and 30.

MDMA also can interfere with temperature regulation and cause acute hyperthermia leading to neurotoxic effects and even death [11].

Opioids Women are more likely to take prescription opioids without a prescription to cope with pain, even when men and women report similar pain levels. Research also suggests that women are more likely to misuse prescription opioids to self-treat for other problems, such as anxiety or tension. From 1999 to 2010, deaths from prescription pain reliever overdoses increased more rapidly for women (400%) than for men (265%) [11].

Sedative-Hypnotics Women are more likely to seek treatment for misuse of sedative-hypnotics. Women are also more likely than men to die from overdoses of medicines for mental health conditions, like antidepressants. Antidepressants and benzodiazepines send more women than men to emergency departments. Because women are also more at risk than men for anxiety, depression, and insomnia, women are prescribed more of these types of medications, thus increasing the risk of misuse, addiction, and overdose [11].

Nicotine Men and women differ in their smoking behaviors. For instance, women smoke fewer cigarettes per day, tend to use cigarettes with lower nicotine content, and do not inhale as deeply as men. Women also smoke for different reasons than men, including regulation of mood and stress. Women may experience more stress and anxiety as a result of nicotine withdrawal than men [11].

Risk of death from smoking-associated lung cancer, chronic obstructive pulmonary disease, heart disease, and stroke continues to increase among women—approaching rates for men. The death ratio of women to men from smoking is over 70%. Some dangers associated with smoking—such as blood clots, heart attack, or stroke—increase in women using oral contraceptives [12].

Diagnosis

Women substance abusers complain more often of a wide range of symptoms, including depression, anxiety, sleeplessness, lethargy, stomach problems, and injuries from accidents or physical abuse. Compared with controls, substance-dependent women report a higher incidence of postpartum depression, irregular menstrual cycles, and amenorrhea.

Women addicts are less likely than men to have problems at work or with the law or to behave violently. They are more inclined than men to report problems with their relationships and children as a result of substance use [13].

In taking a drug history, additional questions specifically appropriate for women include "Do you ever carry an alcoholic beverage in your purse?," "Does your drug use vary with your menstrual cycle?," "Has your drinking or drug taking had any effect on the regularity or quantity of your menstrual periods?," "What effect do you think your drug abuse has had on your children?," and "Has there been physical violence in your home (spouse abuse or child abuse)?" [14].

Screening Questionnaires

Alcohol

Traditional alcohol-screening questionnaires, such as the Michigan Alcoholism Screening Test (MAST) and the CAGE, are less effective in identifying drinking problems among young women than among men. The T-ACE and TWEAK were designed for pregnant women.

T-ACE Questionnaire

The T-ACE questionnaire was the first validated screen for pregnancy-risk drinking (defined as alcohol consumption of 1 oz or more per day) developed for use in obstetric-gynecologic practices. An obstetrician developed the T-ACE after observing that asking patients about their tolerance to the intoxicating effects of alcohol did not trigger denial. It has a sensitivity of 69% and a specificity of 89%. The sensitivity is well above

Table 19.1 T-ACE questionnaire (From Sokol [15]. Approved with permission, American Journal of Obstetrics and Gynecology)

T	Tolerance: how many drinks does it take to make you feel high?
A	Have people annoyed you by criticizing your drinking?
C	Have you ever felt you ought to cut down on your drinking?
E	Eye opener: have you ever had a drink first thing in the morning to steady your nerves or get rid of a hangover?

that of the CAGE and the MAST. The T-ACE questions are given in Table 19.1 [15].

A reply of "more than two drinks" to question T is considered a positive response and scores two points. A yes answer to question A, C, or E scores one point each. A total score of two or more points indicates a positive result.

A positive screen is an opportunity for the physician and patient to discuss prenatal alcohol exposure. The discussion may lead the physician to refer the patient for a detailed diagnostic assessment, or the physician may offer a brief intervention (short counseling sessions) if the patient does not have a severe alcohol problem. Brief interventions may be effective in this population.

TWEAK Questionnaire

The TWEAK is a five-item screening tool that includes questions from the MAST, CAGE, and T-ACE. It is designed to detect alcoholism or heavy drinking. TWEAK questions are given in Table 19.2 [16].

The TWEAK is used to screen for pregnancy-risk drinking, defined as the consumption of 1 oz or more of alcohol per day while pregnant. A positive response to question T of more than five drinks or question W yields two points each; a yes reply to question E, A, or K scores one point each. A total score of two or more points indicates a positive outcome for pregnancy-risk drinking.

The sensitivity and specificity of the TWEAK are 79% and 83%, respectively. The TWEAK does not appear to offer any significant advantages over the T-ACE.

Table 19.2 The TWEAK questionnaire (From Chan [16]. Approved with permission, Alcoholism: Clinical and Experimental Research)

T	tolerance: how many drinks can you hold?
W	Have close friends or relatives worried or complained about your drinking in the past year?
E	Eye opener: do you sometimes take a drink in the morning when you get up?
A	Amnesia: has a friend or family member ever told you about things you said or did while you were drinking that you could not remember?
K	Do you sometimes feel the need to cut down on your drinking?

As with men, the diagnosis of substance dependence in women depends on the DSM-5 criteria discussed in Chap. 1.

Other Drugs

To my knowledge there are no questionnaires dealing with other drugs specifically for women. CAGE-AID and DAST-10 can be used (see Chap. 14).

Treatment

Women, like men, are at risk for developing alcoholism, prescription drug addiction, and addiction to illicit drugs. Women, however, can directly affect other human beings, their unborn fetuses, by their drug use.

Women have unique needs that should be addressed during alcohol or other drug treatments. Special issues related to hormones, menstrual cycle, fertility, pregnancy, breastfeeding, and menopause can impact women's struggles with drug use. In addition, women themselves describe unique reasons for using drugs, including controlling weight, fighting exhaustion, coping with pain, and self-treating mental health problems.

Effective treatment should incorporate approaches that recognize sex and gender differences, understand the types of trauma women sometimes face, provide added support for women with childcare needs, and use evidence-based approaches for the treatment of pregnant women [17, 18].

Many women with young children do not seek treatment or drop out of treatment early because they have no one to take care of their children. They may also fear that authorities will remove their children from their care. The combined burdens of work, home care, childcare, and other family responsibilities, plus attending treatment, can be overwhelming for many women. They may also fear that authorities will remove their children from their care if they admit to a substance use disorder [11].

Alcoholic women are more likely than nonalcoholic women to have alcoholic husbands or lovers and are at increased risk for domestic violence. Frequently, women addicts are victims of incest, child or spouse abuse, or rape or are daughters of alcoholic parents. To be most effective, a treatment program for substance-dependent women must address their practical needs, such as childcare and job training. Unfortunately, because of their lower socioeconomic status in our society, many women addicts are unable to afford treatment.

Low self-esteem seems to be an important feature of all addiction, but particularly for female addicts. How a woman feels about herself depends on developmental, psychological, and societal factors. Self-esteem for many depends on occupation. The lesser value assigned to tasks normally identified as women's work and the lower salaries women earn are important factors in their self-esteem. Housekeeping and childcare in the United States are assigned little or no economic value. Most married women in the work force still carry the major responsibility for housecleaning, shopping, cooking, laundry, and childcare in addition to their outside employment. Both as a factor in her illness and her recovery, the importance of occupation should be explored individually with each substance-dependent woman. Vocational rehabilitation, more adequate childcare, and changes in family attitudes and behavior will be indicated in many cases [19].

Women are more likely than men to encounter barriers that prevent them from seeking or following through with treatment. They are more likely to experience economic barriers to treatment. Women are more likely to have difficulty attending regular treatment sessions because of family responsibilities.

Providing comprehensive services, such as housing, transportation, education, and income support, reduces posttreatment substance use among both men and women, but greater numbers of women need such services. Women are more likely to report feeling shame or embarrassment because they are in substance abuse treatment. Anxiety or depressive disorders, which tend to be more prevalent and severe among women, may prevent women from seeking help with substance abuse problems [2].

Because women are usually responsible for the care of children and because substance-dependent women are frequently separated or divorced, female addicts entering treatment are far more often the heads of single-parent families than the substance-dependent men. As a result, childcare is a major need in the treatment of substance-dependent women. Women cannot benefit maximally from treatment if they are concerned about the welfare of their children. Guilt for being a failure as a mother may be a major problem.

The most useful categorization of alcoholism is the distinction between primary alcoholism (no preexisting emotional disorder) and secondary alcoholism (preexisting emotional disorder). Most patients who undergo treatment are of the primary type. Among men, the most common form of secondary alcoholism is associated with antisocial personality disorder. This is true of other drug addictions as well. In women the most common secondary type is associated with depression. Diagnosis of primary depression must be based on a careful life history, since the presence of depressive symptoms early in treatment will not differentiate between primary and secondary alcoholism. Once a woman is identified as a secondary alcoholic, long-term treatment should include, in addition to alcoholism treatment, attention to possible recurrence of depression. Early treatment of such recurrence may help women maintain sobriety. Women alcoholics attempt suicide or make suicide gestures more frequently than alcoholic men.

Societal pressures exert more of an influence on drinking patterns in women than they do in men. The society traditionally considers alcoholism less acceptable in women than in men; low self-esteem is a common finding in female alcoholics. Feelings of guilt and embarrassment lead to efforts to conceal drinking, and women often drink at home than do men. They are also more likely to have alcoholic spouses or lovers and to copy their spouses' or lovers' drinking patterns.

Women are more likely than men to drink in response to stress in their environment. The most frequent stressors include recent loss of a loved one, family crisis, an unrewarding marriage, domestic and economic factors, and depression [20].

Family or interpersonal crises more often cause alcoholic women to seek treatment for their alcoholism than work or health-related problems do. Alcohol use increases the risk of suicide, and alcoholic women outnumber alcoholic men in both attempted and completed suicides.

A woman is often defined through her relationship to others. She is someone's daughter, someone's wife, someone's mother, or even someone's ex-wife. Some women's dependence on men may be a treatment issue. Helping alcoholic women confront their feelings about themselves as independent individuals is an important part of treatment [14].

It is important for all female addicts to structure their lives. If they go back to the unstructured world of housework and childcare, they run a greater risk of relapse, especially if they do not prefer those roles. Woman should explore educational goals, whether that means getting a high school equivalency diploma, a college degree, or a postgraduate degree. Trade schools should be used as resources.

Some alcoholic women relate drinking episodes to their menstrual cycles, particularly in the premenstrual period. Strategies for relief or prevention of dysmenorrhea, such as ibuprofen (Motrin), attending extra AA meetings, and calls from AA sponsors should be planned with patients to help them negotiate this difficult period [21]. Female treatment issues are summarized in Table 19.3 [22].

Table 19.3 Female treatment issues (From Milhorn [22]. Approved with permission, Springer)

ACOA issues	Guilt
Assertiveness	Incest
Child abuse	Job training
Childcare	Life structuring
Depression	Premenstrual drinking or drug using
Divorce or separation	Relationship with spouse or significant other
Eating disorders	Self-esteem
Feelings about being an independent individual	Spouse abuse
Fetal concerns	Unhealthy dependence on male relationships

Women are a minority in most treatment programs. As a result, many substance-dependent women find themselves in treatment programs designed for men. They need to feel comfortable with themselves and are reluctant to discuss many of their problems, such as rape or spouse abuse, in mixed company. Hence, attending all-women groups is important for most women addicts, especially in early recovery [17, 18].

Women-only treatment centers are located in many places around the United States. Addiction treatment for women can be relaxing to those who may have trouble with men or have the need to feel connected with other women. These facilities help women work together to support a drug-free lifestyle. If the program is not for women only, it should offer extensive gender-specific treatment sessions [21].

The Pregnant Addict

Although drug use of all types, including drinking alcohol, appears to be increasing in this country, it appears to be increasing faster in women than in men, and the overwhelming majority of drug-using women are reproductively active. It is now abundantly clear that gestational abuse of any mood-altering substance can cause serious maternal and perinatal problems. Many women addicts use more than one drug, commonly combining, for instance, alcohol, marijuana, cocaine, and nicotine. Evaluating risk factors for pregnant addicts and their newborns must take into consideration all of these drugs. Identifying pregnant addicts, however, is difficult. They often attempt to conceal their addiction by obtaining medical treatment for an array of somatic complaints, such as headaches, anxiety, or low back pain. Although they usually deny illicit drug use, most substance-dependent pregnant women will admit to using legal drugs (caffeine, nicotine, alcohol).

A mother's continuing drug use after delivery puts her child at risk for neglect, physical abuse, and malnutrition [23–25].

Medical Problems

A 40–50% incidence of medical complications among illicit drug-dependent women has been reported. The most frequently reported complications include anemia, endocarditis, phlebitis, cellulitis, hepatitis, hypertension, urinary tract infection, and venereal disease. In addition, pregnant intravenous drug users are at increased risk for contracting AIDS. Regardless of the route of drug administration, the economic necessities of supporting drug addiction may lead to illegal means (theft, prostitution) of obtaining them; secondary malnutrition and the associated unhealthy personal and family psychosocial environment further complicate maternal well-being and prenatal care [25].

Obstetrical Concerns

During pregnancy, the drugs used by the mother can enter the baby's bloodstream and in some cases cause serious problems.

Health Risks Associated with Drug Use

When a pregnant woman uses drugs, she and her unborn child may face serious health problems. During pregnancy, the drugs used by the mother can enter the baby's bloodstream. The most serious effects on the baby can be HIV infection, prematurity, low birth weight, sudden infant death syndrome (SIDS), small head size, stunted growth, poor motor skills, and behavior problems. Some of the health risks of both mother and baby are given in Table 19.4.

Table 19.4 Health risks associated with drug use (Based on [4])

Mother	Baby
Depression	Birth defects
Early delivery	HIV/AIDS
High blood pressure	Infections
HIV/AIDS	Learning disabilities
Low self-esteem	Low birth weight
Low weight gain	Neurological problems
Physical abuse	Poor motor skills
Poor nutrition	Prematurity
Preterm labor	Small head size
Rapid heartbeat	Stunted growth
Sexually transmitted disease	Sudden infant death syndrome

Some women report using marijuana to treat severe nausea associated with their pregnancy. Smoking tobacco or marijuana, taking prescription pain relievers, or using illegal drugs during pregnancy is associated with double or even triple the risk of stillbirth.

Maternal Detoxification

Detoxification of pregnant women should be individualized according to the primary drug used and the stage of gestation. Detoxification before 14 weeks of gestation is not advocated because of the risk of inducing abortion. Likewise, during the last trimester of pregnancy, detoxification is not advised because of the risk of provoking preterm labor or fetal distress [25].

CNS Depressants Detoxification from alcohol can be accomplished with hospitalization and a tapering dose of a benzodiazepine, as can withdrawal from barbiturates and benzodiazepines themselves. Withdrawal from benzodiazepines may be prolonged, and delayed seizures sometimes occur [24].

Opioids Whether to detoxify for opioid dependence at any time during pregnancy remains controversial. Traditionally, most patients were switched from their abused opioids to methadone to avoid the danger of relapse and repeated intoxication and withdrawal cycles. Mother and baby were then individually detoxified from methadone after birth. Methadone maintenance for opioid-addicted pregnant women removes them from the drug-seeking environment, eliminates the illicit behavior associated with it, prevents vacillations in maternal (and fetal) drug levels, improves maternal nutrition, and involves them in prenatal care and psychological/social rehabilitation [21].

Buprenorphine has become a popular maintenance medication for pregnant women. When compared with methadone use in utero to treat opioid dependence in the mother, buprenorphine use resulted in fewer infants requiring withdrawal treatment. In addition, of infants who did require treatment, those exposed to buprenorphine spent fewer days in the hospital compared with those exposed to methadone [26].

When it is absolutely essential for pregnant opioid addicts to be detoxified from methadone during pregnancy, it should be done by decreasing the dose by 5 mg every other week between the 14th and 28th week of gestation [27].

Other Drugs Detoxification of pregnant women from other drugs of abuse (CNS stimulants, cannabinoids, hallucinogens, phencyclidines, inhalants) is associated with few or no withdrawal symptoms and does not present any special maternal concerns.

The Fetus

Because approximately 85% of drug-addicted women are of childbearing age, there is a corresponding increase in the number of infants at risk for a complicated prenatal and postnatal course, including congenital defects and withdrawal symptoms [28].

Congenital Defects

During the embryonic period (second to eighth week after conception), each organ system in the body undergoes a sensitive stage in its development during which adverse influences can cause congenital anomalies. During the fetal period (9 weeks after conception to delivery), the fetus has concluded new organ development and is, therefore, less likely to develop congenital malformations. Instead, after that point, the fetus may suffer altered skeletal growth, growth retardation, alteration of external genitalia, and central nervous system defects. The affected child may have behavioral and psychological disturbances later in life [24].

Stillbirth Risks

The stillbirth risk with tobacco use in pregnancy is 1.8–2.8 times greater than nonsmokers, with the highest risk found among the heaviest smokers. With marijuana use the risk is 2.3 times greater. Passive exposure to tobacco smoke increases the risk of stillbirth 2.1 times greater than those not exposed [29].

Specific Drug Effects

Severity of newborn withdrawal from substances depends on the drugs and the frequency and magnitude of use by the mother during pregnancy.

Alcohol Effects In 1748, a British physician noted that when gin became cheap, more mothers gave birth to babies that were physically defective or mentally retarded. In 1759, the London College of Physicians petitioned the British Parliament to reinstate taxes on gin, so that it would be less available and constitute less of a risk to pregnant women and their offspring. Fetal alcohol syndrome (FAS) was identified in 1973.

Clinical findings in a newborn with FAS include a characteristic pattern of facial anomalies with short palpebral fissures, a thin upper lip, and a long, smooth philtrum. Other findings may include a flat midface, ptosis of the eyelids, epicanthal folds, an upturned nose with a flat nasal bridge, underdeveloped ears ("railroad track" appearance), clinodactyly of the fifth fingers, camptodactyly, "hockey stick" palmar creases, hirsutism, and cardiac defects. Prenatal or postnatal growth retardation typically results in a height or weight below the 10th percentile for age and race. Microcephaly is common, as are structural brain anomalies. To date, full-blown FAS has been seen only in children of women who were very heavy drinkers during pregnancy [30, 31].

Fetal alcohol syndrome is the leading preventable congenital birth defect and occurs in 1.9 in 1000 births. Among all birth defects, it ranks third behind Down syndrome and spina bifida. Raising a physically and mentally handicapped child presents problems, particularly to a mother who cannot cope with her own problems.

Less severe but significant birth defects, including some that are subtle, may occur in offspring of women who drink lesser amounts of alcohol, including social drinkers. Neuropsychological testing of children of drinking mothers has found IQ scores lower than controls, as well as retarded development of concept formation and practical reasoning. Emotional instability, hyperactivity, distractibility, and short attention span were also significantly more prevalent in children of drinking mothers. For every child born with FAS, as many as ten others may be born with fetal alcohol effects (FAE). In addition, the risk of spontaneous abortion is increased [21].

A safe level of alcohol consumption has not been established. The best advice for pregnant women is to abstain from alcohol [32].

Benzodiazepine Effects Maternal benzodiazepine use may result in teratogenic effects on fetuses, including dysmorphic features, growth aberrations, and central nervous system abnormalities. The dysmorphic features resemble those of FAS, although greater focal involvement of cranial nerves may occur. The infants at birth may appear to have a sullen and expressionless face and to have little vitality [33, 34].

Phenobarbital Effects Phenobarbital abuse has been associated with fetal facial dysmorphia and congenital malformations [23].

Opioid Effects Common metabolic disturbances in opioid-addicted neonates include hyperbilirubinemia, hypoglycemia, hypocalcemia, and hypomagnesemia. Convulsions may occur, and even with prompt and early attention, the mortality rate may be increased. Most deaths are associated with low birth weight. Respiratory problems such as aspiration pneumonia, in particular from meconium, are commonly reported. Thrombocytosis and increased circulating platelet aggregation can occur and may persist for over 16 weeks, causing local infarcts and subarachnoid hemorrhage. Prolonged exposure to opioid drugs may cause irreversible damage to an infant's central nervous system, resulting in mental retardation. Intrauterine growth retardation appears to be highest for pentazocine (Talwin) abuse [34, 35].

Cocaine Effects Cocaine abuse can produce a variety of neonatal effects, including growth retardation in utero, smaller head circumference, and premature rupture of the membranes. There is an increased incidence of abruptio placenta, prematurity, stillbirth, and spontaneous abortion. Infants may have depressed interactive behavior and impaired organizational abilities after birth, as well as increased tremulousness and startle response.

Infants born to cocaine-abusing mothers may suffer meconium aspiration leading to neurological damage or death. They also tend to have low birth weight and heart defects, and they may have seizures [36]. Although the mechanism for cocaine teratogenicity is not known, it is hypothesized that cocaine-induced vasoconstriction, acute hypertension, and cardiac arrhythmias interrupt the interoplacental blood supply causing fetal hypoxia [35, 36].

Nicotine Effects Nicotine causes a dose-related decrease in birth weight and head circumference. Congenital defects may occur. A permanent long-term effect on linear growth of infants born to mothers who smoke has been documented. Early in life, infants of smoking mothers appear to be less alert and by age seven may be hyperactive. By age 11, children suffer decreases in general abilities, most evident in reading comprehension and mathematics [34] .

Marijuana Effects Marijuana is a commonly abused substance, with greater than 25% of women in their reproductive years admitting to past or current marijuana use. Although marijuana use during pregnancy has been associated with few short-term or long-term effects on the exposed neonate, its risks are dose dependent. A dose-related decrease in birth weight and head circumference has been documented. An increased incidence of SIDS has been seen in infants born to heavy users [35, 36].

Phencyclidine Effects Virtually all phencyclidine abusers are multiple drug users. Hence, it has been difficult to determine fetal effects of phencyclidine alone. Phencyclidine-addicted infants have sudden outbursts of agitation, rapid changes in level of consciousness, increased lability, poor consolability, coarse arm flapping, tremors, nystagmus, and roving eye movements. They may have respiratory depression at birth. There does not seem to be an effect on weight or length [34]).

Inhalant Effects Because of high lipid solubility, solvents and aerosols readily cross the placenta and cause fetal anomalies, including growth retardation, microcephaly, narrow bifrontal diameter, hypoplastic midface, and blunt fingertips. This syndrome closely resembles the physical findings of fetal alcohol syndrome and has been called *fetal solvent syndrome*. Increased rates of spontaneous abortion have been reported. Deficits in speech and cognitive skills may occur as the child gets older [34].

Sniffing of volatile hydrocarbons containing toluene during pregnancy may result in a syndrome of prenatal and postnatal growth retardation, microcephaly, CNS dysfunction, and cranial, facial, limb, and renal anomalies. The facial features consist of short palpebral fissures, deep-set eyes, narrow midface, ear anomalies, and narrow forehead [19].

Neonatal Abstinence Syndromes

Dependence can develop in the fetus as well as the mother. The type and severity of an infant's withdrawal symptoms depend on the drug(s) used, how long and how often the birth mother used them, how her body breaks the drug down, and whether the infant was born full term or premature.

The use of alcohol, barbiturates, benzodiazepines, and caffeine during pregnancy may cause the infant to show withdrawal symptoms at birth. Symptoms of neonatal withdrawal are often present at birth but may not reach a peak for 3–4 days of life; however, they may peak as late as 10–14 days after birth for some drugs [35].

Opioids

Neonatal opioid abstinence syndrome consists of central nervous system, gastrointestinal, autonomic, and respiratory effects (Table 19.5 [37]).

Withdrawal from opioids can persist in a subacute form for 4–6 months after birth, with a peak in symptoms around 6 weeks of age. High doses of maternal methadone (80–120 mg per day) produce a severe and prolonged abstinence syndrome in newborns. This complication is avoided when the pregnant woman is placed on low-dose methadone maintenance, especially if the third trimester dose is less than 20 mg per day [28].

Table 19.5 Neonatal opioid abstinence syndrome (Based on Bio [37])

Central nervous system	Autonomic nervous system
Abnormal sucking reflex Excessive or high-pitched crying High-pitched cry Hyperactive reflexes Hyperactivity Hypertonicity Increased muscle tone Irritability Seizures Sleep disturbances Sleep problems Tremor	Blotchy skin coloring Dermatological system Fever Frequent yawning Increased heart rate Nasal congestion Salivation Sneezing Stuffy nose and sneezing Sweating
Gastrointestinal system	**Respiratory system**
Diarrhea Poor feeding Vomiting	Respiratory distress Tachypnea

Methadone withdrawal symptoms typically appear within 48–72 h, but may not start until the infant is aged 3 weeks. This is particularly true for infants whose mothers took excessively higher doses [26].

Buprenorphine withdrawal symptoms typically occur within the first 72 h. Typically, fewer postnatal complications are reported compared with methadone, but 10% of infants exposed to buprenorphine are delivered prematurely compared with 7% of infants who are not exposed [38].

Other Drugs

Abstinence syndromes in neonates exposed to nonnarcotic drugs in utero have been described for a variety of drugs. Withdrawal from these drugs does not appear to result in symptoms as severe as for withdrawal from opioids. In general, these infants are irritable, restless, feed poorly, cry, and have impaired neurobehavioral abilities [28, 39]. Signs and symptoms of infants born to mothers addicted to nonopioid psychoactive drugs are given in Table 19.6.

Table 19.6 Signs and symptoms of infants born to mothers addicted to nonopioid psychoactive drugs (Based on Hudak [23])

Drug	Signs/symptoms
Alcohol	Hyperactivity, crying, irritability, poor sucking, tremors, seizures, poor sleeping patterns, hyperphagia, and diaphoresis
Barbiturates	Irritability, severe tremors, hyperacusis, excessive crying, vasomotor instability, diarrhea, restlessness, increased tone, hyperphagia, vomiting, disturbed sleep
Benzodiazepines	Irritability, tremors, hypotonia, poor sucking, hyperreflexia, vomiting, hyperactivity, tachycardia
Cocaine	Tremors, high-pitched cry, irritability, excessive sucking, hyperalertness, apnea, and tachycardia
Nicotine	Fine tremors and variations in tone; recent data have shown that maternal smoking was associated with subtle neonatal behaviors, such as poor self-regulation and an increased need for handling
Caffeine	Jitteriness, vomiting, bradycardia, tachypnea
Marijuana	Mild opiate-like withdrawal syndrome has been observed. Signs may include fine tremors, hyperacusis, and a prominent Moro reflex; however, these symptoms rarely require treatment
Phencyclidine	Jitteriness, hypertonia, vomiting, lethargy, vertical nystagmus

Estimated Times of Onset of Withdrawal Symptoms

Estimated times of onset of withdrawal symptoms are given in Table 19.7 [40].

Neonatal Detoxification

Initial treatment of the neonate experiencing withdrawal should be primarily supportive, because pharmacologic therapy may prolong hospitalization and subject the infant to exposure to the side effects of medications that may not be indicated. Supportive care includes swaddling to decrease sensory stimulation, frequent small feedings to supply the caloric requirements, and observation of sleeping habits, temperature stability, weight gain or loss, and change in clinical status that might suggest another disease process. Intravenous fluids and replacement electrolytes may be necessary to stabilize the infant's condition in the acute stage.

Indications for drug therapy are seizures, poor feeding, diarrhea, and vomiting resulting in excessive weight loss and dehydration, inability to sleep, and fever unrelated to infection [41].

Opioids The mainstay of therapy for opioid-addicted newborns is sedation and gradual reduction of the dose and lengthening the intervals

Table 19.7 Estimated times of onset of withdrawal symptoms (Based on [40])

Drug	Estimated time of withdrawal onset
Alcohol	3–12 h
Barbiturates	4–7 days but can range from 1–14 days
Sedatives	1–3 days
Heroin	Within 24 h
Other opioids	
Short acting	1–3 days
Long acting	2–6 days
Methadone	3 days but up to 5–7 days
Methamphetamines	Usually no withdrawal signs but sometimes neurobehavioral abnormalities that occur at 48–60 and last several months
Cocaine	Usually no withdrawal signs but sometimes neurobehavioral abnormalities (decreased arousal and physiologic stress) occur at 48–60 h and dysregulation can potentially last for several months
Marijuana	Usually no clinical withdrawal signs

between administrations according to response. Morphine, methadone, phenobarbital, buprenorphine, and clonidine have been used for neonatal detoxification. Buprenorphine combined with naloxone, compared to a morphine taper, is equally safe for treating babies born with neonatal abstinence syndrome [42].

Other Drugs Neonatal abstinence syndromes also occur with other drugs, with most intensity being from CNS depressant drugs (including alcohol). Gradually tapered doses of phenobarbital are usually effective if needed [22].

Nonpharmacologic Methods

Nonpharmacologic methods to aid with detoxification include [40]:

- Swaddling
- Skin to skin with parent
- Rocking
- Rooming in
- Minimal sensory or environmental stimulation
- Maintain temperature stability
- Providing baby with a pacifier for non-nutritive sucking
- Breast milk feedings when appropriate can help reduce the need for pharmacological intervention
- Feeding (consider alternating breast/bottle and pacifier during feed to compensate for excessive sucking and possibly prevent emesis)

Breastfeeding

Some substances, such as marijuana, alcohol, nicotine, and certain medicines, can be found in breast milk. However, little is known about the long-term effects on a child who is exposed to these substances through the mother's milk.

Women in a methadone treatment program should be allowed to breastfeed; however, more research is needed to determine the efficacy of breastfeeding when women are receiving buprenorphine. Breastfeeding should not be recommended in women who abuse heroin recreationally until more information is known about the actual amount of morphine present in the breast milk.

In general, it's probably not a good idea for breastfeeding women to use alcohol, nicotine, or illicit drugs until more research has been done and we have some definitive answers [43].

Aftercare

There are many ways for women to stay vigilant and continue improving their lives while reducing the risk of relapse. Some forms of aftercare involve professional help and are paid services; others are free services in the community. Aftercare for women might include: follow-up meetings with the rehabilitation center staff, attending local support groups (Narcotics Anonymous, Alcoholics Anonymous, SMART Recovery, Women for Sobriety), individual or family therapy, and medication if the woman has a co-occurring condition. Lifestyle changes are extremely important.

Summary

Equality for women has included greater freedom to drink. Women are particularly at risk for becoming dependent on prescription drugs. Women substance abusers complain more often of a wide range of symptoms, including depression, anxiety, sleeplessness, lethargy, stomach problems, and injuries from accidents or physical abuse. Compared with controls, substance-dependent women report a higher incidence of postpartum depression, irregular menstrual cycles, and amenorrhea. Low self-esteem seems to be an important feature of all addiction, but particularly for female addicts.

The T-ACE questionnaire was the first validated screen for pregnancy-risk drinking (defined as alcohol consumption of 1 oz or more per day) developed for use in obstetric-gynecologic practices. The TWEAK is used to screen for pregnancy-risk drinking, defined as the consumption of 1 oz or more of alcohol per day while pregnant.

Women, like men, are at risk for developing alcoholism, prescription drug addiction, and addiction to illicit drugs. Women, however, can directly affect other human beings, their unborn fetuses, by their drug use. Gestational abuse of any mood-altering substance can cause serious maternal and perinatal problems. Detoxification of pregnant women should be individualized according to the primary drug used and the stage of gestation.

Because approximately 85% of drug-addicted women are of childbearing age, there is a corresponding increase in the number of infants at risk for a complicated prenatal and postnatal course, including congenital defects and withdrawal symptoms.

The type and severity of an infant's withdrawal symptoms depend on the drug(s) used, how long and how often the birth mother used them, how her body breaks the drug down, and whether the infant was born full term or premature. Indications for drug therapy for infant detoxification are seizures, poor feeding, diarrhea, and vomiting resulting in excessive weight loss and dehydration, inability to sleep, and fever unrelated to infection.

References

1. Schmidt L, Wiesner C. The emergence of problem-drinking women as a special population in need of treatment. In: Galanter M, editor. Recent developments in alcoholism, vol. 12: alcoholism and women. New York: Plenum Press; 1995. p. 309–34.
2. Green CA. Gender and use of substance abuse treatment services. Alcohol Res Health. 2006;29(1):55–62.
3. Rubin A, Stout RL, Longabaugh R. Gender differences in relapse situations. Addiction. 1996;91(Suppl):S111–20.
4. Women and drug abuse. Department of Health and Human Services: Public Health Service: National Institutes of Health (NIH): National Institute on Drug Abuse. *NIH Publication.* 1994; 94–3732.
5. Sex and gender differences in substance use. National Institute on Drug Abuse (NIDA) website. https://www.drugabuse.gov/publications/research-reports/substance-use-in-women/sex-gender-differences-in-substance-use. September 2015.
6. Back SE, Contini R, Brady KT. Substance abuse in women: does gender matter? *Psychiatric Times,* December 31, 2006.
7. Royce JE. Alcoholics anonymous. In: Alcohol problems and alcoholism. London: Free Press; 1981. p. 242–55.
8. Alcohol: a women's health issue. U.S. Department of Health and Human Services: National Institutes of Health (NIH): National Institute on Alcohol Abuse and Alcoholism (NIAAA). *NIH Publication.* 2015; 15–4956.
9. Smith CG, Asch RH. Drug abuse and reproduction. Fertil Steril. 1987;48:355–73.
10. Griffe ML, Weiss RD, Mirin SM, Lange U. A comparison of male and female cocaine abusers. Arch Gen Psychiatry. 1989;46(2):122–6.
11. Substance use in women: sex and gender differences in substance use. National Institute on Drug Abuse (NIDA) website. https://www.drugabuse.gov/publi-

cations/research-reports/substance-use-in-women/sex-gender-differences-in-substance-use. September 2016.
12. Are there gender differences in tobacco smoking? National Institute on Drug Abuse (NIDA) website. https://www.drugabuse.gov/publications/research-reports/tobacco/are-there-gender-differences-in-tobacco-smoking. July 2012.
13. Holliday A, Bush B. Women and alcohol abuse. In: Barnes HN, Aronson MD, Delbanco TL, editors. Alcoholism: a guide for the primary care physician. New York: Springer-Verlag; 1987. p. 176–80.
14. Blume S. Women and alcohol. In: Bratter TE, Forrest GG, editors. Alcoholism and substance abuse: strategies for clinical intervention. New York: Free Press; 1985. p. 623–38.
15. Sokol RJ, Martier SS, Ager JW. The T-ACE questions: practical prenatal detection of risk-drinking. Am J Obstet Gynecol. 1989;160(4):868–70.
16. Chan AWK, Pristach EA, Welte JW, Russell M. Use of the TWEAK test in screening for alcoholism/heavy drinking in three populations. Alcohol Clin Exp Res. 1993;17(6):1188–92.
17. Cohen S. Alcoholism and women. In: The substance abuse problems: volume one. New York: Haworth Press; 1981. p. 341–6.
18. Royce JE. Alcoholism problems and alcoholism: a comprehensive survey. New York: Free Press; 1981. p. 65–8.
19. Reed BG. Drug misuse and dependency in women: the meaning and implications of being considered a special population. Int J Addict. 1985;20(1):13–62.
20. Hennecke L, Fox V. The woman with alcoholism. In: Gitlow SE, Peyser HS, editors. Alcoholism: a practical treatment guide. New York: Grune and Stratton; 1980. p. 181–91.
21. Gearhart JG, Beebe DK, Milhorn HT, Meeks GR. Alcoholism in women. Am Fam Physician. 1991;44(3):907–13.
22. Milhorn HT. Alcohol dependence: diagnosis, treatment, and prevention. New York: Springer-Verlag; 1990.
23. Hudak ML, Tan RC. Neonatal drug withdrawal. Pediatrics. 2012;129(2):e540–60.
24. Martin JN, Martin RW, Hess LW, McColgin SW, McCall JF, Morrison JC. Pregnancy-associated substance abuse and addiction: current concepts and management. J Miss State Med Assoc. 1988;29:369–74.
25. Matteo S. The risk of multiple addictions: guidelines for assessing a woman's alcohol and drug abuse. West J Med. 1988;149(6):741–5.
26. Wang M. Perinatal drug abuse and neonatal drug withdrawal clinical presentation. Medscape website. http://emedicine.medscape.com/article/978492-clinical. January 29, 2014.
27. Williams A. When the client is pregnant: information for counselors. J Subst Abus Treat. 1985;2(1):27–34.
28. Chesnoff I. Drug use in pregnancy: parameters of risk. Pediatr Clin N Am. 1988;35(6):1403–12.
29. Tobacco, drug use in pregnancy can double risk of stillbirth. National Institutes of Health (NIH) website. https://www.nih.gov/news-events/news-releases/tobacco-drug-use-pregnancy-can-double-risk-stillbirth. December 11, 2013.
30. Cohen S. The fetal alcohol syndrome: alcohol as a teratogen. In: The substance abuse problems: volume one. New York: Haworth Press; 1981. p. 245–50.
31. Wattendorf DJ, Muenke M. Fetal alcohol spectrum disorders. Am Fam Physician. 2005;72(2):279–82, 85.
32. The effects of alcohol on pregnancy outcome. Alcohol and health. Fifth special report to the U.S. Congress from the secretary of health and human services. Rockville: National Institute on Alcohol Abuse and Alcoholism (DHHS);1983. p. 69–82.
33. Laegreid L, Olegard R, Walström J, Conradi N. Teratogenic effects of benzodiazepine use during pregnancy. J Pediatr. 1989;114(1):126–31.
34. Hill RM, Tennyson LM. Maternal drug therapy: effect on fetal and neonatal growth and neurobehavior. Neurotoxicology. 1986;7(2):121–39.
35. Silverman S. Interaction of drug-abusing mother, fetus, types of drugs examined in numerous studies. J Am Med Assoc. 1989;26:1689–90.
36. Wolman I, Niv D, Yovel I, Pausner D, Geller E, David MP. Opioid-addicted parturient, labor, and outcome: a reappraisal. Obstet Gynecol Surv. 1989;44:592–7.
37. Bio LL, Siu A, Poon CY. Update on the pharmacologic management of neonatal abstinence syndrome. J Perinatol. 2011;31(11):692–701.
38. Oro A, Dixon SD. Perinatal cocaine and methamphetamine exposure: maternal and neonatal correlates. J Pediatr. 1987;111(4):571–8.
39. Farid WO, Dunlop SA, Tait RJ, Hulse GK. The effects of maternally administered methadone, buprenorphine and naltrexone on offspring: review of human and animal data. Curr Neuropharmacol. 2008;6(2):125–50.
40. Neonatal Abstinence Syndrome: best practices guidelines. Indian Health Service (IHS) website. http://www.ihs.gov/odm/includes/themes/newihstheme/display_objects/documents/NAS-Guidelines-Recommendation.pdf
41. Neonatal drug withdrawal. American Academy of Pediatrics (AAP): committee on drugs. Pediatrics. 1998;101(6):540–560.
42. Medical consequences of drug abuse: prenatal effects. National Institute on Drug Abuse (NIDA) website. https://www.drugabuse.gov/publications/medical-consequences-drug-abuse/prenatal-effects. December 2012.
43. Substance use while pregnant and breastfeeding. National Institute on Drug Abuse (NIDA) website. https://www.drugabuse.gov/publications/research-reports/substance-use-in-women/substance-use-while-pregnant-breastfeeding. September 2016.

20 Adolescents

Adolescence has been defined as the period between 13 and 18 years of age. It is the period following the onset of puberty during which time a young person develops from a child into an adult.

Key Chapter Points

- The teenage years are a critical period of vulnerability to substance use disorders because the brain is still developing, and some brain areas are less mature than others.
- The overwhelmingly predominant reason adolescents give for recurrent drug use is that drugs make them feel good and that they experience no adverse consequences from them.
- Unfortunately, parents often are caught up in adolescent denial and develop a denial system of their own.
- During the using stage, behavior controls the drug; in the dependence stage, the drug controls behavior, and addicts no longer have a choice in using the drug.
- The key to the difficult process of diagnosing adolescent substance dependence is a persistent, careful, and comprehensive assessment.
- The interviewer should start with the least threatening and move to increasingly sensitive subjects.
- The CRAFFT questionnaire is designed specifically for adolescent screening for alcohol or other drug problems.
- With adolescents, the psychosocial assessment is usually more helpful than the medical assessment.
- A good inpatient treatment program uses a multifactorial approach to treatment which includes assessment, treatment plan development, rehabilitation, and discharge planning.
- Because of the deep-seated denial that substance dependent adolescents develop, many authorities believe that outpatient treatment alone cannot be effective.

The Normal Adolescent

During adolescence, physiological and psychological development is in transition. The teenage years are a critical period of vulnerability to substance use disorders because the brain is still developing, and some brain areas are less mature than others. The parts of the brain that process feelings of reward and pain are the first to mature during childhood. The prefrontal cortex and its connections to other brain regions remain incompletely developed until the individual is in his or her mid-20s.

The adolescent brain is often likened to a car with a fully functioning gas pedal, the reward system, but weak brakes, the prefrontal cortex. Teenagers are highly motivated to pursue pleasurable rewards and avoid pain, but their judgment and decision-making skills are limited. This affects their ability to weigh risks accurately and

H.T. Milhorn, *Substance Use Disorders*, DOI 10.1007/978-3-319-63040-3_20

to make sound decisions, including decisions about using alcohol or other drugs [1].

Hormonal changes accelerate physical growth and sexual maturation, and as a result adolescents may feel awkward and insecure. They frequently feel inadequate about their appearance, popularity with peers, school achievement, and ultimate prospects of functioning as independent adults. Because adolescence is a time of frustration, it is also a time of anger and rebellion [2].

Peer affiliation and peer acceptance are hallmarks of adolescence. Young people have intense needs for acceptance, praise, and approval. These needs are more profound during adolescence than at any other time in life. Adolescents test limits and manipulate others. They need to experiment with extremes of values and behaviors and are often confused and scared. One minute they demand total independence, and the next minute they cry out for protection from themselves and the world they live in. They often experience free-floating anxiety and identity crises. They commonly act out, expressing unacknowledged internal conflicts. Adolescence is a period of exploratory, risk-taking, and sensation-seeking behavior. Experimenting with chemicals is a part of this world [3].

The Substance-Dependent Adolescent

When substance use disorders occur in adolescence, they affect key developmental and social transitions, and they can interfere with normal brain maturation. These potentially lifelong consequences make addressing adolescent drug use an urgent matter. Chronic marijuana use in adolescence, for example, has been shown to lead to a loss of IQ points that are not recovered even if the individual quits using in adulthood. Impaired memory or thinking ability and other problems caused by drug use can derail a young person's social and educational development and hold him or her back in life [1].

Prevalence of Use

In this country, on average, boys first use psychoactive substances at 11.9 years of age and girls at 12.7 years of age. Drug use has become an integral part of coming of age in American culture. Prevalence of past-year nonmedical drug use among 12th graders for 2015 is given in Table 20.1 [4].

A survey of drug use and attitudes among American 8th, 10th, and 12th graders showed decreasing use of alcohol, cigarettes, and many illicit drugs over the last 5 years. It showed no increase in the use of marijuana among teens, decreasing use of synthetic drugs, and decreasing misuse of prescription drugs. However, the survey highlighted continuing concerns over the high rate of e-cigarette use and softening of attitudes around some types of drug use, particularly a continued decrease in perceived harm of marijuana use [5].

The use of e-cigarettes remained high among teens with 6.2% of 8th graders, 14.0% of 10th

Table 20.1 Prevalence of past-year nonmedical drug use among 12th graders for 2015 (percent) (From [4])

Drug	Prevalence	Drug	Prevalence
Alcohol	58.2	Hallucinogens	4.2
Marijuana/hashish	34.9	OxyContin	3.7
Amphetamines	7.7	Sedatives	3.6
Adderall	7.5	MDMA (ecstasy)	3.6
Snus	5.8	LSD	2.9
Narcotics other than heroin	5.4	Hallucinogens (other than LSD)	2.9
Synthetic cannabinoids	5.2	Cocaine	2.5
Tranquilizers	4.7	Ritalin	2.0
Cough medicine	4.6	Inhalants	1.9
Vicodin	4.4	Salvia	1.9

graders, and 16.2% of 12th graders reporting using e-cigarettes in the past month [6].

Past-month use of smoked marijuana remained steady among 8th graders at 6.5%, 10th graders at 10.3%, and 12th graders at 12.4%. Six percent of 12th graders report daily use of marijuana. The majority of high school seniors do not think occasional marijuana smoking is harmful, with only 31.9% saying that regular use puts the user at great risk compared to 78.6% in 1991. The recent legalizing of marijuana by several states undoubtedly played a role in this [5].

Overall, past-year use of illicit drugs was reported by 23.6% of 12th graders. Past-month use of alcohol was 9.7%, 21.5%, and 35.3% of 8th, 10th, and 12th graders, respectively.

These data are somewhat conservative, because students who drop out of school before their senior year are not included. Drug use among this group is expected to be higher than among their in-school peers [6].

Substance abuse can lead to significant problems, such as poor schoolwork, loss of friends, problems at home, and legal problems. Alcohol and other drug use is a leading cause of teenage death or injury related to car crashes, suicides, violence, and drowning.

Many illegal drugs today are made in home labs, so they can vary greatly in strength. These drugs also may contain bacteria, dangerous chemicals, and other unsafe substances.

Substance use before age 18 is associated with an eightfold greater likelihood of developing substance dependence in adulthood [7].

Consequences

Accidents are the leading cause of death among teenagers. Of the nearly 13,000 accidental deaths among them annually, 2270 teens in the United States ages 16–19 were killed in motor vehicle crashes. Homicide is the second leading cause of death among adolescents at 17% (2200). Suicide accounts for 14% (1800) of the deaths. Alcohol and other drug use is a leading, if not the leading, cause of death among teenagers. Less dramatic but more insidious are the developmental, emotional, and social costs of adolescent substance use [8].

Substance abuse can increase the risk of pregnancy and sexually transmitted infections, including HIV because of unprotected sex.

Why Adolescents Use Drugs

We live in a drug-taking society, surrounded by images of people using drugs. Television advertisements depict drug use in two ways. Some link drinking to having fun; others link drug use (medication) to getting relief. Both give viewers the message that there is a drug to alter every human feeling and mood and that it is acceptable to use drugs for this purpose. Most adolescents who experiment with drugs or use them socially do not become substance dependent. Unfortunately, some do [2].

Adolescents have many reasons for beginning to use drugs. They use them for recreation, to help them socialize more easily, and as a rite of passage into adulthood. They try drugs because the use represents a new experience and because they produce pleasure. Adolescents use drugs to rebel, in response to an impulse, and as part of self-exploration. They use them to conform to their peers; to prove sexuality; to reduce stress; to relieve anxiety, fatigue, or boredom; and to solve their personal problems.

MacKenzie and Jacobs identified 14 reasons why adolescents use drugs (Table 20.2).

Other reasons adolescents use drugs are that they want to fit in with friends or certain groups, and they believe it makes them more grown up. The overwhelmingly predominant reason adolescents give for recurrent drug use is that drugs

Table 20.2 Why adolescents use drugs (Based on MacKenzie [9])

As recreation	In self-exploration
As a rite of passage	To conform
As a socializer	To prove sexuality
For a new experience	To reduce stress
For pleasure	To relieve anxiety, depression, or fatigue
In rebellion	To relieve boredom
In response to an impulse	To solve personal problems

make them feel good and that they experience no adverse consequences from them. They simply don't believe adults who tell them otherwise. Their peers confirm to them on a daily basis that their way of thinking is the correct one [9].

Differences from Adult Substance Dependence

Substance dependence among adolescents differs in several aspects from that of adults. Adolescents lack adult coping skills, and most have not separated completely from their parents. They are developing physiologically and psychologically, and many feel sexually insecure. They have not yet experienced meaningful, loving, bonding relationships. Most still live at home and are not responsible for their financial support or for the financial support of others. Parents seldom withdraw food and shelter, so that adolescents do not suffer the same consequences as adults. Whereas adult alcoholics may get cited for driving under the influence, for example, adolescents may not suffer this consequence simply because they have not yet begun to drive [10].

Unlike adults, substance-dependent adolescents in treatment must undergo habilitation rather than rehabilitation—that is, they must learn, not relearn.

Denial

The Adolescent

Most substance-dependent people, and particularly adolescents, undergo denial, which results from the substance dependence. It leaves adolescents unable to perceive themselves or others as they really are. Because of this self-deception, adolescents begin to deceive others. They lie about their behaviors and feelings and hide them from those who might confront them about their drug use. They avoid people who might make them aware of their fear of loss of control over the chemical.

Adolescents in denial lie about substance use; guard supplies of chemicals; appear in public in altered states of consciousness; hide drugs; are preoccupied with chemicals; continue to use despite punishment, warnings, or advice; self-prescribe; frequently visit emergency rooms or their physicians; have dysfunctional emotional involvements with others; feel anger, rage, and defensiveness about their drug use; blame others for their problems; pity themselves; attempt to control others; intellectualize; withdraw; isolate; and are chronically irresponsible. In a vicious cycle, denial produces greater drug use that, in turn, causes greater denial.

Adolescents use the same mechanisms of denial as adults (Chap. 1). These include rationalization, projection, repression, suppression, isolation, and minimization [11].

The Parents

Unfortunately, parents are often caught up in adolescent denial and develop a denial system of their own. Typical statements parents make in denying their child's drug use include [12]:

- "This is just a phase of rebellion. All teenagers go through this."
- "He is just shy."
- "My child makes poor grades because he does not like school."
- "He doesn't drink all the time."
- "He will grow out of it. All he needs is more time."
- "It's his friends. My child just picks the wrong friends. It's their fault."
- "All I need to do is spend more time with him and everything will be alright."
- "He only drinks beer. At least my child is not shooting heroin."
- "He has so many pressures in school and with friends."
- "He just doesn't have enough willpower."

Diagnosis

Careful distinction must be made between drug use and dependence. During the using stage, behavior controls the drug; in the dependence stage, the drug controls behavior, and addicts no longer have a choice in using the drug. Drug use becomes controlled by deeper, more primitive, centers of the brain, and compulsion to use drugs precludes rational and logical thought [11].

Assessment

The key to the difficult process of diagnosing adolescent substance dependence is a persistent, careful, and comprehensive assessment. The assessment consists of a drug use history obtained from the patient or family members, the use of a screening questionnaire, a psychosocial assessment, a family history, a physical examination, and some lab work, including a drug screen.

Assessment is difficult because adolescents often deny that they have any problems related to drinking alcohol or using other drugs. They typically withhold accurate information about drinking or other drug use. Consequently, physicians often must obtain information from others who know the adolescent. The cooperation of family members is essential for this process. Open-mindedness is important in determining whether an adolescent is addicted. Substance dependence is not the cause of every behavior disorder; the diagnosis of substance dependence must be made on factual information.

It is important to interview the patient without the presence of a parent for at least part of the visit. The physicians must assure patients of their concern for privacy if a trusting relationship is to be developed. Each state has laws that establish confidentiality rules, and states vary in their laws allowing minors to give consent for substance abuse treatment. Physicians should be aware of their state's laws when providing health care to adolescents.

The physician might ask adolescents what their friends do for fun—if they experiment with alcohol or other drugs or if they feel pressure from their peers to experiment. Physicians can listen and encourage adolescents to maintain positive peer relationships and avoid friends who make poor choices. The longer adolescents defer experimentation, the less likely they are to develop long-term substance use problems [7].

Behavioral Signs and Symptoms

The behavioral signs and symptoms of adolescent substance dependence are numerous. Substance-dependent teenagers drink and use drugs to get high, to escape (not simply for the elation or euphoria they once pursued), and to block emotional pain and discomfort. They gradually change friends to include drinking and drug-using peers. Blackouts may occur.

With the progression of substance use, difficulties occur more frequently at home, and family conflict increases. Adolescents may be suspended at school, and their grades may decline. They may be verbally abusive and rebellious, fight, and be sexually promiscuous. They believe they can stop using drugs anytime they choose and that they can stop by themselves.

For drug-using adolescents, life becomes centered around alcohol and other drugs. Their peer groups change dramatically, so that eventually all their friends are exclusively drug users. They attempt to stop drinking or using other drugs, but the fact that they can cut down or stop for a limited period of time leads them mistakenly to believe they can control their drug use.

Drug-using adolescents may deteriorate physically—in appearance or health. They may feel increasingly lonely and isolated, feelings that may be profound and dramatic. Parents, teachers, and even friends begin to express concern. Adolescents have a lot of accidents and frequently visit physicians and emergency departments. They may make psychosomatic complaints.

Gradually, adolescents lose self-esteem, increase their denial, and become angrier and more depressed. Serious family conflicts occur. Persistent substance use by adolescents may lead to repeated institutionalization, incarceration, or even death [11].

Progression of substance dependence in adolescents is much more rapid than in adults, and it delays the emotional maturation of adolescents. It is not unusual to deal with an 18-year-old in treatment who thinks and behaves as a 15-year-old [2, 13].

Treatment with ADHD medication, like Ritalin or Adderall, does not increase a child's risk for developing a substance use disorder [14].

Drug-Use History

The interviewer should start with the least threatening and move to increasingly sensitive subjects. Because drugs from legitimate prescriptions are necessary and socially approved, this is a good place to start. The next step is to ask about the adolescent's use of over-the-counter medicines. The interviewer can then progress to tobacco products, including cigarettes, smokeless tobacco, e-cigarettes, and then to alcohol use, prescription drug abuse, and marijuana use. Finally, the interviewer should ask about other illicit drugs [10].

Keep in mind that many adolescents abuse substances that are not usually considered to be drugs. These substances may include glues, paint thinners, mushrooms, Liquid Paper, and Scotchgard. Also, keep in mind that adolescents may drink over-the-counter substances, like mouthwash, because they are too young to buy alcohol legally and some of these products contain up to 70% alcohol (140 proof). For example, I had one 15-year-old patient who drank several ounces of Dr. Tichenor's, an antiseptic high in alcohol content, every morning on her way to school. Her reasoning was very logical. She stated that she drank the Dr. Tichenor's because she was too young to buy alcoholic beverages [12].

Screening Questionnaire

The CRAFFT questionnaire is designed specifically for adolescent screening for alcohol or other drug problems (Table 20.3 [15]). It consists of a series of six questions developed to screen adolescents for high-risk alcohol and other drug disorders.

Each "yes" answers gets one point. Two or more positive items indicate the need for further assessment.

Table 20.3 CRAFFT screening questionnaire (From [15]. Approved with permission, CeASAR)

C – Have you ever ridden in a CAR driven by someone (including yourself) who was "high" or who had been using alcohol or drugs?
R – Do you ever use alcohol or drugs to RELAX, feel better about yourself, or fit in?
A – Do you ever use alcohol or drugs while you are ALONE?
F – Do you ever FORGET things you did while using alcohol or drugs?
F – Do your family or FRIENDS ever tell you that you should cut down on your drinking or drug use?
T – Have you gotten into TROUBLE while you were using alcohol or drugs?

If screening indicates the possibility of substance use, the physician can conduct a more in-depth evaluation in the office or refer the patient to a physician specializing in addiction medicine. It is important also to evaluate the adolescent for co-occurring mental illness. A family history of substance use and psychiatric disorders should be taken.

Psychosocial Assessment

With adolescents, the psychosocial assessment is usually more helpful than the medical assessment. A general psychosocial assessment of an adolescent provides the basis for addressing substance use and the foundation for determining whether he or she behaves dysfunctionally. It should include an assessment of home and family relationships, the young person's functioning at school, peer relationships, legal difficulties, leisure activity, employment, and self-perception. Sensitive issues, such as violence and child abuse or risk of suicide, should be identified and addressed. Many adolescents who abuse drugs have a history of physical, emotional, and/or sexual abuse or other traumas. If abuse is suspected, referrals should be made to social and protective services, following local regulations and reporting requirements [10]. A psychosocial history should include the information given in Table 20.4.

Table 20.4 Psychosocial assessment (Based on Milhorn [12])

Personal functioning
Has his personal appearance and hygiene deteriorated? Does he lie, steal, and cheat? Does he have losses of money or possessions? Does he, for some unexplained reason, possess large sums of money? Does he wear clothing with drug-related slogans? Does he act secretively, for example, whispering on the phone? Does he spend a lot of time in his room alone when at home? Does he spend a lot of time in the bathroom with the door locked? Has he had episodes of not remembering things? Does he frequently use incense in his room? Does he say that he can quit using drugs anytime? Does his dress reflect an "offbeat" attitude? Does he seem to feel that the rest of the world is out of step? Is he preoccupied with drugs? Does he binge drink? Have you smelled alcohol on his breath? Does he wear sunglasses even in the house? Does get into fights? Has he tried to stop using drugs before and failed? Have you found drugs or drug paraphernalia in his room? Has he run away from home? Does he smoke (adolescents who smoke are at a higher risk for drug dependence than those who don't)?
Family relationships
Have relationships with family members deteriorated? Is he verbally abusive? Is he generally rebellious? Does he seem to be involved in a lot of family conflict? Does he stay out late at night, refusing to give accurate information about his activities or give flippant answers? Have siblings or relatives expressed concern about his behavior or drug use? Have items of value disappeared from the house?
Peer relationships
Has he changed friends to a less desirable crowd? Are most or all of his friends drug users? Have friends expressed concern about his behavior or drug use? Is he sexually promiscuous?
School functioning
Have his grades declined? Does he skip school? Has he been in trouble with school authorities? Has he been suspended from school? Has he dropped out of school? Has a teacher or school counselor expressed concern about his behavior or drug use?
Leisure activities
Has he stopped doing things he really used to enjoy? Does he seem to want just to "hang out" with friends all the time rather than participate in other activities? Is he overly into heavy rock music?
Employment problems
Has he been fired from a job because of tardiness, missing work, or a bad attitude? Has a boss or fellow employee ever expressed concern about his behavior or drug use?
Legal problems
Has he been in trouble with the law for driving under the influence; possession of alcohol, marijuana, or other controlled substances; drunk and disorderly behavior; or petty crimes?
Psychological functioning
Does he seem to be on edge a lot? Does he seem angry all the time? Is he withdrawn or depressed? Does he seem to have a poor self-image? Does he undergo rapid mood changes? Is his behavior unpredictable? Does he seem to have lost the ability for goal-directed drives (amotivational syndrome)? Has he made suicide threats, gestures, or attempts?

Physical Examination

Physical addiction and withdrawal symptoms do occur in adolescents, but with much less frequency than in adults. Alcoholic hepatitis is uncommon in adolescents, and cirrhosis of the liver is rare. Some physical findings that might be found in adolescent substance users are given in Table 20.5.

Family History

Attention should be paid to the family history. Alcoholism and probably other drug addictions tend to run in families. A strong family history of addiction increases the likelihood that the adolescent is drug addicted.

Laboratory Tests

Laboratory evidence of substance dependence in the adolescent is not very helpful. Elevated liver

Table 20.5 Some physical findings that might be found in adolescent substance users (Based on Milhorn [12])

Gastrointestinal problems due to alcohol irritating the stomach wall
Hallucinations and pupillary dilation may occur with hallucinogen use
Needle tracks on the arms, cellulitis, and abscesses from opioid injections may be present. Addicts tend to wear long sleeve shirts, even in the summertime, to cover needle tracts
Nystagmus, paranoid delusions, and delusions of extreme strength may result from phencyclidine use
Pupillary constriction and constipation from opioid use may be present
Rashes around the mouth or nose and on the hands may indicate inhalant use
Rhinitis, nasal bleeding, sinus problems, nasal septal perforation may be present due to cocaine or nasal inhaler use
Suspiciousness, paranoia, or outright psychosis may result from amphetamine, cocaine, or phencyclidine use
The eyes may be red and a chronic cough may be present due to marijuana smoking. They may wear sunglasses to cover up their eyes, even indoors
Untidiness in personal appearance and habits is common

enzymes due to alcoholic hepatitis are uncommon. A drug screen, when positive, is helpful but not diagnostic. It only proves that the adolescent has used the drug at least once. A home drug-screening test provides immediate, early information about whether a urine sample contains drugs such as amphetamine, cocaine, or marijuana.

If, prior to the drug screen, the adolescent was adamant about never having used drugs, a positive result may have the effect of breaking through the denial and forcing the adolescent to be honest about his drug use.

A negative drug screen does not rule out drug dependence. For many drugs it may mean that the adolescent has not used drugs for the past 2 or 3 days. For other drugs, it may mean that the drug wasn't screened for. Lysergic acid diethylamide (LSD) is a popular adolescent drug that is not on routine drug screens. If it, or other drugs not on the drug screen, is suspected, it can be added to the drug screen.

Many adolescents are aware that a urine drug screen can be made to give a falsely negative result by substituting their urine with someone else's or by adulterating their sample. Commonly used adulterants are vinegar, lemon juice, and chlorine bleach. Ingesting large amounts of water or diuretics may dilute the drug in the urine to such that a level that is not detectable. Substances can be purchased on the Internet to affect a urine drug screen. Drug screens were discussed in detail in Chap. 14.

Testing adolescents for sexually transmitted diseases like HIV, as well as hepatitis B and C, is an important part of drug treatment. Adolescents who use drugs, whether injecting or using orally, are at an increased risk for diseases that are transmitted sexually as well as through the blood. All psychoactive substances alter judgment and decision making, increasing the likelihood that adolescents will engage in unprotected sex and other high-risk behaviors, including sharing contaminated needles. Unsafe tattooing and body piercing practices are potential routes of virus transmission [16].

Getting the Adolescent into Treatment

Tough Love and Intervention by Confrontation

Useful tools for getting adolescents into treatment are tough love and intervention as described in Chap. 18.

Court Order

In many if not most states, adolescents can be court ordered to treatment for evaluation. If they are found to have a substance use disorder, they are committed to treatment.

Treatment

Substance abuse in adolescents is undertreated in the United States. Approximately 1 in 11 who needs care for a substance use disorder receives it. Primary care physicians are well positioned to recognize substance use in their patients and to take steps to address the issue before use escalates. Common mental disorders among adolescents with substance abuse include depression, anxiety, conduct disorder, and attention-deficit/hyperactivity disorder.

Inpatient Treatment

Programs offering inpatient treatment are usually in psychiatric hospitals or free-standing treatment centers. These programs offer intense courses of treatment, providing a structured residential stay that is usually 4–6 weeks long. They consider substance dependence to be a disease, may use the 12 steps of Alcoholics Anonymous, and are committed to total abstinence from psychoactive substances as a way of life.

Staffing is multidisciplinary and includes physicians, nurses, and substance dependence counselors. Fewer than 5% of adolescents admitted for treatment require medication for detoxification. Healthy activities are explored to replace substance use. Inpatient programs often have elaborate rules with some sort of behavioral privilege system. Patients may not be allowed to send or receive telephone calls or e-mails or have visitors for the first week. The Internet is off limits as well [17].

If adolescents perceive the treatment setting as one simply imposed on them by adults, they resent it and it is ineffective. Preaching, lecturing, and scolding are not effective. Positive peer influence is a powerful force. When this approach is used, peers replace adults, at least in part, as authority figures [2].

Patient government groups serve several functions. They promote responsibility and accountability. Group leaders are in charge of unit meetings and act as positive role models for other patients; unit secretaries record the minutes of meetings and post duties on the bulletin board; and other patients are elected to make coffee, clean lounges, act as buddies to new patients on the unit, and buy necessities for patients without shopping privileges. Indirectly, patient government groups build confidence and improve patient self-esteem [6].

Adolescents have a higher energy level than most adults and are often bored. Treatment programs need to incorporate this energy into program activities and so must make sufficient recreational activities available to patients.

Visits by program graduates are well received by adolescent patients. Graduates may return to a facility on regularly scheduled visits, perhaps once a month, and conduct Alcoholics Anonymous or Narcotics Anonymous meetings or informal discussions. They are able to speak with credibility about the kinds of problems patients will face after they complete treatment. They serve as living examples of adolescents in recovery [2].

Some programs require 6 weeks of partial day-care following discharge from an inpatient stay. Following this, once-weekly aftercare, extending for 6 months, may be required. Continued academic training is extremely important. Maintaining academic performance may increase an adolescent's self-esteem and sense of responsibility [17].

A good inpatient treatment program uses a multifactorial approach to treatment which includes assessment, treatment plan development, rehabilitation, and discharge planning [12].

Assessment

Assessment includes medical assessment, psychological assessment, and social assessment.

Medical Assessment An ASAM- or APA-certified addictionist uses information provided by the family and referring physician as well as information obtained from his own physical examination, drug and medical histories, and psychosocial assessment to verify the diagnosis. A detoxification plan is formulated if one is felt to be necessary. Fortunately, most adolescents who use drugs do not have significant withdrawal symptoms on cessation of drug use. However, because drug-addicted adolescents often minimize their drug use, they are observed by nursing personnel for withdrawal symptoms for the first 24 h. Detoxification medication if needed is prescribed. Medical problems when present are treated.

Psychological Assessment Psychological assessment is done early in the treatment process. It consists mainly of testing. The Minnesota Multiphasic Personality Inventory-Adolescent (MMPI-A) [18] is a psychological test that assesses personality traits and psychopathology of adolescents. It is the most widely used personality inventory for adolescents. It is a self-report instrument designed to aid in the assessment of a wide range of clinical conditions. There are eight validity scales and ten basic clinical or personality scales scored in the MMPI-A [19].

An IQ test, such as the Kaufman Adolescent and Adult Intelligence Test (KAIT), is also given. KAIT is an individually administered general intelligence test appropriate for adolescents and adults aged 11 to over 85 years [20].

Social Assessment Social assessment involves collecting data from the patient, family members, friends, teachers, and employers on the patient's level of social functioning. It includes the adolescent's educational level, history of childhood abuse, legal history, childhood role models, family life, and a detailed lifelong drug history [10].

Treatment Plan Development

Finally, a treatment plan is developed based on the medical, psychological, and social assessments. The addictionist and the patient's counselor work together to formulate a list of identified problems that are placed on a master treatment list. Individual problems may be dealt with in treatment, may be noted and merely monitored, may be dealt with after treatment, or may require no action.

For each problem that is to be dealt with in treatment, a treatment plan that sets forth specific goals and objectives for resolving the problem is developed. The treatment plan includes a projected time course for the resolution of the problem. For example, denial of having a drug problem and poor coping skills are two common problems encountered and dealt with in treatment.

Each patient is assigned a primary counselor on admission to guide his day-to-day activities and a treatment team, which usually meets weekly to discuss the adolescent's progress on each problem on the list and to update the treatment plan [12].

Rehabilitation

The rehabilitation process in many aspects is like that of adults (Chap. 15). The process may include education, individual therapy, group therapy, family treatment, life story, peer assessment, recreational therapy, coping skills and relaxation therapy, support group attendance, and spirituality [12].

Education Despite significant experience with a variety of drugs, adolescents in general possess little factual information about them. To correct this, patients attend lectures or view films daily on such diverse subjects such as the disease concept of addiction, adverse effects of drugs on the body, psychological and social aspects of drug use, cross addiction, various steps of AA or NA (if in a 12-step treatment program), recovery process, and how to prevent relapse. From time to time, they are given specific reading assignments. Regular school studies are continued.

Individual Therapy Problems inappropriate for group therapy or problems better dealt with on a one-to-one basis are addressed in individual therapy. Cognitive behavioral therapy may be part of this. Writing or reading assignments may be made in individual therapy; the work is then presented and then discussed.

Group Therapy Group therapy involves from 10 to 15 adolescents and a group leader who is usually a certified alcohol/drug counselor. It provides an opportunity for patients to deal with a variety of issues, aided by other group members.

Group therapy helps patients identify feelings, see how their addictions have hurt them and others, and begin to see the need for change. It allows them to share feelings they usually have suppressed and helps them identify the defense mechanisms they habitually use to hide their feelings.

Group therapy helps young people discover who they are by listening to what other adolescents share with them about the behaviors that they have observed.

Life Story Early in treatment, adolescents are asked to write their life stories. Life stories include information about their childhoods, family relationships, school, legal problems, any previous treatment, and their thoughts about their futures.

Peer Assessment A special kind of group called "peer assessment" gives patients an opportunity to contribute constructively to the therapy of another adolescent who is having difficulty in treatment. Patients identify problem areas, like dishonesty, defensive behavior, not participating in treatment, and other undesirable behaviors.

One at a time they get the opportunity to present their information to the problem patient.

The patient is not allowed to respond defensively to these discussions. Quite often, peer pressure has a positive effect on improving attitude and behavior.

Recreational Therapy Drug-using adolescents typically do not exercise. Since adolescents have a high energy level and often become bored, sufficient recreational activities must be made available. These activities may include playing basketball, volleyball, and racquetball, walking or running, and swimming. Exercise improves depression, gives a sense of well-being, and promotes a good night's sleep.

Coping Skills and Relaxation Therapy Many drug-using adolescents use drugs to relax and cope with stress. Now they have to learn to do these things without drugs. Role-playing stressful situations to learn appropriate ways to handle them is a helpful tool. Patients learn to relax by means other than drugs—deep breathing, relaxation tapes, exercise, and other techniques.

Support Group Attendance Attendance and participation in a 12-step support group, such as Alcoholics Anonymous, Cocaine Anonymous, or Narcotics Anonymous, is a part of most treatment programs. These meetings are held among patients in the treatment facility. Visits by program graduates exert a positive influence. They usually return to the facility periodically to conduct support group meetings or have informal discussions. They are able to speak with credibility and serve as living examples of adolescents in recovery.

Attendance of support group meetings while in treatment is important because it introduces adolescents to the groups and familiarizes them with their operation and function. After discharge, patients are expected to continue attending support group meetings in their home towns for the rest of their lives. The disease of addiction never goes away.

Spirituality Spirituality is an elusive concept; it is not religion. In the treatment of substance dependence, it is used in a much broader sense. It has been defined as being in contact with yourself, with those around you, and with a power greater than you. It is that which enables the growth of positive and creative development in a human being. It involves honesty, humility, humor, and hope. It is seeing the beauty that is around us. Working within the Alcoholics Anonymous program is a spiritual process, as is taking the time to stop and smell some flowers.

A spiritual identity crisis may ensue with the onset of adolescence. Prior to this time, they had passed through childhood accepting the values they received in the home, churches, and schools. Their acceptance of these values was automatic and comforting.

Substance-dependent adolescents are particularly bankrupt when it comes to spirituality. Sobriety, by contrast, brings a positive and creative lifestyle to counter their previous destructive and negative existence [12].

Typical Daily Activity Schedule

A typical activity schedule for adolescents in inpatient treatment is given in Table 20.6.

Family Treatment

Most family members do not realize the extent to which their responses to the addicted adolescent—isolation, enabling, depression, anxiety, and even physical illness—have resulted from their own dysfunctional behavior. Therefore, it is important that family members go through a treatment process just like the adolescent does. Treatment of the family helps set the groundwork for leading a normal, healthy life during the adolescent's recovery, not only for the adolescent but for the rest of the family as well. Addiction is truly a family disease.

Four useful treatment resources are available for the family: (1) family week, (2) family therapy, (3) codependent treatment, and (4) support groups [12].

Family Week In some treatment programs, family members join the adolescent the last week in the treatment facility. A typical family week includes interviews to determine each member's understanding of drug dependence. Presentations on such subjects such as the disease concept of addiction, various steps of Al-Anon and Alateen if it is a 12-step program, and information about healthy family functioning follow. Group therapy is an important part of family week.

Table 20.6 A typical activity for adolescents in inpatient treatment (Based on Milhorn [12])

Morning	
6:30–7:00	Wake up, hygiene, make beds
7:00–7:30	Breakfast
7:30–8:00	Devotional/community meeting
8:00–9:00	Lecture
9:00–9:30	Break
9:30–11:00	Group therapy/individual therapy
11:00–12:00	School (on the adolescent unit)
Afternoon	
12:00–12:30	Lunch
12:30–1:30	Peer assessment
1:30–2:30	Coping skills/relaxation therapy
2:30–3:00	Break
3:00–4:00	Recreational therapy
4:00–5:00	School (on the adolescent unit)
Evening	
5:00–5:30	Dinner
5:30–6:00	Free time
6:00–7:00	Study time
7:00–8:00	Support group attendance
8:00–9:30	Study time
9:30–10:30	Free time
10:30	Lights out

Family Therapy Family therapy involves group treatment of members of an individual family or group treatment of several families. Family therapy groups include the addicted adolescent. Sessions with members of several families are helpful for sharing experiences, for recognizing that the adolescent's problem is truly a problem that adversely affects every family member, and for breaking through family denial.

Properly supervised confrontation between the adolescent and the other family members is helpful for releasing long-standing anger and resentment. Commonly, family therapy sessions are conducted weekly for up to 6 months after the adolescent has returned home.

Codependency Treatment Since codependence is common in substance-dependent families, some treatment programs offer codependent treatment for family members who have been adversely affected by the adolescent's drug use. A codependent is a person who is psychologically dependent in an unhealthy way on someone who is addicted to alcohol or another drug. Codependency treatment usually follows inpatient treatment and lasts 4–6 weeks, meeting in the evenings. Treatment consists of identifying and learning to deal with their own problems and issues.

Support Group Attendance Family members are introduced to a 12-step program which has been adapted from that of Alcoholics Anonymous, and they are expected to attend support groups such as Al-Anon, Alateen, Nar-Anon, and Codependents Anonymous. Non-AA-related support groups may be preferred by some if such programs are available locally. The treatment premise is that the family can get well whether the addicted adolescent does or not.

Discharge Planning

Assessing the needs adolescents are expected to have after discharge is called *discharge planning.* Part of discharge planning involves making a decision about whether the adolescent will be ready to return home or should be transferred to a less intense level of non-hospital treatment, that is, residential treatment.

Discharge planning also includes decisions about aftercare meetings and support group attendance once the adolescent is discharged. The patient and the aftercare coordinator sign a contract spelling out the terms of aftercare [12].

Extended Care

Many authorities believe that adolescents need a longer length of stay than adults spend in inpatient treatment programs. Therefore, many adolescent programs last 46–60 days. Regardless of the length of inpatient treatment, most programs feel that follow-up care is extremely important. Extended care is thought to be necessary for adolescents because their age, immaturity, lack of nonchemical coping skills, and emotional development lag behind from prolonged drug use during a period when adolescents normally mature emotionally. [12].

Outpatient Treatment

Patients in outpatient treatment do not live at treatment facilities and are free to maintain their daily school schedule. A typical outpatient program might require a patient to attend three evening sessions a week at the treatment center and two or three support group meetings a week in the community.

Because of the deep-seated denial that substance-dependent adolescents develop, many authorities believe that outpatient treatment alone cannot be effective. Instead, it is used for adolescents who have not yet developed dependence to keep them from reaching that stage. It can also be used to support an adolescent returning home from an inpatient treatment program. An adolescent should meet two criteria to be a candidate for primary outpatient treatment. First, the patient must come from a functionally healthy family. The family plays an important role in outpatient treatment. Second, the adolescent must be in the use stage, not yet having reached full-blown dependence [2]. Other details of outpatient treatment were discussed in Chap. 15.

Residential Treatment

Therapeutic communities constitute one form of residential treatment. These programs stress open and frank communication and emphasize acceptance of one's responsibility with the group. They tend to use a relatively high proportion of paraprofessional staff. A traditional therapeutic community may have only one or two professional counselors.

Another type of residential treatment, half-way houses, are not intended as primary treatment facilities. They are structured settings from which recovering adolescents can reenter the community before returning home from inpatient treatment. They offer places for newly recovering adolescents to give one another support [18]. Other details of therapeutic communities and half-way houses are discussed in Chap. 15.

Aftercare

A very small number of adolescent patients complete treatment with the insight, determination, and courage needed for successful recovery. Therefore, a well-developed aftercare plan is essential. Concerns to be addressed in aftercare include maintaining sobriety, continued involvement with community support groups and sponsors, educational priorities, vocational goals, and psychological counseling. Also included in the aftercare plan are goals for having fun while remaining clean and sober and a no-use contract. This is an agreement between the patient and the family that the adolescent will not use alcohol or other drugs [2].

Adolescents recovering from substance use disorders may experience relapse. Triggers associated with relapse can include mental stress and social situations linked with prior drug use. It is important to identify a return to drug use early before an undetected relapse progresses to more serious consequences. A relapse signals the need for more treatment or a need to adjust the individual's current treatment plan to meet better his needs [1].

Summary

Adolescence has been defined as the period between 13 and 18 years of age. Peer affiliation and peer acceptance are hallmarks of adolescence. Young people have intense needs for acceptance, praise, and approval. The teenage years are a critical period of vulnerability to substance use disorders because the brain is still developing, and some brain areas are less mature than others. The overwhelmingly predominant reason adolescents give for recurrent drug use is that drugs make them feel good and that they experience no adverse consequences from them. Unfortunately, parents often are caught up in adolescent denial and develop a denial system of their own.

During the using stage, behavior controls the drug; in the dependence stage, the drug controls behavior, and addicts no longer have a choice in using the drug. The key to the difficult process of diagnosing adolescent substance dependence is a persistent, careful, and comprehensive assessment. The interviewer should start with the least threatening and move to increasingly sensitive subjects. The CRAFFT questionnaire is designed specifically for adolescent screening for alcohol or other drug problems.

With adolescents, the psychosocial assessment is usually more helpful than the medical assessment. A good inpatient treatment program uses a multifactorial approach to treatment, which includes assessment, treatment plan development, rehabilitation, and discharge planning.

Part of discharge planning involves making a decision about whether the adolescent will be ready to return home or should be transferred to a less intense level of non-hospital treatment, that is, residential treatment.

References

1. Principles of drug addiction treatment: a research-based guide. 3rd ed. National Institute on Drug Abuse (NIDA) website. https://www.drugabuse.gov/publications/principles-drug-addiction-treatment-research-based-guide-third-edition/acknowledgments. December 2012.
2. Heaslip J, Van Dyke D, Hogenson D, Vedeers L. Young people and drugs: evaluation and treatment. Center City: Hazelden Education Materials; 1989.
3. Cohen S. Coming of age in America – with drugs: contemporary America. In: The substance abuse problems, volume two. New York: Haworth Press; 1985. p. 203–7.
4. DrugFacts: high school and youth trends. National Institute on Drug Abuse (NIDA) website. https://www.drugabuse.gov/publications/drugfacts/monitoring-future-survey-high-school-youth-trends?hootPostID=851244dc58fec3b952f61590a3b2e9d8. December 2016.
5. Monitoring the future survey, overview of findings 2015. National Institute on Drug Abuse (NIDA) website. https://www.drugabuse.gov/related-topics/trends-statistics/monitoring-future/monitoring-future-survey-overview-findings-2015. December 2015.
6. Schonberg SK, editor. Substance abuse: a guide for professionals. Elk Grove Village: American Academy of Pediatrics; 1988.
7. Griswold KS, Aronoff H, Kernan JB, Kahn LS. Adolescent substance use and abuse: recognition and management. Am Fam Physician. 2008;77(3):331–6.
8. Teen Drivers: get the facts: how big is the problem?. Center for Disease Control and Prevention (CDC). https://www.cdc.gov/motorvehiclesafety/teen_drivers/teendrivers_factsheet.html. October 13, 2016.
9. MacKenzie RG, Jacobs EA. Recognizing the adolescent drug abuser. Adolesc Med. 1987;14:225–35.
10. Anglin TM. Interviewing guidelines for the clinical evaluation of adolescent substance abuse. Pediatr Clin N Am. 1987;4:381–99.
11. Morrison MA, Smith QT. Psychiatric issues of adolescent chemical dependence. Insight. 1987;3:3–10.
12. Milhorn HT. Drug and alcohol abuse: the authoritative guide for parents, teachers, and counselors. New York: Da Capo Press; 2003.
13. Royce JE. Special groups. In: Alcohol problems and alcoholism. New York: Free Press; 1981. p. 103–18.
14. Does treatment of ADHD with stimulant medications like Ritalin® and Adderall® increase risk of substance abuse later in life? Principles of adolescent substance use disorder treatment: a research-based guide. National Institute of Drug Abuse (NIDA) website. https://www.druga-

buse.gov/publications/principles-adolescent-substance-use-disorder-treatment-research-based-guide/frequently-asked-questions/does-treatment-adhd-stimulant-medications-ritalinr-adderallr-increase-risk-substance-abuse-later-in. January 2014.
15. The CRAFFT screening tool. The Center for Adolescent Substance Abuse Research (CEASAR) website. 2016. http://www.ceasar-boston.org/CRAFFT/index.php
16. Semlitz L, Gold MS. Adolescent drug abuse: diagnosis, treatment, and prevention. Pediatr Clin N Am. 1986;9:455–73.
17. Blum RW. Adolescent substance abuse: diagnosis and treatment issues. Pediatr Clin N Am. 1987;34:523–37.
18. Wheeler K, Malinquist J. Treatment approaches in adolescent chemical dependency. Pediatr Clin N Am. 1987;34:437–47.
19. Minnesota Multiphasic Personality Inventory (MMPI). Scribd website. https://www.scribd.com/doc/2890384/Minnesota-multiphasic-personality-inventory
20. Kaufman Adolescent and Adult Intelligence Test (KAIT). Encyclopedia of Mental Disorders website. http://www.minddisorders.com/Kau-Nu/Kaufman-Adolescent-and-Adult-Intelligence-Test.html

The Elderly

21

Key Chapter Points

- As a person grows older, physiological changes tend to extend the life of drugs in the body and enable them to have more powerful effects.
- In addition to physiological alterations, concurrent disease may also alter a drug's effect.
- Few older Americans use street drugs. However, they do have problems with prescription medications and alcohol.
- Alcohol is the number one drug of abuse of older Americans.
- Elderly alcoholics can be divided into two major groups: hardy survivors and late-onset group.
- Older adults are at risk for prescription drug abuse because they take more prescription medicines than other age groups.
- Diagnosing substance dependence in the elderly can be difficult. Seniors who abuse alcohol or other drugs tend to go undetected.
- The SMAST-G has been specifically developed as an alcohol-screening tool for the elderly.
- Inpatient treatment is often needed to address such issues as detoxification, depression, poor nutrition, weight loss, treatment of acute and chronic medical problems, and polypharmacy.
- The goal of planning aftercare is to have elderly patients living at their highest level of functioning and lowest level of care.

Most developed world countries have accepted the chronological age of 65 years as a definition of elderly. Older individuals represent an increasing proportion of the US population. Persons 65 years of age and older now number 46.2 million in the United States. They represent 14.5% of the population or about one in every seven Americans. People 65 and older are expected to represent 21.7% of the population by 2040, and it is estimated that by 2060, there will be 98 million older individuals, more than twice the current number [1].

Only about 5% of the elderly are living in institutions; this means that 95% are living with the rest of the society.

Of men and women over 65, 86% have at least one or more chronic ailments. Thus, elderly people are more likely to take several prescription and over-the-counter medications, as well as to self-medicate with alcohol or other drugs. Many prescription medications have the potential for addiction as well as for synergistic action among themselves and with alcohol and other drugs [2].

Although alcohol and drug abuse is harmful at any age, it is more harmful on the elderly. The impact of alcohol- and drug-related injuries is much more severe, the risk of harmful medication interactions is much greater, and the general physical effects of alcohol and drugs are more debilitating.

H.T. Milhorn, *Substance Use Disorders*, DOI 10.1007/978-3-319-63040-3_21

Prevalence of Use

There are 2.5 million older adults with an alcohol or drug problem. Fourteen percent of elderly emergency room admissions, 6–11% of elderly hospital admissions, and 20% of elderly psychiatric hospital admissions are a result of alcohol or drug problems. Widowers over the age of 75 have the highest rate of alcoholism in the United States. Nearly 50% of nursing home residents have alcohol-related problems [3].

Pathophysiology of Aging

As a person grows older, physiological changes tend to extend the life of drugs in the body and enable them to have more powerful effects. Physiological changes in the elderly are given in (Table 21.1 [4]).

Disease

In addition to physiological alterations, concurrent disease may also alter a drug's effect. A number of abnormalities are common among the elderly, including congestive heart failure, renal disease, dehydration, hypotension, hypertension, diabetes, malnutrition, and cirrhosis. Such disorders can further reduce the functions of vital organs and thereby alter drug absorption, distribution, metabolism, and excretion. In addition, the central nervous system's sensitivity to alcohol and other drugs increases with age.

The renal elimination of drugs is altered by aging, although there is significant variation between individuals for any given decade. Drug excretion does correlate with creatinine clearance, which declines by 50% by age 75. However, because lean body mass decreases with aging, the serum creatinine level tends to overestimate the creatinine clearance of older adults [5].

As a result of physiological and pathological changes of aging, an extreme variability occurs in older adults' responses to drugs. As a general principle, a physician should expect an increased and prolonged drug effect in the elderly. Tolerance levels for alcohol and other drugs decrease with age. This means that the elderly can experience increasingly negative effects even when they are only using these substances at the same level as in the past [4].

Table 21.1 Physiological changes in the elderly (Based on Shlafer [4])

Physiological change	Pharmacokinetic alteration
Increased gastric pH	Decreased absorption of drugs that are normally nonionized at low pH
Increased body fat	Decreased fat-soluble drug concentration in the blood
Decreased body water	Increased fat-soluble drug concentration in the blood
Decreased serum albumin	Increased unbound drug, leading to increased drug activity
Decreased cardiac output	Decreased metabolism of drugs
Decreased renal blood flow	Decreased excretion of drugs
Decreased splanchnic blood flow	Decreased absorption of drugs taken orally, decreased metabolism
Decreased liver mass and hepatic blood flow	Decreased metabolism of drugs

The Elderly Addict

Few older Americans use street drugs. However, they do have problems with prescription medications and alcohol. Most elderly patients admitted for treatment of substance abuse are dependent on alcohol alone (86%); most of the remainder are dependent on prescription drugs alone or in combination with alcohol (14%) [6]. They rarely use illicit drugs like cocaine and methamphetamine.

There are many reasons why elderly people may turn to alcohol or other drugs in later life, including loneliness, grief due to the death of loved ones, boredom, health concerns, reduced cognitive functioning, lack of meaningful employment, chronic pain, fear of getting old, family problems, and financial hardship. Other reasons the elderly use alcohol and other drugs include being separated or divorced, having abused substances when they were younger and carried it into older age, feeling disappointed with their achievements in life, mental health problems, and feeling socially isolated.

Older people are far more likely to suffer physical and mental damage as a result of alcohol or other drug use. They suffer falls as a result of intoxication and are more likely to suffer serious injury [7].

Alcohol

Alcohol is the number one drug of abuse of older Americans. Alcohol abuse among the elderly is a hidden national epidemic. It is believed that about 10% of this country's population abuses alcohol, but as many as 17% of the over-65 adults have an alcohol problem. It has been found that 2.5 million older adults and 21% of older hospital patients have alcohol-related problems [8].

Recommended Drinking Limits

The National Institute on Alcohol Abuse and Alcoholism (NIAAA) recommends that people over age 65 should have no more than seven drinks a week and no more than three drinks on any 1 day. If they are taking certain medicines, they may need to drink less or not drink at all [9]. Binge drinking in the elderly is defined as drinking four or more drinks during a single drinking day for men or three or more drinks during a single day for women.

Groups

Elderly alcoholics can be divided into two major groups: (1) hardy survivors and (2) late-onset group.

Hardy Survivors Hardy survivors comprise almost two-thirds of older alcoholics and have an early onset of alcohol abuse. Although most alcoholics die at an earlier age, survivors have beaten the odds. Most of them have numerous medical problems, including cirrhosis, organic brain syndrome, and psychiatric problems. They are more likely to be men (67%) and to have long-standing behavioral problems, more physical problems, and numerous attempts at treatment. They have personality characteristics similar to young alcoholics and more often drop out of treatment than the late-onset group [8].

Late-Onset Group The late-onset group, also known as reactors, start drinking relatively late in life. To them, alcoholism is secondary to the stresses of aging, the death of a spouse or other person close to them, retirement, loneliness, reduced income, poor health, or geographic relocation. Because of the late onset of drinking, reactors show fewer physical consequences and fewer lifestyle disruptions than hardy survivors. With abstinence from alcohol and good nutrition, recovery from the physical effects of alcoholism can be complete. Nearly a third of elderly alcoholics fall into this group. Alcoholics in this group are more likely to be women. They may have physical impairments and diminished social support; however, they are more likely to undergo successful treatment.

Some add a third category, the *binge drinker*. These individuals do not drink regularly but occasionally go on binges, drinking relatively large amounts of alcohol over a few days or weeks. Intermittent stress (depression, loneliness, anxiety) is a common ingredient in initiating these episodes. Binge drinkers represent only a small percentage of elderly alcoholics [8].

Health Consequences

One of the most important pathological consequences of alcoholism in the elderly is its effect on the cardiovascular system. Alcohol impairs cardiac function, resulting in decreased cardiac output. It may deaden angina pain, a warning sign leading to myocardial infarction. Alcohol can also cause worsening of hypertension and adversely affect pulmonary function. Alcohol abuse can cause a decrease in respiratory drive, resulting in mental confusion in elderly people who have chronic obstructive pulmonary disease. Alcoholism also can lead to adverse nutritional effects in the elderly, including deficiency of thiamine and other nutrients. Gastrointestinal disorders (gastritis, peptic ulcer disease, diarrhea) are common among elderly alcoholics, as are neurological disorders (neuropathy, decreased coordination, decreased seizure threshold) [4, 5].

Elderly individuals are more apt to develop cognitive impairment from the use of alcohol than younger ones. They tend to become forgetful and to have more difficulty with reasoning. They may become stubborn because of a lack of understanding or angry and agitated as they become confused. Dementia due to alcoholism in the elderly is mostly two types—Wernicke-Korsakoff syndrome and alcoholic dementia.

Wernicke-Korsakoff syndrome is a stage of brain dysfunction characterized by general cloudiness of the mind and gross confusion. Some ataxia and nystagmus may occur. When treated with thiamine, many of the acute symptoms clear. What is left after about 3 days is called Korsakoff's psychosis. It is characterized by an inability to learn, a loss of immediate memory, and confabulation. With proper nutrition, absence of alcohol, and time, the condition usually clears or improves. Most improvement is seen in the first 3 months, but may continue up to 5 years.

Alcoholic dementia is characterized by a gradual intellectual decline due to long-term alcohol abuse and is irreversible. Progression ceases with abstinence from alcohol [10].

The combined effects of alcoholism and aging are additive, placing older alcoholics at increased risk of premature dementia and decreasing their potential for recovering [11].

Other Drugs

The elderly spend over $500 million yearly on medications. Combining medications and alcohol frequently results in significant adverse reactions. The consequences of drug misuse by the elderly are dramatic [8].

Older adults are at risk for prescription drug abuse because they take more prescription medicines than other age groups. People over 60 account for 40% of all drug reactions; one-sixth of hospital admissions for patients over 70 result from adverse drug reactions, and nearly one-fourth of hospital admissions for the elderly are due to taking prescriptions incorrectly. Factors that contribute to prescription drug misuse among older Americans include poor communication between older patients and physicians, pharmacists, and nurses; complex regimens that require them to take a number of drugs at the same time; treatment by several different physicians, all of whom may be prescribing medicine; a lack of awareness that a drug's effects can be magnified or reduced in aging bodies; an inability to take medicines as prescribed because of vision, hearing, and memory loss or other changes associated with aging; and poor compliance (not taking a prescribed drug at all, discontinuing the drug prematurely, or purposefully altering consumption of it) [12, 13].

The high rates of comorbid illnesses in older populations, age-related changes in drug metabolism, and the potential for drug interactions may make any of these practices more dangerous than in younger populations. Further, a large percentage of older adults also use OTC medicines and dietary supplements, which (in addition to alcohol) could compound any adverse health consequences resulting from prescription drug abuse.

Among the elderly, a significant prescription drug abuse problem exists, one that is often referred to as American's hidden problem. The drugs elderly people abuse are almost invariably ones that depress the central nervous system, as these people withdraw from frustrating existences and evade stress. There is a great variability in the response among older people to mood-altering substances; they may be hypersensitive to even average amounts of chemical substances and suffer mental confusion or fluctuating delirium as a result [14, 15].

Commonly prescribed drugs with abuse potential include those for anxiety, pain, and insomnia, such as benzodiazepines, opiate analgesics, and skeletal muscle relaxants [16].

Due to a reduction in blood flow to the liver and kidneys in the elderly, there can be a 50% decrease in the rate of metabolism of some medications, especially benzodiazepines. Additionally, chlordiazepoxide (Librium) and diazepam (Valium) have such long half-lives in the elderly that prolonged sedation from these drugs, combined with the sedative effects of alcohol, can increase the risk of serious falls and fractures. The benzodiazepine user may become confused and take extra doses or other medications, causing overdose or death.

Caffeine is frequently a component of OTC medications and can cause anxiety and insomnia. Often, mixing alcohol and the OTC medications increases the occurrence of side effects and can intensify negative consequences.

Nicotine dependence is also a significant problem in the elderly. Use early in life sets the stage for morbidity and mortality from this addiction in later life. Elderly smokers not only continue to impair their respiratory systems but also are also more apt to die from cardiovascular disease.

Aging drug addicts can be divided into two groups: surviving street addicts and prescription addicts [17].

Surviving Street Addicts

There are few street addicts over the age of 60. Most have either died from the consequences of injecting unsterile material for years, accidental overdoses, suicide, or trauma. Some opioid addicts over 60 can be found in methadone maintenance clinics [17].

Prescription Addicts

Prescription drug abuse is defined as a person using prescription medication not prescribed for that person or using the medication in a way that was not prescribed by a doctor. Prescription drug abuse is a term usually reserved for improper use of medicines that are categorized as controlled substances by the FDA, such as opioids, benzodiazepines, and Z drugs. A person who abuses prescription drugs may take more medicine than their doctor prescribed, take medicine when it is not needed, or mix the medicine with alcohol or other drugs.

Older adults are at risk for prescription drug abuse because they take more prescription medicines than other age groups. Americans 65 years of age or older make up only 14.5% of the US population, yet they consume approximately 33% of all prescription drugs.

Older adults are also at risk for prescription drug abuse because they often take more than one prescription medicine each day. This increases the risk for mistakes when taking the medicines and for drug interactions.

Signs of prescription drug abuse include requests for drug refills that indicate use out of proportion to objective signs and symptoms or more rapid use than directed; requests for refills of controlled substances prescribed by another physician; requests for refills before the original prescriptions are finished; requests for specific usually very potent drugs, when other less potent drugs in the same class are said to be ineffective or cause adverse reactions; and undue familiarity with many potent psychoactive drugs, their appearances, side effects, and formulations. They may be uncomfortable or defensive when asked about the medicine being abused, they may store extra pills in their purse or in their pocket, or they may sneak or hide medicine.

A person can abuse any type of prescription drug, but elderly adults commonly take three types of medicines that have a high potential for addiction—opioids, benzodiazepines, and Z drugs [18].

Diagnosis

Diagnosing substance dependence in the elderly can be difficult. Seniors who abuse alcohol or other drugs tend to go undetected. Those who live alone find it easier to hide their substance abuse. When the symptoms of abuse become evident, they may be misdiagnosed as the effects of aging. The elderly are also far less likely to encounter legal difficulties as a result of their substance abuse.

Physicians use many rationalizations for not confronting elderly addicts. Family members and physicians may accept an ongoing alcohol or other drug problems as a justifiable response to the stress of aging. Another obstacle to recognizing addiction in the elderly is the stereotype of the skid row bum. Because elderly patients usually do not fit this picture, addiction to alcohol or other drugs may not be suspected. In addition, the elderly may not come to the attention of those who might suspect they have a problem. When behavioral problems develop in the elderly, causes other than drug use are often considered first. The effects of alcohol and other CNS depressants may produce a syndrome indistinguishable from senile dementia [5].

Drug-related health problems in the elderly may be more difficult to separate from chronic illness and the effects of medication than in younger populations. When elderly patients have problems with controlling gout, diabetes mellitus, hypertension, angina, or incontinence, alcohol abuse should be considered. Temperature regulation may be impaired, increasing the age-related risk of hypothermia. The diuretic effect of alcohol may be significant in the frail elderly. Arrhythmias and decreased left ventricular function are potential cardiac side effects [19].

Clues in the history and physical examination that may indicate substance dependence in the elderly include insomnia or changes in sleep patterns, abrupt confusion, inability to function, gastrointestinal problems, palpitations, gait abnormalities and frequent falls, bruises, fractures, burns, or sprains. Self-neglect, poor grooming, or malnutrition also may indicate a problem with alcohol or other drugs. Noticeable behavioral changes, such as social isolation, depression, paranoid behavior, increased family quarrels, or estrangement from family or friends should be investigated [5, 7].

Alcohol withdrawal is commonly overlooked during elderly patients' hospitalizations because transient confusion is so common in this population. It may be confused with delirium or dementia [19].

A problem with allowing the elderly to report their own level of drinking is setting a cutoff level for heavy drinking. A few drinks a day may be relatively benign for a healthy young person, but the same intake could be disastrous for any elderly person who is in poor health, has decreased tolerance, or is taking several prescription medications.

Most measures of substance dependence were standardized on nonelderly men. Such measures include problems with family or friends, employment or legal problems, drinking and driving problems, financial problems, and neglecting responsibilities. Physical aggression, breaking the law, driving a car, and being employed tend to characterize men more than women but characterize the elderly least of all [20].

Indicators of drug use more appropriate for the elderly might include housing problems, falls or accidents, poor nutrition, inadequate personal care or care of clothing or living quarters, lack of physical activity, and social isolation [21].

Being suspicious of and questioning the elderly about substance dependence can make their care more appropriate and effective.

Other signs that might indicate a substance abuse problem include irritability, changes in eating habits, wanting to stay alone much of the time, not staying in touch with family or friends, and lack of interest in usual activities. In addition, they may experience secretive behavior, loss of interest in activities they once enjoyed, inability to concentrate, neglect of personal grooming and hygiene, and irrational behavior [22].

Screening Tools

The SMAST-G has been specifically developed as an alcohol-screening tool for the elderly (Table 21.2 [23]). Each "yes" answer gets one point. A score greater than or equal to two points indicates an alcohol problem. The extra question should not be calculated in the final score, but should be asked. To the author's knowledge, there are no screening questionnaires specifically for the nonalcoholic elderly addict; however, the CAGE-AID and the DAST-10 can be used, probably with somewhat less accuracy than for younger individuals.

Family members have important roles in the treatment of elderly alcoholics and should have access to support and education about alcoholism. Frail elderly patients may benefit from compre-

Table 21.2 SMAST-G: geriatric screening tool for alcoholism (From Blow [23]. Approved with permission, Alcoholism: Clinical and Experimental Research)

1. When talking with others, do you ever underestimate how much you drink?
2. After a few drinks, have you sometimes not eaten or been able to skip a meal because you didn't feel hungry?
3. Does having a few drinks help decrease your shakiness or tremors?
4. Does alcohol sometimes make it hard for you to remember parts of the day or night?
5. Do you usually take a drink to calm your nerves?
6. Do you drink to take your mind off your problems?
7. Have you ever increased your drinking after experiencing a loss in your life?
8. Has a doctor or nurse ever said they were worried or concerned about your drinking?
9. Have you ever made rules to manage your drinking?
10. When you feel lonely, does having a drink help?
Extra question: Do you drink alcohol and take mood or mind altering drugs, including prescription tranquilizers?

hensive geriatric assessment and referral to appropriate community agencies for home care, nutritional programs, transportation, and other services. Nursing home placement may be the most appropriate treatment option for some refractory, long-term alcoholics with dementia [24].

Treatment

Unfortunately, only a fraction of substance-dependent elderly people ever receive treatment for their disease. Inpatient treatment is often needed to address such issues as detoxification, depression, poor nutrition, weight loss, treatment of acute and chronic medical problems, and polypharmacy. Individual counseling and support are crucial in alleviating patients' guilt, frustration, and depression [25].

The initial treatment of older addicted adults often requires more intensive medical support than is necessary in younger patients. Withdrawal is typically more difficult and dangerous for older adults. In addition, social and psychological withdrawal, as well as behavior modification, can also be more strenuous for older patients [26].

Evaluation

Patients' abilities to function and to solve problems must be evaluated early in treatment. If problems are detected in these areas, evaluations should be repeated periodically to look for improvement. Senility may have developed to so great a point in some elderly patients that they simply cannot benefit from treatment—other than by learning to abstain from alcohol and other drugs and to develop better nutrition. They may be better suited for nursing home care. Some may need legal or financial guardians, and their families must make such decisions in these situations. Those with mild or moderate memory impairment should be taught to keep notes and a daily schedule [10].

Detoxification

Detoxification generally takes longer in the elderly. Benzodiazepines with a short half-life, such as oxazepam (Serax) or lorazepam (Ativan), are preferable to the longer-acting ones such as diazepam (Valium) or chlordiazepoxide (Librium). The dosages should be one-half to two-thirds those used in younger adults [26].

Thiamine and screening for dietary deficiencies (folate, vitamin B_{12}, magnesium) are advised. Signs and symptoms of concomitant barbiturate, benzodiazepine, or opioid abuse may complicate the picture. Benzodiazepine addiction in particular may prolong the detoxification period [19].

Rehabilitation

Elderly people, in general, tend to hold very definite ideas. They feel that things should look good on the surface and therefore tend not to make waves but instead comply. They tend to be offended by coarse language, sloppy clothes, and long hair, which are attitudes physicians and counselors should deal with openly and with respect. To them, family secrets should not be aired in public, but what they consider to be personal secrets may not be the same things people of different generations consider to be secret.

They may, for example, sometimes consider divorce in the family a secret. The elderly feel that authority should be respected and usually have rigid ideas on male and female roles. Elderly women tend to be dependent and look for people to defend them; elderly men have been taught to be protectors. This rigidity should be recognized.

The immortality view of substance dependence has been deeply engraved in older people. They have been raised to view alcoholism as sinful and the alcoholic as weak, and it is very difficult for them to accept the disease concept of addiction. Finally, many elderly people were brought up with deep religious beliefs but have strayed from church over the years. Sometimes their return to church may help their spiritual progress [10].

The elderly deny abuse much more so than other age groups do. Many of today's elderly grew up at a time when drinking was frowned on, and they may be reluctant to admit even limited consumption [21].

Frequently, elderly addicts need to deal with deaths, divorces, or other significant losses that happened years ago and that they have not dealt with because of their substance abuse. This is especially true of the late-onset alcoholic, whose heavy drinking may have been initiated by such a loss [10].

Vocational rehabilitation is generally inappropriate for the elderly. However, social services are especially relevant for older recovering addicts because they often live alone and have few social resources [26].

Unlike younger people, the elderly are not likely to return to work or to child-rearing. They should be helped to look at the need to improve their physical health and to make sure that their living conditions meet their needs. Reestablishing broken ties with lost family members, and thus improving social support systems, should be pursued.

Counselors should address such relevant issues as retirement, free time, volunteer work, and interactions with grown children. Often, the elderly are concerned about the costs of retirement. They should be told that treatment for substance dependence is paid for by Medicaid and Medicare.

Physical activity is a great healer of depression. Regular walking stimulates people physically, emotionally, and psychologically and should be recommended. Relaxation therapy is well received in this age group and helps to improve their general sense of well-being.

The best approach to treat the elderly is that of gentle support and loving encouragement. Heavy confrontation has no place in this age group. They do not need judgment or punishment, which they tend to provide themselves. They need kind acceptance, gentle support, encouragement that things can change for the better, and reassurance of their importance as people [10].

Elderly patients treated in the special peer group program remain in treatment significantly longer and are more likely to complete treatment than those treated in mixed-age groups [27].

Aftercare

The goal of planning aftercare is to have elderly patients living at their highest level of functioning and lowest level of care. This may involve living independently at home, living at home with local social support systems, and living in halfway houses or institutionalized care.

In the elderly, long-term addiction often results in feelings of loneliness and isolation that are deeper and stronger than those felt by younger people. The elderly may feel extremely unworthy and feel the need to have people around them. They need to find creative use of their leisure time and need to revive old interests. Volunteer work serves a need in this age group.

AA and aftercare meetings are very helpful. Daytime meetings are important because many elderly do not like to be out after dark, and night driving is more difficult for many of them. Transportation may be a problem for some; if so, arrangements should be made prior to discharge from treatment [10].

The elderly are more faithful than younger people in attending support group meetings, but they prefer and receive greater benefit from smaller groups. Older patients complain about the noise, rough language, and cigarette smoke that are often associated with larger meetings [4].

The opiate antagonist naltrexone (Revia, Vivitrol) reduces cravings for alcohol and is intended to be prescribed as adjunctive treatment to psychosocial support to reduce the risk of alcohol relapse. A dosage of 50 mg/day is safe in older individuals with alcohol dependence [15].

Generally, disulfiram (Antabuse) should not be prescribed for the elderly because of the increased risk of delirium and other serious adverse effects [28].

Acamprosate (Campral) may be safer and more effective for patients with liver dysfunction; however, it should be used cautiously in elderly patients with impaired renal function [29].

Sublingual buprenorphine/naloxone (Suboxone) must be administered with caution in the elderly because of the increased risk of respiratory depression and sedation. Lower dosages in the elderly are recommended [30].

Summary

Most developed world countries have accepted the chronological age of 65 years as a definition of elderly. As a person grows older, physiological changes tend to extend the life of drugs in the body and enable them to have more powerful effects. In addition to physiological alterations, concurrent disease may also alter a drug's effect.

Few older Americans use street drugs. However, they do have problems with prescription medications and alcohol. Older people are far more likely to suffer physical and mental damage as a result of alcohol or other drug use. Alcohol is the number one drug of abuse of older Americans. Elderly alcoholics can be divided into two major groups: hardy survivors and late-onset group. Older adults are at risk for prescription drug abuse because they take more prescription medicines than other age groups.

Diagnosing substance dependence in the elderly can be difficult. Seniors who abuse alcohol or other drugs tend to go undetected. The SMAST-G has been specifically developed as an alcohol-screening tool for the elderly.

Inpatient treatment is often needed to address such issues as detoxification, depression, poor nutrition, weight loss, treatment of acute and chronic medical problems, and polypharmacy. Detoxification generally takes longer in the elderly. Benzodiazepines with a short half-life, such as oxazepam (Serax) or lorazepam (Ativan), are preferable to the longer-acting ones such as diazepam (Valium) or chlordiazepoxide (Librium). The goal of planning aftercare is to have elderly patients living at their highest level of functioning and lowest level of care.

References

1. Aging statistics. Administration on aging: U.S. Department of Health and Human Services (DHHS) website. https://aoa.acl.gov/Aging_Statistics/Index.aspx. May 24, 2016.
2. Many older people use both prescription drugs and dietary supplements. National Institute on Drug Abuse (NIDA) website. https://nccih.nih.gov/research/results/spotlight/071509.htm. January 30, 2015.
3. Alcohol, Drug Dependence and Seniors. National Council on Alcoholism and Drug Dependence (NCADD) website. https://www.ncadd.org/about-addiction/seniors/alcohol-drug-dependence-and-seniors. June 26, 2015.
4. Shlafer M, Marieb EN. Age and other patient-related factors that alter drug response. In: The nurse, pharmacology, and drug therapy. Redwood City: Addison-Wesley; 1989. p. 90–108.
5. Olsen-Noll CG, Bosworth MF. Alcohol abuse in the elderly. Am Fam Physician. 1989;39(4):173–9.
6. Abrams RC, Alexopoulos GS. Substance abuse in the elderly: alcohol and prescription drugs. Hosp Commun Psychiatry. 1987;38(12):1285–7.
7. Elderly and substance abuse. Alcohol Rehab website. http://alcoholrehab.com/drug-addiction/elderly-and-substance-abuse
8. Elderly alcohol and substance abuse. Office of Alcoholism and Substance Abuse Services (OASAS) website. http://www.oasas.ny.gov/AdMed/FYI/FYIInDepth-Elderly.cfm

9. Alcohol use in older people. National Institute on Aging (NIA) website. https://www.nia.nih.gov/health/publication/alcohol-use-older-people#much. March 2012.
10. Walker B, Kelly P. The elderly: a guide for counselors. Center City: Hazelden; 1981.
11. Stirling JS, Largen JW, Shaw T. Interactions of normal aging, senile dementia, multi-infarct dementia, and alcoholism in the elderly. In: Hartford JT, Samorajaski T, editors. Alcoholism in the elderly: social and biomedical issues. New York: Raven Press; 1984. p. 227–51.
12. Basca B. The elderly and prescription drug misuse and abuse. Center for Applied Research Solutions website. http://www.cars-rp.org/publications/Prevention%20Tactics/PT09.02.08.pdf.
13. Prescription drug abuse in the elderly. Family Doctor website. https://familydoctor.org/condition/prescription-drug-abuse-in-the-elderly. October 2015.
14. Misuse of prescription drugs: older adults. National Institute on Drug Abuse (NIDA) website. https://www.drugabuse.gov/publications/research-reports/prescription-drugs/trends-in-prescription-drug-abuse/older-adults. August 2016.
15. Substance abuse among older adults: Treatment Improvement Protocol (TIP) Series 26. Rockville: Substance Abuse and Mental Health Services Administration (SAMHSA): Center for Substance Abuse Treatment; 1998.
16. Cohen S. Special groups and situations. In: The substance abuse problems: volume one. New York: Routledge/Taylor and Francis Group; 1981. p. 313–63.
17. Bogunovic O. Substance abuse in aging and elderly adults. Psychiatric Times website. http://www.psychiatrictimes.com/geriatric-psychiatry/substance-abuse-aging-and-elderly-adults. July 27, 2012.
18. Cusack BJ, Vestal RE. Clinical pharmacology: special considerations in the elderly. In: Calkins E, Davis PJ, Ford AB, editors. The practice of geriatrics. Philadelphia: WB Saunders; 1986. p. 115–31.
19. Hesse K, Savitsky J. The elderly. In: Barnes HN, Aronson MD, Delbanco TL, editors. Alcoholism: a guide for the primary care physician. New York: Springer-Verlag; 1987. p. 167–75.
20. Whitcup SM, Miller F. Unrecognized drug dependence in psychiatrically hospitalized elderly patients. J Am Geriatr Soc. 1987;35(4):297–301.
21. Graham K. Identifying and measuring alcohol abuse among the elderly: serious problems with existing instrumentation. J Stud Alcohol. 1986;47(4):322–6.
22. Milhorn HT, Gardner LC. When to suspect alcoholism: how to help when you do. Sr Patient. 1990;2(7):41–5.
23. Blow F, et al. Brief screening for alcohol problems in elderly populations using the Short Michigan Alcohol Test-Geriatric Version (SMAST-G). Alcohol Clin Exp Res. 1998:22(Suppl):131A, 20–5.
24. Rigler SK. Alcoholism in the elderly. Am Fam Physician. 2000;61(6):1710–6.
25. Alcohol use disorder. National Institute on Drug Abuse (NIDA) website. https://niaaa.nih.gov/alcohol-health/overview-alcohol-consumption/alcohol-use-disorders
26. Bienenfeld D. Alcoholism in the elderly. Am Fam Physician. 1987;36(2):163–9.
27. Kofoed LL, Tolson RL, Atkinson RM, Toth RL, Turner JA. Treatment compliance of older alcoholics: an elder-specific approach is superior to mainstreaming. J Stud Alcohol. 1987;48(1):47–51.
28. Rogers J, Wiese BS. Geriatric drinkers: evaluation and treatment for alcohol overuse. B C Med J. 2011;53(7):353–6.
29. Acamprosate (Oral route). Mayo Clinic website. http://www.mayoclinic.org/drugs-supplements/acamprosate-oral-route/before-using/DRG-20066802. April 1, 2015.
30. Suboxone: Indications and usage for Suboxone. Drugs.com website. https://www.drugs.com/pro/suboxone.html. June 2016.

22 Other Groups

Key Chapter Points

- Race refers to a person's physical characteristics, such as bone structure and skin, hair, or eye color. Ethnic describes a group of people sharing a common background, language, and identity.
- American Indians and Alaska Natives experience some of the highest rates of substance abuse compared to other US racial or ethnic groups.
- Asian Americans, who make up less than 2% of the population of the United States, have low levels of alcohol and drug use.
- Abuse of alcohol and other drugs is most common among urban African American males.
- Hispanic men have relatively high rates of alcoholism, while Hispanic women have high rates of abstention.
- About a third of all people experiencing mental illnesses also suffer from substance dependence.
- Primary substance use disorder must be differentiated from secondary substance use disorder.
- The LGBT community suffers from a higher rate of substance use disorders than the heterosexual population.
- HIV and AIDS patients suffering concurrent substance use issues need immediate intervention and treatment.

This chapter will discuss four other groups: (1) ethnic minority groups, (2) co-occurring disorder patients, (3) LGBT patients, and (4) HIV-positive patients.

The Ethnic Minority Groups

The United States has a racially and ethnically diverse population. Race refers to a person's physical characteristics, such as bone structure and skin, hair, or eye color. Ethnic describes a group of people sharing a common background, language, and identity. Members may have similar characteristics, but more importantly, they share beliefs and behaviors that differ from other ethnic groups. When an ethnic group is not allowed full participation in society and reacts to this discrimination, it is classified as a minority group. Population size is not a part of this definition.

Ethnic minorities make up about a third of the population of the United States and are expected to become a majority by 2050. These diverse communities have unique behavioral health needs and experience different rates of substance use disorders and treatment access.

The four primary ethnic racial categories are (1) American Indians/Alaska Natives, (2) Asian/Pacific Islanders, (3) African Americans, and (4) Hispanic Americans. The definitions for the four categories are as follows [1]:

- **American Indian/Alaska Natives**. A person having origins in any of the original peoples of North America who maintains cultural identification through tribal affiliations or community recognition.

H.T. Milhorn, *Substance Use Disorders*, DOI 10.1007/978-3-319-63040-3_22

- **Asian/Pacific Islanders**. A person having origins in any of the original peoples of the Far East and Southeast Asia, the Indian subcontinent, and the Pacific Islands.
- **African Americans**. A person having origins in any of the racial groups of Africa.
- **Hispanic Americans**. A person of Mexican, Puerto Rican, Cuban, Central or South American, or other Spanish culture or origin regardless of race.

American Indians/Alaska Natives, Asian/Pacific Islanders, African Americans, and Hispanic Americans constitute over 40% of total admissions to treatment programs, even though they represent only 33% of the population. Despite this, our knowledge of the use of alcohol and other drugs among America's ethnic minority populations is incomplete, and most of what we know is limited to information about minority youth. Less information exists about ethnic adults, the elderly, and families. Any attempt to deal with substance dependence in people of a particular culture must show sensitivity to the language, the customs, and the thinking of that culture [1].

American Indians/Alaska Natives

There are about 5.2 million American Indians and Alaska Natives in the United States, which are about 1.7% of the total population. They belong to hundreds of tribes representing many distinct cultural traditions. Roughly half of these remain on reservations; the other half live primarily in cities.

American Indians and Alaska Natives experience some of the highest rates of substance abuse compared to other US racial or ethnic groups. Alcohol and drug abuse is believed to be a significant problem among American Indians. The rate of illegal drug use in the last month among American Indians and Alaska Natives ages 12 and up in 2014 was 14.9%.

American Indians and Alaska Native youth ages 12–20 in 2014 reported past-month alcohol use at a rate of 21.9%, compared with the national average of 22.8%. Past-month underage binge drinking was 14.3% for American Indian and Alaska Native youth, while the national average was 13.8%. In 2010, Native Americans had the highest rate of drug-induced death (17.1%).

Most research on Indian substance abuse has been conducted on reservations—virtually none has been done on urban Indians. We know that Indians began to drink centuries ago after they came into contact with European traders. Alcohol continues to be their drug of choice.

By their ninth birthday, 12% of Indian children regularly drink beer, wine, or liquor; 97% of them use alcohol by the eleventh grade. Heavy drinking is the main reason one in two Indian students never finishes high school. In some tribes, rates of male alcoholism may be as high as 80–85% and female alcoholism 35–55%. Alcohol is a factor in 75% of Indian deaths, in 80% of suicides, and in contributing to a homicide rate three times the national average.

Indians have high rates of cirrhosis and other alcohol-related problems. American Indian women appear to be susceptible to alcohol-related problems. Although they drink less than men, they account for nearly half of American Indian cirrhosis deaths and seem to be at particular risk for fetal alcohol syndrome.

The use of other drugs (marijuana, inhalants, heroin, cocaine, minor tranquilizers, sleeping pills) among Indian youth is higher than among non-Indian youth.

American Indian values stress the family unit, cooperation, humility, and avoidance of individual recognition. Indians are less likely to talk about their feelings and may be uncomfortable in group therapy. They may view confrontational techniques as hostile acts. They tend to be stoic, and, as a result, the severity of their problems may be underestimated [1–3].

Asian/Pacific Islanders

There are about 18.2 million people who identify themselves as Asian American. There are also 1.4 million Native Hawaiians or other Pacific Islanders in the United States.

Asian Americans, who make up less than 2% of the population of the United States, have low levels of alcohol and drug use in general. However, Asian American youth appear to use drugs at a rate equal to, if not higher than, the national average.

In 2014, among people ages 12 and up, the rate of illegal drug use in the last month was 4.1% among Asian Americans and 15.6% among Native Hawaiians or other Pacific Islanders.

The rate of binge alcohol drinking was lowest among Asian Americans ages 12 and up (14.5%). The binge alcohol use rate was 18.3% among Native Hawaiian or other Pacific Islanders. The past-month, binge alcohol use rate for youth ages 12–20 was 6.7% for Asian Americans compared with the national average of 13.8%.

The rate of substance dependence was 4.5% for Asian Americans and 10% for Native Hawaiians or other Pacific Islanders.

It is often assumed that Asian Americans have similar drinking and drug-using patterns regardless of their national origin. However, Asian Americans have a great diversity of backgrounds, with origins in China, Japan, the Philippines, Korea, India, Vietnam, Cambodia, and other Asian countries.

There appear to be significant differences in psychoactive substance use among Asian Americans of different origins. The diversity of subgroups within this ethnic group adds complexity to the drug abuse effort. Furthermore, findings from a sample of Japanese Americans who have lived in the United States for several generations are very different from those obtained from a group of recent Japanese immigrants.

Similarly, findings obtained from a group of Asian American students in a large university are very different from those obtained from a group of young men of similar age who have recently arrived in the United States as refugees from Southeast Asia. The language problems are formidable.

In general, Asians value academic and occupational accomplishments that bring honor to the family. Failure brings them shame.

Asian patients may be uncomfortable expressing emotions openly. They don't like to talk directly about personal problems and may describe these as educational or physical issues.

Gender and age roles tend to be more traditional, and it may take some time for them to become comfortable in family sessions.

Male Asians who are recent immigrants lose status if they have to assume jobs of lower rank than they had in their original communities; their feeling of shame over this may disrupt their families. Many Asians, therefore, respond well to counseling that has a vocational or educational theme [1, 2].

African Americans

There are about 44.5 million African Americans in the United States. The largest ethnic group in the United States, African Americans, make up about 12% of the total population and 92% of the nonwhite population.

The rate of illegal drug use in the last month among African Americans ages 12 and up in 2014 was 12.4%, compared to the national average of 10.2%. The rate of binge drinking (drinking five or more drinks on a single occasion for men) among African Americans ages 12 and up was 21.6%—compared with the national average of 23%.

African American youth ages 12–20 in 2014 reported past-month alcohol use at a rate of 17.3%, compared with the national average of 22.8. Past-month underage binge drinking was 8.5% for African American youth, while the national average was 13.8%.

In 2014, 3.8% of African American adults ages 18 and older had a past-year mental illness and a substance use disorder, while the national average was 3.3%.

Abuse of alcohol and other drugs is most common among urban African American males.

African Americans tend to drink heavily or not at all.

Among drinkers, African American men are less likely to be heavy drinkers than Caucasian men; the reverse is true of female drinkers—African American women are more likely to be heavy drinkers than Caucasian women. However, both African American men and women have higher rates of abstention. African American women over 60 use few psychoactive substances of any kind. African American alcoholics often feel uncomfortable at Alcoholics Anonymous meetings dominated by Caucasians, and the AA program is most successful for them when developed within African American communities.

Twice as many African American senior high school students abstain from drugs as Caucasians students. Furthermore, African American students who do drink consume less alcohol and drink less frequently than Caucasian students. However, more of the African American abstainers do report using marijuana than the white abstainers.

African Americans, especially African American males, are at high risk for certain alcohol-related illnesses, particularly cirrhosis of the liver, fatty liver, and hepatitis. They have an extremely high incidence of cancer of the esophagus, with incidence rates several times those of whites. Alcohol is considered to be a major causal factor in this type of cancer [1, 2, 4].

Hispanic Americans

There are about 52 million Hispanics in the United States, about 16.7% of the total population. Hispanic youth are the fastest growing ethnic minority age group in America.

Hispanic Americans are a heterogenous group with diverse cultural, national, and racial backgrounds. They come from Columbian, Cuban, Dominican, Puerto Rican, and Mexican backgrounds.

The rate of illicit drug use in the past month among Hispanic individuals ages 12 and up was 8.9%, while the national average was 10.2%. The rate of binge alcohol use among Hispanics within this age group was 24.7%. Alcohol use in the last year among Hispanic youth ages 12–17 was 23.9%. About 3.3% of this population had a co-occurring mental health and substance use disorder. Hispanic youth often drop out of school because of substance abuse.

Hispanic men have relatively high rates of alcoholism, while Hispanic women have high rates of abstention. Psychoactive drug use among Hispanic women increases with age; those over 60 tend to use minor tranquilizers more than other women and to use them with greater frequency. Mexican American men have both the highest rate of abstention and the highest level of heavy drinking when compared with Hispanics of Cuban, Puerto Rican, or other Latin American origin. Mexican American women also drink more heavily than women in other groups but also have a high rate of abstention [1, 2, 5].

Diagnosis

Diagnosis of substance dependence in ethnic minority groups obeys the principles outlined in Chap. 13. It may be somewhat complicated by language barriers and by cultural influences among the various ethnic groups and subgroups. Remember that many of the assessment instruments and psychological tests in use today were developed on white, middle-class adult norms and may not be as reliable when used with other populations [6].

Treatment

Treatment of individuals belonging to ethnic minority groups obeys the principles outlined in Chap. 14. Treatment, like diagnosis, may be somewhat complicated by language barriers and by cultural factors. The use of written assignments may be a problem if a patient's English is poor.

The typical family session and group process must be adapted when necessary to cultures in which the young do not speak out in front of elders or in which women and men do not easily discuss their problems together.

Many minority members feel strongly about discrimination and prejudice, and their attitudes may influence their interactions with members of the treatment team. It should be kept in mind that each patient who is a member of an ethnic minority group is an individual. That individual's ethnic beliefs should be assessed and not merely assumed [6–8].

Recovery

The same recovery principles apply to ethnic minority groups as the general population, as discussed in Chap. 15. In certain neighborhoods, 12-step group meetings are often geared toward a particular ethnic or racial group. This phenomenon occurs because of the density of that group living in the area.

Physicians should realize that substance abuse is a significant problem in all cultures, be willing to work with patients and their families to get patients into treatment despite the barrier that language difficulty and cultural differences may pose, and be a part of patients' long-term recovery.

Co-occurring Disorder Patients

Co-occurring disorders, formerly known as dual diagnosis, refers to patients who have both a substance use disorder and a psychiatric disorder that is independent of the substance use. Patients with substance use disorders and a psychiatric disorder resulting from the substance use are not considered to have a co-occurring disorder.

About a third of all people experiencing mental illnesses also suffer from substance dependence. Men are more likely to develop a co-occurring disorder than women are. Other people who have a particularly high risk of co-occurring disorder include individuals of lower socioeconomic status, military veterans, and people with more general medical illnesses [9, 10].

Secondary Versus Primary Psychiatric Disorders

All psychoactive substances affect the brain and change patients' levels of functioning. Therefore, it is not surprising that alcohol and other drugs can produce alterations in mood and interfere with the ability to reason and with the content of thinking. Patients abusing alcohol or other drugs may be depressed, anxious, confused, or psychotic. The problem is to decide if these disorders occur secondarily to the substance use or if they occur independently of it. Psychiatric disorders occurring independently of substance abuse are said to be primary disorders. The distinction between primary and secondary psychiatric disorders is made by the history of the time course of the disorders. The one that appeared first is called primary, and the one that appeared second is called secondary. When the first disorder is substance dependence, it is highly likely that psychiatric symptoms will improve rapidly within a few days to weeks after patients stop using alcohol or other drugs.

A protracted withdrawal syndrome can occur, with psychiatric and other symptoms persisting for months after cessation of use. Benzodiazepines are the most notable drug for inducing prolonged withdrawal effects, with symptoms sometimes persisting for up to a year after cessation of use [11–16].

Primary Psychiatric Disorders

Co-occurring mental illness and substance dependence involve people with mental illness who also use alcohol or other drugs. Co-occurring mental health conditions and substance use disorders affect nearly 7.9 million Americans each year. Of those, only 7.4% receive appropriate treatment. Of all people diagnosed with a primary mental illness, 29% abuse either alcohol or other drugs. Conversely, 37% of alcohol abusers and 53% of those who abuse other drugs also have at least one serious primary mental illness [17].

Common examples of co-occurring disorders include major depression with cocaine dependence, panic disorder with alcohol dependence, schizophrenia with polydrug dependence, and borderline personality disorder with benzodiazepine dependence.

The self-medication theory suggests that people with severe mental illnesses misuse substances to relieve a specific set of symptoms or counter the negative side effects of antipsychotic medication. Nicotine dependence highlights the striking relationship between addiction and mental illness. Mentally ill individuals are about twice as likely to smoke as others are; although they comprise an estimated 28% of the population, they consume about 44% of all cigarettes smoked. Rates of smoking are particularly high (75–95%) among people with schizophrenia [18].

Diagnosis

Primary care physicians need to differentiate between primary and secondary disorders because the overall course of the illness is best predicted by its primary diagnosis. Primary alcoholism, for instance, has a better prognosis than primary antisocial personality disorder. If possible, the physician should wait for the secondary disorder to clear before making the diagnosis of a primary psychiatric disorder and initiating treatment [19].

The mental health problems that most commonly co-occur with substance dependence are depression, anxiety disorders, and bipolar disorder.

Schuckit recommends the following steps when confronted with a patient who fulfills criteria for a psychiatric disorder and who, at the same time, meets the criteria for substance dependence [20]:

1. Gather the best information possible from the patient and from resource people.
2. Try to establish whether the psychiatric disorder occurred before the onset of the substance abuse or was present during a period of extended abstinence.
3. If the psychiatric disorder is seen only in the context of substance abuse, the chances are ten to one that, with abstinence, the symptoms will markedly improve within a matter of days to weeks.
4. When the psychiatric disorder does not disappear with time or when there is evidence that it is independent of substance abuse, treatment of the psychiatric syndrome must be considered.
5. Patients with primary psychiatric disorders, such as manic-depressive illness or schizophrenia, will require psychiatric medication for an extended period of time.

Treatment

At one time, treatment for substance dependence was considered to be separate from treatment for mental health disorders, and care was delivered at different facilities using different therapeutic approaches. As a result, many people who suffered from depression, schizophrenia, obsessive-compulsive disorder, bipolar disorder, or other serious psychiatric conditions never received treatment for their substance abuse. Similarly, many people who suffered from substance dependence never received adequate treatment for their mental illness.

Having a disorder like bipolar disorder, depression, or schizophrenia as well as a substance dependence problem is no longer considered a reason for excluding patients from substance dependence treatment. At the same time, patients who abuse alcohol or other drugs should not be excluded from needed psychiatric treatment because of the substance use disorder. Today, addiction specialists and mental health clinicians view co-occurring disorders treatment as a unique field in its own right. Ideally, the two conditions should be treated together.

After making a definite diagnosis of a primary psychiatric disorder with a secondary substance use disorder, treatment should be initiated with antidepressants, lithium, or other appropriate drugs. When their psychiatric symptoms are under control, patients can participate in treatment for substance dependence as outlined in Chap. 15.

Treatment for co-occurring disorders begins with a complete neuropsychological evaluation to determine the patient's needs, identify his personal strengths, and find potential barriers to recovery. Using this information, the treatment team can develop a plan of care that addresses the patient's substance abuse and mental illness concurrently.

Some patients already may be aware of having a psychiatric diagnosis when they are admitted to a treatment facility. Others may receive a diagnosis of mental illness for the first time.

To treat both conditions successfully, a facility's mental health and recovery services must be integrated. A patient with a serious mental illness who is treated only for addiction is likely either to drop out of treatment early or to experience a relapse of either psychiatric symptoms or substance abuse.

Integrated recovery plans are designed to overcome the negative side effects of the psychiatric disorder, such as a reduced attention span, a low level of motivation, and a fear of socializing with others. Medication therapy is more effective when the pharmacological plan addresses the psychiatric disorder as well as the substance dependence disorder. The traditional hesitations about prescribing psychotherapeutic medications are no longer an issue.

Group therapy for people with co-occurring disorders offers a stronger support network for individuals who are struggling with psychiatric disorders as well as substance dependence. It allows patients to address their unique relapse triggers, such as depression, mood swings, and panic attacks.

Psychotherapy is almost always a large part of an effective co-occurring disorder treatment plan. Education on the person's illness, and how his beliefs and behaviors influence his thoughts, improves the symptoms of both the psychiatric disorder and the substance use disorder.

Cognitive behavioral therapy in particular is effective in helping people with co-occurring disorders to learn how to cope and to change ineffective patterns of thinking [21–24].

Aftercare

Aftercare for both the psychiatric disorder and the substance use disorder is crucial. Finding one support group that satisfies both needs may not be possible. Some individuals attend one of the 12-step support groups for their substance dependence and a therapist-facilitated support group for their psychiatric disorder.

Although not widely available, support groups for individuals with co-occurring disorders can be very helpful. One such support group is Double Trouble in Recovery.

Double Trouble in Recovery (DTR) is a support group that follows a 12-step approach to recovery, which has evolved from the original Twelve Steps of Alcoholics Anonymous. Only Step 1 and Step 12 are changed.

Step 1. "We admitted we were powerless over mental disorders and substance abuse—that our lives had become unmanageable."

Step 12. "Having had a spiritual awakening as the result of these steps, we tried to carry this message to other dually-diagnosed people and to practice these principles in all our affairs."

People with co-occurring disorders can benefit from attending peer support groups, and they also can benefit from connecting with others who have these co-occurring disorders and are in recovery [25].

LGBT Patients

The true number of people who identify themselves as lesbian, gay, bisexual, and transsexual individuals is not known. Because of a lack of research focusing on the LGBT population and the mistrust that makes many LGBT people afraid to be open about their identity, reliable data are difficult to obtain. However, in the United States, it is estimated that 9.8% of men and 5% of women report some same-gender sexual behavior since puberty and 2.8% of men and 1.4% of women report a homosexual or bisexual identity. The data on the number of transgender people are even more limited [26].

Not every person with a homosexual or bisexual orientation, as indicated by his or her fantasies, engages in homosexual behavior.

The LGBT community suffers from a higher rate of substance use disorders than the heterosexual population. An estimated 55% of gay men struggle with substance use. Twenty to twenty-five percent of gay men and lesbians are heavy alcohol users (compared with three to ten percent of the heterosexuals).

Although LGBT persons use alcohol and other drugs, certain drugs seem to be more popular in the LGBT community than in the majority community. Gay men and men who have sex with men are significantly more likely to have used marijuana, psychedelics, hallucinogens, stimulants, sedatives, cocaine, barbiturates, and MDMA and are much more likely to have used nitrites (poppers). Abuse of methamphetamine has increased dramatically in recent years among some segments of the LGBT community. Party drugs, such as MDMA, ketamine, and GHB, are increasing in popularity among some segments of the LGBT population. Party drugs are often used during circuit parties and raves, and they can impair judgment and result in risky sexual behaviors.

Some LGBT methamphetamine users inject the drug, putting them at risk for HIV and hepatitis C [27].

LGBT Issues

Many factors contribute to the role of substance use in LGBT people. Legal prohibitions against LGBT behavior and discrimination have limited LGBT people's social outlets to bars, private homes, or clubs where alcohol and drugs often play a prominent role. Growing up in a society that says they should not exist and certainly should not act on their sexual feelings, LGBT patients may have internalized this homophobia. LGBT people may be victims of antigay violence and hate crimes, such as verbal and physical attacks.

It is important that substance abuse counselors have training and education to deal with problems associated with emotional challenges, such as rejection and isolation surrounding the process of coming out; fears of physical violence, prejudice, and discrimination; and strong sense of shame, particularly among those LGBT individuals who lack family support and have low self-esteem from feeling different or not being accepted by friends and family.

Counselor training and education should include the ability to deal with problems associated with pressure to fit into the LGBT party scene or subculture; past emotional trauma, often in the form of physical, sexual, or verbal abuse; bullying and harassment by peers, especially during adolescence; and high rates of depression and anxiety, often prompted by the stigma of being gay.

Patients who used substances to medicate their negative feelings about being gay or lesbian may need help to work through those feelings. Since many LGBT individuals struggle with depression, anxiety, and addictions, dual diagnosis treatment is an important part of the recovery process.

Counselors may be the first people to tell individual gays who abuse substances that they are okay and that an important part of recovery may be to explore who they are.

Patients with issues related to HIV/AIDS may need a facility that provides medication management and additional therapeutic support.

You cannot tell if someone is transgender just by looking at him or her. Transgender people do not all look a certain way or come from the same background, and many may not appear visibly trans. It is not possible to look around a room and see if there are any transgender people. You should assume that there may be transgender people at any gathering. Don't make assumptions about a transgender person's sexual orientation. Gender identity is different than sexual orientation.

Sexual orientation is about whom a person is attracted to; gender identity is about the person's own personal sense of being male or female (or someone outside that binary). Transgender people can be gay, lesbian, bisexual, or straight [28, 29].

Avoid backhanded compliments like [30]:

- "I would have never known you were transgender. You look so pretty."
- "You look just like a real woman."
- "She's so gorgeous, I would have never guessed she was transgender."
- "He's so hot, I'd date him even though he's transgender."
- "You're so brave."

- "You'd pass so much better if you wore less/ more makeup."
- "You'd pass so much better if you had a better wig."
- "Have you considered a voice coach?"

In short, be professional.

Diagnosis

The diagnosis of substance dependence in an LGBT individual is the same as for a heterosexual individual as discussed in Chap. 14.

Treatment

The most effective drug rehabilitation programs for lesbian, gay, bisexual, and transgendered individuals are gay-friendly programs that offer specialized support. The ideal program is culturally sensitive, employs LGBT-sensitive staff, honors a culture of diversity, and has contacts with LGBT self-help support groups and related resources.

By participating in an LGBT-friendly drug rehabilitation program, patients are more likely to feel understood, supported, and accepted and are less likely to leave treatment early.

There are a number of centers that are gay friendly, but one may not be available locally. These centers incorporate all of the traditional drug rehabilitation components, such as counseling, life skills training, relapse prevention planning, and aftercare, but with an emphasis on personal identity, family dynamics, a social support network, and the internal turmoil that leads to substance abuse [31, 32].

HIV-Positive Patients

An estimated 1.2 million people in the United States were living with HIV at the end of 2013, the most recent year for which this information is available. Of those people, about 13% did not know they were infected. In 2015, 39,513 people were diagnosed with HIV infection in the United States. The number of new HIV diagnoses fell 19% from 2005 to 2014. In 2014, there were 12,333 deaths of people with diagnosed AIDS [33].

Most cases of HIV infection have occurred through one of four routes. The most common mode of transmission is sexual contact, which is responsible for 75% of AIDS cases. Transmission by intravenous drug use occurs through contaminated needles or paraphernalia. Blood and blood products can also transmit the infection, as can infected mothers to newborns.

HIV and AIDS patients suffering concurrent substance use issues need immediate intervention and treatment. Continuing substance use increases the transmission of HIV through risky sexual and drug-taking behaviors, as well as exacerbating the psychological challenges facing these patients.

Patients with HIV/AIDS and substance use disorders present complex challenges to addiction professionals. However, treatment needs to take place with an understanding of the unique issues and challenges of substance users with HIV and AIDS [34].

The Centers for Disease Control and Prevention (CDC) recommends that people who inject drugs or engage in other behaviors that put them at increased risk for becoming infected with HIV get tested for HIV at least once every year. The CDC also recommends that sexual partners of those who inject drugs get tested at least once per year [35].

It has become clear that drug treatment programs can play an important role in reaching HIV-positive individuals. However, for them to be successful, program staff members must overcome their fears of AIDS through education about the disease, sharing feelings with colleagues, learning from other programs, finding and using all available resources, and remembering that fear is usually of the unknown. Practical experience with the feared agent generally reduces the fear or eliminates it [36].

Risk Factors

HIV-infected blood can get into drug solutions used for injection by reusing blood-contaminated syringes to prepare drugs; reusing water used to rinse the syringes; reusing bottle caps, spoons, or other containers ("cookers") to dissolve drugs and to heat drug solutions; and reusing small pieces of cotton or cigarette filters to filter out particles that could block the needle.

Street sellers of syringes may repackage used syringes and sell them as sterile syringes. For this reason, people who inject drugs should get syringes from reliable sources of sterile syringes, such as pharmacies or needle exchange programs.

It is important to know that sharing a needle or syringe for skin popping or injecting steroids, hormones, or silicone can put a person at risk for HIV and other blood-borne infections.

The use of amyl nitrite (poppers) also has been associated with increased HIV risk. Poppers are sometimes used in anal sex because they relax the anal sphincter. They have long been linked to risky sexual behaviors, illegal drug use, and sexually transmitted infections among gay and bisexual men [37].

Substance Dependence Treatment

The substance-dependent, HIV-positive patient must deal with two potentially fatal diseases. One cannot be adequately treated without dealing with the other. Standard treatment techniques should be used for substance dependence.

The involvement of outside case workers and doctors will need to be incorporated into the treatment plan, and there needs an awareness of the pharmaceutical requirements of these patients, as well as any pharmaceutical side effect issues.

Confidentiality, critical to all aspects of substance dependence treatment, is particularly important with these patients. They must continue their HIV/AIDS medications in treatment [9].

Treatment goals for HIV-positive individuals include clarifying their particular HIV status, impelling change to reduce the risk of their transmitting the virus to others and to reduce the progression of their disease, and instilling in them a hope for lives with quality.

Patients who are known to be HIV positive or those in whom the diagnosis is made after they are admitted to treatment program should be assessed for their understanding of what their particular condition does and does not mean, their awareness of safe and unsafe interactions with others, and their knowledge of healthy living strategies [37].

An important aspect of treating substance-dependent patients who are HIV positive includes an education about the history of AIDS, how transmission occurs, how the virus works, the difference between the carrier state, the progression of the disease, testing information (ELISA and Western blot), viral load test, and how to prevent HIV infection.

Counseling HIV-positive patients involves assessment, developing treatment goals, treating the psychosocial aspects of the condition, and planning for referral to community resources [9].

Developing Treatment Goals

Treatment goals for HIV-positive individuals include clarifying their particular AIDS-related condition and impelling change to reduce the risk of their transmitting the virus to others and to reduce the progression of their disease [37]. Substance dependence treatment goals are the same as for non-HIV-positive patients as discussed in Chap. 15.

Psychosocial Treatment

Upon learning of seropositive test results, patients tend to progress through three adjustment stages: (1) the initial crisis stage, (2) a transitional stage, and (3) the acceptance stage [38].

Crisis Stage The *crisis stage* occurs when patients first learn that they are seropositive. This is essentially a state of shock and denial. Another characteristic of this stage is the disruptive impact it has on patients' supportive relationships. The diagnosis of HIV infection may force people to disclose previously undisclosed drug use or sexual orientation, as well as subjecting patients to the stigma associated with having AIDS. For most patients in drug treatment programs, family relationships are already strained, if not severed.

Patients in crisis tend to have difficulty hearing and retaining information and may distort what they hear about their condition. For this reason, they should be assessed later for how much knowledge about HIV infection they have retained, and the information should be repeated if they have forgotten or confused some of it. The primary treatment goal of the crisis stage is to guide patients through denial, allowing it to run its course. The main treatment strategies are empathy, education, and reassurance. For preventive reasons, health-care workers address the question of whom should be informed about the patients' HIV infection; usually this involves patients' sex partners, physicians, and dentists.

Transitional Stage The *transitional stage* begins when alternating waves of anger, guilt, self-pity, and anxiety supersede denial. Treatment during this stage focuses on helping patients deal with these reactions. The strategy used is to allow patients to freely ventilate their distress and confusion and to be guided through these feelings. Empathy and reassurance continue to be appropriate.

Acceptance Stage The *acceptance stage* occurs when patients come to accept the limitations that their HIV status impose on them and realize that they can still manage their lives by reacting more with reason than emotion. They accept their condition and begin to integrate it into their lives.

Recovery

Long-term sobriety and harm reduction best occur when recovering HIV patients continue with comprehensive aftercare under the supervision of a case management worker. The best aftercare regimen continues to be peer group and individual therapy with case management that may include social assistance, such as housing and employment, when appropriate. Support group attendance is also important for this group. Keeping physician appointments is extremely important [9].

Risk Reduction

Patients should be encouraged to stay in treatment and lead lives of recovery. If they should relapse, they should avoid intravenous drugs. If they use IV drugs, they should not share needles, syringes, or paraphernalia. If they share needles, they should sterilize them before each use with alcohol or diluted household bleach and rinse them with clean water. They should avoid shooting galleries.

Patients should avoid sex with promiscuous individuals, should use condoms for intercourse, should avoid anal sex, and should limit the number of sex partners.

General health practices include being cautious about exposure to HIV, improving nutrition, getting proper exercise and rest, and reducing stress. Women at high risk for HIV infection, including sexual partners of risk-group men, should avoid pregnancy unless they seek HIV testing and medical advice first [37–39].

Community Resources

Once patients are in treatment for substance dependence, treatment staff should plan to get them to needed resources in the community. Physicians who specialize in infectious diseases should be consulted. Mental health care for patients suffering severe depression or suicidal tendencies should be arranged. It may be necessary to help AIDS patients arrange for financial assistance through Supplemental Security Income (SSI). In addition, many patients upon discharge will need help with housing, and some will need legal counsel. For example, divorced or separated partners may deny patients' child visitation rights, or unknowledgeable employers may dismiss them on learning of test results even if patients can perform their jobs and have acceptable work histories. Finally, patients should be put in touch with various community support groups for AIDS-related conditions [37].

Patient Needs

Critical to patients' progress is their significant others' knowledge about AIDS-related conditions, the course of the disease, how the virus is transmitted, and practices to ensure safe contact. For a patient's continued health, family members may need to make behavior changes to support patient treatment goals. Family members should be assessed for their understanding the patient's condition, making needed behavioral changes, coping with the array of adjustment reactions, capabilities of supporting the treatment plan outlined for the patient, and assisting with medical and other community resources. A primary strategy is to involve a key support person at the earliest possible opportunity [37].

Family Needs

Family includes not only conventional members by virtue of blood or legal connection but also such others as ongoing sexual and/or drug-using partners, living mates, and friends with whom patients have established meaningful bonds. These individuals will be affected by a patient's condition. Issues will center on patient needs for family support and family needs resulting from the patient's condition.

Needle-sharing associates and sex partners of HIV-infected patients should be assessed for likely risk of past exposure with HIV antibody testing. Family members may need to make behavior changes to support patient treatment goals for the patient's continued health.

Family members should be assessed for their potential for their understanding of the patient's condition, ability to make needed behavioral changes, ability to cope with the array of adjustment reactions, capabilities of supporting the treatment plan outlined for the patient, and assisting with medical and other community resources.

Goals for the family include promoting behavioral change toward healthy, non-risky practices and developing the ability to cope psychosocially with a patient's condition and their response to it [37].

Summary

Race refers to a person's physical characteristics, such as bone structure and skin, hair, or eye color. Ethnic describes a group of people sharing a common background, language, and identity.

American Indians and Alaska Natives experience some of the highest rates of substance abuse compared to other US racial or ethnic groups. Most research on Indian substance abuse has been conducted on reservations—virtually none has been done on urban Indians.

Asian Americans, who make up less than 2% of the population of the United States, have low levels of alcohol and drug use. There appear to be significant differences in psychoactive substance use among Asian Americans of different origins.

Abuse of alcohol and other drugs is most common among urban African American males. Twice as many African American senior high school students abstain from drugs as Caucasian students.

Hispanic men have relatively high rates of alcoholism, while Hispanic women have high rates of abstention. Psychoactive drug use among Hispanic women increases with age; those over 60 tend to use minor tranquilizers more than other women and to use them with greater frequency.

About a third of all people experiencing mental illnesses also suffer from substance dependence.

Primary substance use disorder must be differentiated from secondary substance use disorder.

The LGBT community suffers from a higher rate of substance use disorders than the heterosexual population. Patients who used substances to medicate their negative feelings about being gay or lesbian may need help to work through those feelings.

The substance-dependent, HIV-positive patient must deal with two potentially fatal diseases. One cannot be adequately treated without dealing with the other. Standard treatment techniques should be used for substance dependence. HIV and AIDS patients suffering concurrent substance use issues need immediate intervention and treatment.

References

1. Drug abuse among racial/ethnic minorities. National Institute on Drug Abuse (NIDA) website. https://archives.drugabuse.gov/pdf/minorities03.pdf. September 2003.
2. Racial and ethnic minority populations. Substance Abuse and Mental Health Services Administration

(SAMHSA) website. https://www.samhsa.gov/specific-populations/racial-ethnic-minority. February 18, 2016.
3. Beauvais F, LeBoueff S. Drug and alcohol abuse intervention in American Indian communities. Int J Addict. 1985;20(1):139–71.
4. Primm BJ. Drug use: special implications for black America. In: The state of black America. New York: National Urban League; 1987. p. 145–58.
5. Schinke SP, Moncher MS, Palleja J, Zayas LH, Schilling RF. Hispanic youth, substance abuse and stress: implications for prevention research. Int J Addict. 1988;20(8):809–26.
6. Spicer J. Counseling ethnic minorities. Center City: Hazelden; 1989.
7. Schmidt L, Greenfield T, Mulia N. Unequal treatment: racial and ethnic disparities in alcoholism treatment services. National Institute on Drug Abuse (NIDA) website. http://pubs.niaaa.nih.gov/publications/arh291/49-54.htm
8. Hanson B. Drug treatment effectiveness: the case of racial and ethnic minorities in America: some research questions and proposals. Int J Addict. 1985;20(1):99–137.
9. Milhorn HT. Chemical dependence: diagnosis, prevention, and treatment. New York: Springer-Verlag; 1990.
10. Dual diagnosis. National Alliance on Mental Illness (NAMI) website. https://www.nami.org/Learn-More/Mental-Health-Conditions/Related-Conditions/Dual-Diagnosis
11. Menicucci LD, Wermuth L, Sorensen J. Treatment physicians' assessment of dual-prognosis patients: diagnosis, treatment, referral, and family involvement. Int J Addict. 1988;23(6):617–22.
12. Schuckit MA. Dual diagnoses: psychiatric pictures among substance abusers. Drug Abuse and Alcoholism Newsletter. Vista Hill Foundation; 1988.
13. Baldacchino A, Balfour DJ, Passetti F, Humphris G, Matthews K. Neuropsychological consequences of chronic opioid use: a quantitative review and meta-analysis. Neurosci Biobehav Rev. 2012;36(9):2056–68.
14. Baldacchino A, Hughes Z, Kehoe M, et al. Cannabis psychosis: examining the evidence for a distinctive psychopathology in a systematic and narrative review. Am J Addict. 2012;21(Suppl 1):S88–98.
15. Baldacchino A, Arvapalli V, Oshun A, Tolomeo S. Substance-induced mental disorders. In: el-Guebaly N, Carrà G, Galanter M, editors. Textbook of addiction treatment: international perspectives. Milano: Springer-Verlag Italia; 2015.
16. Substance or medication induced psychotic disorder. In: Arlington: American Psychiatric Association (APA); 2013.
17. Saisan J, Smith M, Segal J. Substance abuse and co-occurring disorders. Help Guide website. https://helpguide.org/articles/addiction/substance-abuse-and-mental-health.htm. December 2016.
18. Addiction and co-occurring mental disorders. National Institute of Drug Abuse (NIDA) website. https://www.drugabuse.gov/news-events/nida-notes/2007/02/addiction-co-occurring-mental-disorders. February 1, 2007.
19. Wilford B. Psychiatric disorders. In: Review course syllabus. New York: American Medical Society on Alcoholism and Other Drug Dependencies; 1987. p. 263–72.
20. Schuckit MA. Evaluating the dual-diagnosis patient. Drug Abuse and Alcoholism Newsletter. Vista Hill Foundation; December 1989.
21. Rozensky RH, Neirick B, Slotnick GM, Morse D. Discriminating between substance abusers with single and dual diagnoses using MMPI profiles and the MacAndrews Alcoholism Scale: Axis I and Axis II subtypes. Psychol Rep. 1988;63(3):985–6.
22. Daley DC, Moss HB, Campbell F. Dual disorders: counseling clients with chemical dependence and mental illness. Center City: Hazelden; 1987.
23. Co-occurring disorders treatment. Dual diagnosis website. http://www.dualdiagnosis.org/co-occurring-Disorders-Treatment
24. Evans K, Sullivan JM. Dual diagnosis, counseling the mentally ill substance abuser. New York: The Guilford Press; 1990.
25. Vogel HS, Knight E, Laudet AB, Magura S. Double trouble in recovery: self-help for people with dual diagnoses. Psychiatr Rehabil J. 1998;21(4):356–64.
26. Basic statistics. Centers for Disease Control and Prevention (CDC) website. https://www.cdc.gov/hiv/basics/statistics.html. November 30, 2016.
27. Michaels S. The prevalence of homosexuality in the United States. In: Cabaj RP, Stein TS, editors. Textbook of homosexuality and mental health. Washington, DC: American Psychiatric Press; 1996. p. 43–63.
28. A physician's introduction to substance abuse treatment for lesbian, gay, bisexual, and transgender individuals. Substance Abuse and Mental Health Services Administration (SAMHSA): Center for Substance Abuse Treatment website. http://store.samhsa.gov/shin/content//SMA12-4104/SMA12-4104.pdf. August 2012.
29. Redding B. LGBT substance use – beyond statistics. Soc Work Today. 2014;14(4):8.
30. Tips for allies of transgender people. GLAAD website. http://www.glaad.org/transgender/allies. May 2015.
31. Green CA. Gender and use of substance abuse treatment services. National Institute on Alcohol Abuse and Alcoholism (NIAAA) website. http://pubs.niaaa.nih.gov/publications/arh291/55-62.htm
32. Grant JE. Substance abuse treatment for lesbian, gay, bisexual, transgender individuals. University of Minnesota School of Medicine website. http://www.888betsoff.com/links/08_presentations/7A.pdf
33. Substance abuse/use. AIDS.gov website. https://www.aids.gov/hiv-aids-basics/prevention/reduce-your-risk/substance-abuse-use/index.html. December 30, 2016.

34. Amin NM. Acquired immunodeficiency syndrome, part 1: epidemiology, history, and etiology. Fam Pract Recertification. 1987;9:36–58.
35. Battjes RJ, Leukefeld CG, Pickens RW, Haverkos HW. The acquired immunodeficiency syndrome and intravenous drug abuse. Bull Narc. 1988;40(1):21–34.
36. Martin EG, Wang KH. Integrating substance abuse treatment into HIV care. J Acquir Immune Defic Syndr. 2013;62(4):421–9.
37. Sulima JP. What every drug abuse counselor should know about AIDS. Washington, DC: Manisses Communications Group; 1987.
38. Stages of HIV infection. AIDS.gov website. https://www.aids.gov/hiv-aids-basics/just-diagnosed-with-hiv-aids/hiv-in-your-body/stages-of-hiv/index.html. August 27, 2015.
39. Jewell ME, Jewell GS. How to assess the risk of HIV exposure. Am Fam Physician. 1989;40(1):153–61.

23 The Impaired Physician

Key Chapter Points

- In 1973, the American Medical Association's Council on Mental Health defined impairment in physicians as "the inability to practice medicine with reasonable skill and safety to patients by reasons of physical or mental illness, including alcoholism or drug dependence."
- Most physicians who abuse substances continue to function fairly well until the problem is far advanced.
- There are six areas in physicians' lives where clues to their chemical dependence can be found: (1) community involvement, (2) family life, (3) employment patterns, (4) physical status, (5) office conduct, and (6) hospital duties.
- Although nearly one-third of physicians are female, nearly 90% of physicians referred for substance use disorder treatment are male.
- Nearly all state medical societies and state licensing boards have a physician health program (PHP) for dealing with impaired physicians.
- The Federation of State Physician Health Programs (FSPHP) is a nonprofit organization that serves as a forum for information exchange among the various state programs.
- The AMA's Code of Medical Ethics states that "physicians have an ethical obligation to report impaired, incompetent and unethical colleagues" and lists several guidelines to follow.
- Typically, the substance-dependent physician is more dysfunctional (physiologically, psychologically, socially, spiritually) than nonphysicians.
- Treatment often is divided into three phases: (1) inpatient, (2) halfway house, and (3) mirror imaging.
- When a structured aftercare program is undertaken, the success rate increases to approximately 90%.

In 1973, the American Medical Association's Council on Mental Health defined impairment in physicians as "the inability to practice medicine with reasonable skill and safety to patients by reasons of physical or mental illness, including alcoholism or drug dependence."

Identification of the impaired physician is essential because patient safety may be at stake, and untreated substance dependence may lead to loss of license, serious health problems, and even death.

Physicians frequently begin using alcohol or other drugs to self-medicate their own stress. They may have compulsive personality traits, marked by a triad of self-doubt, guilt over perceived deficiencies, and an excessive sense of responsibility. These traits are often combined with a low intrinsic sense of self-worth because physicians typically identify their self-worth with what they do rather than who they are [1].

Most of the risk factors for physician substance abuse are similar to those of the general public. However, among the strongest physician-specific predispositions to developing substance

H.T. Milhorn, *Substance Use Disorders*, DOI 10.1007/978-3-319-63040-3_23

abuse are (1) self-treatment with prescription medications, (2) high stress or long hours of practice, and (3) easy or constant access to controlled substances [2].

Prevalence of Use

The prevalence of substance dependence among physicians is difficult to ascertain and probably will remain that way since many impaired physicians are not identified and treated and some have entered treatment voluntarily and confidentially, never coming to the attention of the licensure board.

Conservative estimates are that 8–12% of physicians will develop a substance abuse problem at some point in their careers. At any given time, as many as 7% of practicing physicians may have a substance use disorder [2].

Alcohol is the most commonly abused substance among physicians. Compared with the general population, physicians have higher rates of prescription drug abuse, particularly benzodiazepines and opioids. This is because of the common practice of self-treatment and the ease of access to many drugs [3].

Minor differences exist in the incidence of abuse in certain medical subspecialties, with emergency medicine, psychiatry, and anesthesiology, having slightly higher rates of abuse than other specialties [2].

Characteristics of the Impaired Physician

Most physicians possess a strong drive for achievement, they tend to be very conscientious, and they have an ability to deny personal problems. Although these attributes are advantageous for success in medicine, they may predispose to impairment.

Most physicians who abuse substances continue to function fairly well until the problem is far advanced. Alcoholics, for instance, can often remain sober during working hours for many years, even though they drink large amounts of alcohol at night and on weekends. Intravenous opioid or cocaine abusers, on the other hand, may go from use to dependence in a matter of weeks to months [2].

Identifying impaired physicians is difficult, primarily because of two factors: (1) the conspiracy of silence among professionals and other people in physicians' lives and (2) self-deception in impaired physicians. Talbott and Benson presented six areas in physicians' lives where clues to their chemical dependence can be found: (1) community involvement, (2) family life, (3) employment patterns, (4) physical status, (5) office conduct, and (6) hospital duties. The areas become involved sequentially, although two or three may seem to be involved simultaneously. The last area affected is the medical setting—hospitals, staff rounds, emergency departments, and medical society meeting [4].

Community Involvement

Isolation and withdrawal from the community and its activities often signal the onset of chemical dependence in physicians. Talbott and Benson described the "*target syndrome*" in which successive rings of involvement (community activities, leisure activities, church, friends, peers, distant family, nuclear family) are peeled away until only the center of the target, the physician, remains. The community and friends gradually lose respect for the physician and lose confidence in his emotional stability.

The impaired physician becomes isolated and withdrawal from community activities, leisure activities and hobbies, church, friends, and peers. He displays embarrassing behavior at clubs or parties and may have arrests for driving while intoxicated and other legal problems. He is unreliable and unpredictable in community and social activities. His behavior is unpredictable. He may develop inappropriate spending habits and excessive involvement in political activities [4].

Family Life

As part of the target syndrome, impaired physicians withdraw from family activities, relationships, and communication. They have unexplained absences from home. They may get into fights and may be guilty of child abuse. The children may become involved in abnormal, antisocial, and illegal behavior. Family fights may occur. The best way to identify impaired physicians is not to ask who drinks alcohol or uses other drugs addictively but instead to look at those physicians who are separated from their families or whose children have serious emotional, legal, or scholastic problems.

The spouse and children may have to assume surrogate roles due to the "absence" of the impaired physician.

Sexual problems—impotence, extramarital affairs, and contracultural sexual behavior—may occur. The spouse may physically leave him, and divorce proceedings may take place [1].

Employment Patterns

The impaired physician may have a history of making numerous job changes in the past 5 years. He may also make frequent geographic relocations for unexplained reasons (geographic cure). Unexplained intervals between jobs can also be a significant clue. Inappropriate jobs for a person's level of training may be another clue.

He may have hospitalizations for drug-related problems. His medical history may be complicated and elaborate. In job applications, he may give indefinite or inappropriate references, and he may be reluctant to let his spouse and children be interviewed. He also may be reluctant to undergo an immediate preemployment physical examination for fear that his liver enzymes will be found to be elevated or other signs of drug dependence will be discovered [4].

Physical Status

Next, physical signs and symptoms of the disease become evident. Poor personal hygiene and unkempt appearance in a previously well-dressed physician are strong clues. Deterioration in his clothing and dressing habits may develop.

Numerous and constant physical complaints, frequent visits to fellow physicians, multiple medications (often self-prescribed), and frequent hospitalizations may provide additional clues.

Repeated automobile accidents or accidents while on vacation or involved in hobbies or leisure activities may also provide evidence of chemical dependence, as may wide mood swings and emotional crises [4].

Office Conduct

Impaired physicians may arrive late or have unexplained and lengthy absences from their offices. They may have frequent "illnesses." They may have disrupted appointment schedules.

They may become angry, hostile, and inconsistent, prompting complaints from patients and, later, office staff. Physicians may give inappropriate orders and frequently lock themselves in their offices or bathrooms to use drugs. Talbott and Benson call this the *locked-door syndrome*.

They may order medications for themselves from local druggists or by mail or email. Patients may complain to the staff about the doctor's behavior [4].

Hospital Duties

The last place impaired physicians' problems become apparent is in the hospital. Making rounds at midnight, writing inappropriate orders, going into the wrong rooms, reading the wrong charts, writing more illegibly than usual, or writing inappropriate orders for medications can all be signs of substance dependence.

The impaired physician's behavior frequently changes, and he may be slow in responding to emergency room calls or not answer them at all. Hospital staff may notice slow, slurred speech and may report smelling alcohol on his breath. Impaired physicians may become involved in malpractice suits and legal sanctions against hospitals. Reports of behavioral changes from hospital personnel ("hospital gossip") may begin [4].

Artecona also compiled a list of characteristics that may help identify the impaired physician (Table 23.1 [5]).

Table 23.1 Characteristics of the impaired physician (Based on Artecona [5])

Altercations with staff, peers, and patients	Irresponsibility
Avoids departmental meetings, CME events, medical social events	Irritability, mood swings
Blackouts	Needle tracks
Bruises	Negative attitude, argumentative
Decreased performance	Odd hours for rounds, volunteers for graveyard shift, absent from doctor's lounge, eats alone
Deviation from standard procedures	Off-duty intoxication
Dilated or constricted pupils	Overreaction to criticism
Disheveled appearance	Personality change
Drug procedures (use of excessive amounts, unwitnessed wasting, insufficient patient analgesia, excessive spillage/breakage)	Prolonged lunch break
Frequent forgetfulness	Red, yellow, or black and blue eyes
Frequent illness	Slurred speech on phone
Frequent malpractice actions	Staff, patient, or peer complaints
Frequent tardiness, frequent absences	Subject of hospital gossip (marital problems, DUI, financial problems, party reputation)
Frequent trips to bathroom	Tremors
Hasty rounds	Unavailable when on call
Heavy drinking at staff or social functions	Unexplained intervals between jobs, frequent job changes, frequent relocations
Inaccessibility	Unusual medical history
Inadequate charting	
Inappropriate anger	
Inappropriate orders	
Indefinite references	

Impaired physicians don't seek help due to shame and guilt, and they are conditioned to maintain emotional control. Time demands of work make it hard to get care. They fear stigma and career impact, and they see themselves as healers—not among those who need healing.

Physicians who are abusing alcohol or other drugs work hard to keep their probable invisible. They become loners, avoiding colleagues and friends who might notice the effects of substance abuse. Suggestions that the physician's behavior or performance has changed are first met with explanations and later with avoidance or anger. The drug-abusing physician will often leave a job rather than risk being identified as impaired [2].

Differentiating substance abuse from clinical depression can also be difficult. A depressed colleague may not be outwardly depressed. As with the substance abuser, there may be irritability, apathy, or interpersonal strife. The physician's quality of work may decline because of sleep problems, fatigue, or poor concentration, and he may fall behind on record keeping and other administrative duties. Attempts to compensate for low productivity may result in working excessive hours or rounding at unusual times. The depressed physician may withdraw from participation in once enjoyable social activities and may exhibit an increased use of alcohol and drugs. Clearly, there is a considerable overlap between impairment by substances and depression [6].

The Impaired Woman Physician

Although nearly one-third of physicians are female, nearly 90% of physicians referred for substance use disorder treatment are male. Female physicians are more likely to suffer major depression and less likely to have a personality disorder or to have criminal consequences of their substance use problem. They are more likely to undergo treatment and more likely to have suffered permanent physical damage from their substance use than their male counterpart.

Female physicians also are more likely to have begun their substance use after a traumatic life event and to have a shorter course between the onset of drug use and the initiation of treatment. They are less likely to use illicit substances. They are more likely to take prescribed opioids and tranquilizers than their male counterparts [1].

Several studies have examined substance-dependent women in medicine. Bissell and Skorina examined the patterns of diagnosis, referral, and help-seeking behaviors of 95 alcoholic women in AA who had at least a year of sobriety. Addiction to drugs other than alcohol was common, with only 40% reporting addiction to alcohol alone. Nearly 77% reported serious suicide ideation prior to sobriety, 27.4% reported suicide ideation after stopping drinking, and 40% had actually made suicide attempts—15.8% of them more than once. Treatment experiences ranged from AA only (21%) to long-term resident treatment of 15 weeks or more (23%). Most had reached treatment by means other than referral by therapists or by impaired physician committees [7].

Martin and Talbott studied 37 female physicians who had been in treatment in the Georgia Impaired Physicians Program. This represented only 4.6% of all physicians in the program, despite the fact that nationally, at that time, women made up 13.4% of all physicians. The physicians tended to be high academic achievers, and many had mates who expected them to fit into traditional social and family roles. Many identified with self-effacing and nonassertive roles rather than with more powerful postures male physicians often identify with [8, 9].

Many of the issues of female physicians in treatment are the same as those of nonphysician women discussed in Chap. 15.

Physician Health Programs

Early Efforts

The American Medical Association (AMA) provided early leadership in the area of physician impairment. In 1972, the AMA House of Delegates adopted a policy statement declaring that any physician who became aware of an apparent problem in a colleague had the ethical responsibility to take affirmative action, that is, to seek treatment or rehabilitation for that physician [10].

In 1974 the AMA drafted model legislation that state legislatures could use in modifying individual medical practice acts to provide for the treatment and rehabilitation of impaired physicians. The response of state medical societies to those initiatives was dramatic [11, 12].

The Programs

Nearly all state medical societies and state licensing boards have a physician health program (PHP) for dealing with impaired physicians. State medical society programs typically offer impaired physicians confidential and nonpunitive assistance. If they refuse to cooperate in their own rehabilitation, some state medical associations report them to the state board of medical examiners. Some PHPs are run by independent nonprofit corporations and others by state medical societies; still others are under the aegis of state medical licensing boards. Some are well funded; others are not.

All shared information is treated confidentially and can be given without fear of retaliation. The PHP can serve as an advocate for the physician before the medical board. After the initial contact is made with the PHP, the organization will arrange for a comprehensive assessment of the physician to help identify a substance abuse problem or psychiatric illness.

If the PHP determines that an intervention is needed, a small group consisting of representatives from the PHP or local physician wellness committee, and sometimes colleagues, will meet with the physician and recommend a formal evaluation be done to determine if any treatment is necessary [11, 13].

Medical societies usually have mechanisms for confidential reporting of impairment. Reports may come from colleagues, hospital administrators, nurses, patients, or physicians' families. Once the information is verified, it is given to a committee member, or members, who is responsible for confronting physicians with evidence of their impairment and persuading them to enter treatment [14].

At the end of treatment, physicians enter into a contract with the PHP, which typically lasts for 5 years for substance dependence. Random urine drug screens are required with declining frequency. Members are required to attend 12-step support group meetings (AA, NA, CA) three to four times per week in the first 3 years and two to three times per week in the last 2 years. They also are required to attend a Caduceus meeting once a week. Group and/or individual therapy or treatment may be required for a minimum of 2 years. Workplace/practice monitoring is required.

Dupont et al. looked at 904 physician participants enrolled in the 16 PHPs. The physicians were predominantly male (86%). The average participant was 44 years old and married (63%).

Family medicine represented 20%, internal medicine 13%, anesthesiology 11%, emergency medicine 7%, and psychiatry 7%. The primary drugs of choice reported by these physicians were alcohol (50%), opioids (33%), stimulants (8%), and other substance (9%).

Fifty percent reported abusing more than one substance, and 14% reported a history of intravenous drug use. Seventeen percent had been arrested for an alcohol or other drug-related offense, and 9% had been convicted on those charges. Thirty-nine percent had a prior experience in addiction treatment, and 14% had experienced disciplinary action by their licensing agency prior to this episode of care [15].

Federation of State Physician Health Programs

The Federation of State Physician Health Programs (FSPHP) is a nonprofit organization that serves as a forum for information exchange among the various state programs.

The Federation of State Physician Health Programs evolved from the initiatives taken by the American Medical Association (AMA) and individual state physician health programs. It focuses on rehabilitation and monitoring of physicians with psychoactive substance use disorders as well as mental and physical illness [16].

Intervention by Confrontation

Directly questioning a physician about his substance abuse is rarely successful and will often lead to counter accusations, such as "You're out to get me" and "You are trying to ruin my practice [2]."

The AMA's Code of Medical Ethics states that "physicians have an ethical obligation to report impaired, incompetent and unethical colleagues" and lists several guidelines to follow. Before reporting impaired physicians to the state licensing board, the guidelines state that doctors should try to get an impaired colleague into a treatment program or contact their hospital's chief of staff [17].

However, in a survey by Terry, only 65% of physicians stated that they would report the impaired physician to the appropriate authorities. Thirty-one percent said they would talk to the physician privately but take no other action. Five percent said that they would ignore the situation [18].

A process that culminates in confrontation, intervention is often necessary to get impaired physicians to go to treatment because they have difficulty reaching out for help. It involves convincing them of the seriousness of their drug problem and helping them enter treatment while protecting their dignity, preserving their anonymity, and sparing them embarrassment. It is not an easy or pleasant task, but it is a necessary one. The two main types of intervention are professional and nonprofessional. Nonprofessional intervention is done most often by family members and/or close friends [4, 11] and was discussed in Chap. 18. Professional intervention is discussed below.

The Intervention Team

The intervention team should consist of at least two persons. The team concept allows the confronters to give each other emotional support. At least one member of the team should be someone in the same specialty, of the same sex, and, if possible, recovering from substance dependence. Members of the team should have nonjudgmental and supportive attitudes and should have experience or training in intervention strategies [11].

Members of the intervention team must have no professional or social association with the impaired physician. Because of the impaired physician's denial, he would use such a relationship to destroy the effectiveness of the intervention [19].

Preparing for the Confrontation

Training of the intervention team begins by examining their attitudes and instilling desirable ones in them. These attitudes include understanding, appreciating, and accepting that substance dependence is a biopsychosocial disease, not a bad habit, moral or ethical fault, or psychological disorder.

Substance dependence is a disease involving the family, which needs to be included and helped.

Response to the intervention team may be anger, threats, hostility, or massive denial; the team must be prepared for this.

The intervention team should have clearly defined goals and objectives for the confrontation. Regardless of its outcome, the team should have a plan of action when they leave the confrontation. Members should anticipate and be prepared to deal with denial, hostility, and other defenses. They should have documentation on paper of the impaired physician's destructive behavior and actions resulting from substance dependence, and they should mobilize support systems, including the spouse and older children and the physician's partners, peers, nurses, or hospital administrator. The team may have to meet two or three times before actually confronting the impaired physician [19].

The Confrontation

When the members of the team feel they are adequately prepared, they contact the impaired physician by telephone, telling him that the caller represents the state medical society and that they need to see him or her immediately on professional business, which is too personal to discuss on the phone. The physician is given a choice of meeting with the team in his office, his home, or in the state medical society office. A date, time, and place for the meeting are then arranged.

At the time of the confrontation, the following procedure is followed [19]:

1. The leader of the intervention team introduces himself or herself as well as the other members of the team and explains why they are there.
2. The leader explains the medical society's program for impaired physicians and its advocacy role. The physician is told that the team is there to help, not hurt.
3. The team member who is a recovering physician discusses his disease and recovery, pointing out that substance dependence is a treatable disease and that the behavior, actions, emotions, and consequences are secondary to the illness. Members emphasize that the impaired physician is suffering from a disease and is not bad, evil, weak, or crazy.
4. Members present the specifics of the physician's drug-abusing behavior in a factual, nonjudgmental manner.
5. Members anticipate the physician's responses, such as denial, anger, or rationalization. They should never argue with the physician or get angry or defensive, even in the face of personal or professional attack.
6. The team should not let the physician sidetrack the discussion.
7. The intervention team shares its assessment of the seriousness of the physician's problem.
8. Members explain what will happen if the physician does not enter treatment.
9. The impaired physician is given specific treatment plans and programs, both local and out of state, but is not allowed to arrange for a friend to treat him. Members advise him that the treatment plans and programs presented are the only ones acceptable to the state medical society [19, 20].

Once a mutually acceptable treatment source is agreed on, arrangements are made for the physician to enter treatment. He is presented a contract that states he will not practice again until cleared according to the advocacy position of the state medical society as it relates to licensure, medical staff positions, and medical standing in the community.

If the team is unsuccessful, it returns in a day or two. If this intervention fails, the physician is told that the intervention committee will abandon its advocacy role and make a report to the impaired physician committee, which in turn may file a report with the state medical association, which can then notify the state examining and licensure board of the physician's problem [19] .

Treatment

Typically, the substance-dependent physician is more dysfunctional (physiologically, psychologically, socially, spiritually) than nonphysicians. They often have been so absorbed in their practices that they have become isolated from other people. Because elaborate denial and defense mechanisms are part of the disease of substance dependence, they go to great lengths to deny that they have a problem and to prove that their lives are under complete control. Another problem with treating physicians is that they adamantly reject the role of patient.

The treatment of physicians with substance dependence problems is different from the treatment of the general public. Short-term outpatient therapy relapse rates are greater than 60%, which is unfavorable, considering physicians will be returning to a workplace where judgment must not be compromised. Extended treatment that lasts 3 to 4 months has better success rates [11].

Treatment of physicians is more successful if it takes place in a center that has a significant number of other physician patients. Unless there are a number of physician patients in the program, the physician in treatment often gets special treatment from other patients and staff, negating some of the benefits of treatment [2]. The sarcastic title "Mdiety" sometimes is given to physicians in this circumstance.

Although there is a relatively low incidence of primary psychiatric disorders among substance-dependent physicians, secondary depression is common. This usually clears in a few days to weeks after detoxification. Physicians tend to minimize their drug use.

Whereas street addicts tend to congregate in a drug culture, physicians tend to use drugs privately for fear that their drug abuse will be discovered [11].

Because of most physicians' high level of denial, inpatient treatment is almost always indicated. Treatment programs vary considerably throughout the country. The format for the Medical Association of Georgia's Impaired Physician Program has become a model for many. Treatment is divided into three phases: (1) inpatient, (2) halfway house, and (3) mirror imaging [21].

Phase I. Inpatient The first phase is inpatient treatment, which lasts 28 days or more and obeys the same principles outlined in Chap. 15. In addition, problems specific to physicians, such as practice and licensure issues, are discussed in groups for impaired health professionals.

Phase II. Halfway House During the second phase, physicians live in halfway houses with other impaired health professionals. During the day, they attend a partial hospitalization (day program). Several evenings a week, they attend AA or NA meetings, and once or twice a week, they attend a Caduceus meeting, which is a support group for health professionals. This phase is about a month long.

Phase III. Mirror Imaging In phase three, physicians participate in a process called mirror imaging. As part of treatment, they may work in treatment centers as associate counselors but not as physicians. Mirror imaging is a method of allowing patients to see other patients whose disease is more advanced than theirs and to realize that "there, but for the grace of God, go I." They continue to live in halfway houses, to attend evening AA or NA meetings and to attend some evening group sessions. They also continue to attend Caduceus meetings. This phase may last 1 to 2 months or more.

There are several prognostic indicators as to whether a physician will do well in treatment and recovery and be able to return to medical practice. These indicators include the following: (1) the physician accepts that he has the disease of substance dependence and has a high motivation for recovery; (2) he has supportive family members, significant others, and close friends; and (3) there are minimal legal complications and problems with license, hospital privileges, or employment.

Aftercare

At the time of discharge from treatment, physicians sign aftercare contracts that may require them to attend three to four AA or NA meetings a week, as well as weekly meetings of local Caduceus clubs. Random drug screens are an integral part of aftercare, which usually lasts for 5 years. During this period, and afterward, Caduceus clubs serve as physician advocates in issues such as licensure and DEA registration [22–24].

Recovery

After treatment, most physicians can return to their prior specialties. For all physicians with substance use impairment, work hours may need to be restricted to allow a gradual return to work that coincides with establishing a steady recovery program.

Recovery for physicians progresses through the same stages as for nonphysicians—pretreatment, stabilization, early recovery, middle recovery, and late recovery. Recovering physicians also may be caught up in partial recovery, and many of the factors contributing to their relapse are the same as for other addicts (Chap. 17).

Many physicians face a temptation nonphysicians do not have to deal with—such as returning to a profession in which mood-altering and addicting drugs are abundant. The anesthesiologist whose drug of choice was fentanyl, for example, must return to the operating room after treatment and actually administer the drug to patients. When relapse does occur, physicians should follow the procedures outlined in Chap. 17.

A factor that may be important to a successful return to practice is the possibility that relapse will entail financial, personal, and professional losses. Modifiable factors that contribute to relapse include failure to understand and accept that substance dependence is an illness, continued denial, a dysfunctional family, poor mechanisms to cope with stress, overconfidence, poor relationship skills, and shame and guilt [25].

For married physicians, spouses usually play major roles in detection, intervention, treatment, and recovery. Families can be physicians' most important resources in recovery. Al-Anon, Alateen, and Nar-Anon can be exceptional sources of information and support for spouses and other family members [26–28].

Success rate for treated substance-abusing physicians is about 70%. However, when a structured aftercare program is undertaken, the success rate increases to approximately 90%. The majority of relapses occur in the first 2 years after treatment. After 5 years of recovery, physicians are less likely to suffer a relapse [2].

Summary

Conservative estimates are that 8 to 12% of physicians will develop a substance abuse problem at some point in their careers. In 1973, the American Medical Association's Council on Mental Health defined impairment in physicians as "the inability to practice medicine with reasonable skill and safety to patients by reasons of physical or mental illness, including alcoholism or drug dependence." Most physicians who abuse substances continue to function fairly well until the problem is far advanced.

There are six areas in physicians' lives where clues to their chemical dependence can be found: (1) community involvement, (2) family life, (3) employment patterns, (4) physical status, (5) office conduct, and (6) hospital duties. Directly questioning a physician about his substance abuse is rarely successful and will often lead to counter accusations, such as "You're out to get me" and "You are trying to ruin my practice." Although nearly one-third of physicians are female, nearly 90% of physicians referred for substance use disorder treatment are male.

Nearly all state medical societies and state licensing boards have a physician health program (PHP) for dealing with impaired physicians.

The Federation of State Physician Health Programs (FSPHP) is a nonprofit organization that serves as a forum for information exchange among the various state programs. The AMA's Code of Medical Ethics states that "physicians have an ethical obligation to report impaired, incompetent, and unethical colleagues" and lists several guidelines to follow.

Typically, the substance-dependent physician is more dysfunctional (physiologically, psychologically, socially, spiritually) than nonphysicians. Treatment often is divided into three phases: (1) inpatient, (2) halfway house, and (3) mirror imaging. When a structured aftercare program is undertaken, the success rate increases to approximately 90%.

References

1. Schorling JB. Physician impairment due to substance use disorders. Medscape website. http://www.medscape.org/viewarticle/582133_1. November 20, 2009.
2. Chicala RS. Substance abuse among physicians: what you need to know. Hosp Physician. 2003:39–45.
3. Johnson BA. Dealing with the impaired physician. Am Fam Physician. 2009;80(9):1007–8.
4. Talbott GD, Benson EB. Impaired physicians: the dilemma of identification. Postgrad Med. 1980;68(7):56–64.
5. Artecona J. The impaired physician: identification and treatment. Tulane University: Phoenix Society website. http://tmedweb.tulane.edu/mu/phoenix/resources/impaired-physicians
6. Boisabin EV, Levine RE. Identifying and assisting the impaired physician. Am J Med Sci. 2001;322(1):31–6.
7. Bissell L, Skorina JK. One hundred alcoholic women in medicine. J Am Med Assoc. 1987;257:2939–44.
8. Martin CA, Talbott GD. Women physicians in the Georgia impaired physicians program. J Am Med Women's Assoc. 1987;42(4):115–21.
9. Martin CA, Talbott GD. Special issues for female impaired physicians. J Am Med Assoc Georgia. 1986;75(8):483–8.
10. The sick physician: impairment by psychiatric disorders, including alcoholism and drug dependence. J Am Med Assoc. 1973;223(6):684–87.
11. Wilford BB. The drug-abusing physician. In: Drug abuse: a guide for the primary care physician. Chicago: American Medical Society; 1981. p. 285–98.
12. Conner SL. Comparison of impaired physicians programs nationwide. Md Med J. 1988;37(3):213–5.
13. Johnson BA. Dealing with the impaired physician. Am Fam Physician. 2009;80(9):1007–8.
14. Spickard WA. The impaired physician. In: Barnes HN, Aronson MD, Delbanco TL, editors. Alcoholism: a guide for the primary care physician. New York: Springer-Verlag; 1987. p. 188–93.
15. DuPont RL, McLellan AT, White WL, Merlo LJ, Gold MS. Setting the standard for recovery: physicians' health programs. J Subst Abus Treat. 2009;36(2):159–71.
16. About FSPHP. Federation of State Physician Health Programs (FSPHP) website. http://www.fsphp.org/about
17. Terry K. Impaired physicians: speak no evil? Medical Economics website. http://medicaleconomics.modernmedicine.com/medical-economics/content/impaired-physicians-speak-no-evil?page=full. 2002;19:110. October 11, 2002.
18. Milhorn HT. Chemical dependence: diagnosis, prevention, and treatment. New York: Springer-Verlag; 1990.
19. Talbott TD. The impaired physician and intervention: a key to recovery. J Fla Med Assoc. 1987;69(9):793–7.
20. Robertson JJ. Confrontation techniques. In: The impaired physician proceedings of the third AMA conference. Chicago: American Medical Association; 1979.
21. Talbott GD, Gallegos K, Wilson PO, Porter TL. The Medical Association of Georgia's impaired physician program. J Am Med Assoc. 1987;257(21):2927–30.
22. Arnold WP, Smith MA, Bedford RF, Garner L. Drug-impaired physicians: identification, intervention, treatment. Va Med. 1987;114(8):467–72.
23. Haynes TL. The physician and chemical dependence. Mich Med. 1988;87(6):326–8.
24. Ross S. Identifying an impaired physician. AMA J Ethics. 2003;5(12). http://journalofethics.ama-assn.org/2003/12/cprl1-0312.html.
25. Yancey JR, McKinnon HD. Reaching out to an impaired physician. Fam Pract Manag. 2010;17(1):27–31.
26. Samkoff JS, Krebs JR. Families and physician impairment. Pa Med. 1989;92:38–9.
27. Samkoff JS, Krebs JR. Treating the chemically impaired medical family. Pa Med. 1989;92(2):32–4.
28. Talbott GD. The impaired physician: the role of the spouse in recovery. J Med Assoc Ga. 1987;76(3):190–2.

Index

H.T. Milhorn, *Substance Use Disorders*, DOI 10.1007/978-3-319-63040-3

MIX
Papier aus verantwortungsvollen Quellen
Paper from responsible sources
FSC® C105338

If you have any concerns about our products,
you can contact us on
ProductSafety@springernature.com

In case Publisher is established outside the EU,
the EU authorized representative is:
Springer Nature Customer Service Center GmbH
Europaplatz 3, 69115 Heidelberg, Germany

Printed by Libri Plureos GmbH
in Hamburg, Germany